Drug Receptor Subtypes and Ingestive Behaviour

Edited by

STEVEN J. COOPER

Department of Psychology, University of Durham
Durham, UK

and

PETER G. CLIFTON

Laboratory of Experimental Psychology, School of Biology
University of Sussex, Brighton, UK

ACADEMIC PRESS

Harcourt Brace & Company, Publishers

London   San Diego   New York
Boston   Sydney   Tokyo   Toronto

ACADEMIC PRESS LIMITED
24–28 Oval Road
LONDON NW1 7DX

U.S. Edition Published by
ACADEMIC PRESS INC.
San Diego, CA 92101

This book is printed on acid free paper

A catalogue record for this book is available from the British Library
ISBN 0-12-187620-9

Typeset by Paston Press Limited, Loddon, Norfolk
Printed in Great Britain by Hartnolls Limited, Bodmin, Cornwall

Drug Receptor Subtypes and Ingestive Behaviour

Contents

Contents ix

A colour plate section appears between pages 336 and 337

Contributors

I. Bednar Department of Clinical Neuroscience and Family Medicine, Division of Applied Neuroendocrinology, Karolinska Institute, Novum S-141 57 Huddinge, Sweden

Richard J. Bodnar Department of Psychology and Neuropsychology Doctoral Sub-Program, Queens College, City University of New York, 65-30 Kissena Boulevard, Flushing, New York 11367-0904, USA

Kenneth D. Carr Millhauser Laboratories, Department of Psychiatry, New York University Medical Center, 550 First Avenue, New York, NY 10016, USA

H. Carrer Instituto de Investigación Médica, M. y M. Ferreyra, Córdoba, Argentina

Peter G. Clifton Laboratory of Experimental Psychology, School of Biology, University of Sussex, Brighton BN1 9QG, UK

Steven J. Cooper Department of Psychology, University of Durham, South Road, Durham DH1 3LE, UK

Eric S. Corp Department of Psychiatry, Cornell University Medical College and The Edward W. Bourne Behavioral Research Laboratory, The New York Hospital–Cornell Medical Center, 21 Bloomingdale Road, White Plains, NY 10605, USA

Paul J. Currie Department of Psychology, Wayne State University, 71 W. Warren Avenue, Detroit, MI 48202, USA

Blake A. Gosnell Department of Psychiatry, University of Wisconsin–Madison, 6001 Research Park Blvd., Madison, WI 53719, USA

Giuliano Grignaschi Istituto di Ricerche Farmacologiche 'Mario Negri', Via Eritrea 62, 20157 Milan, Italy

Suzanne Higgs Department of Psychology, University of Durham, South Road, Durham DH1 3LE, UK

Helen C. Jackson Knoll Pharmaceuticals Research Department, Thane Road West, Nottingham NG2 3AA, UK

A. E. Johnson Department of Psychiatry, Ulleråker, University of Uppsala, S-750 17 Uppsala, Sweden

J. M. Kaplan Department of Psychology, University of Pennsylvania, Philadelphia, PA 19104, USA

Allen S. Levine Departments of Psychiatry and Food Science and Nutrition, University of Minnesota, St Paul, MN 55417, USA and Veterans Administration Medical Center, Minneapolis, MN, USA

H. Mamoun Department of Renal Medicine, Karolinska Institute, S-141 86 Huddinge, Sweden

Timothy H. Moran Department of Psychiatry and Behavioral Sciences, Johns Hopkins University School of Medicine, 720 Rutland Avenue/Ross 618, Baltimore, MD 21205-2196, USA

Paolo Nencini Institute of Medical Pharmacology, University of Rome 'La Sapienza', P. le A. Moro 5, 00185 Rome, Italy

Stelios Nicolaïdis Neurobiologie des Régulations, C.N.R.S. URA 1860, Collège de France, 11 place Marcelin-Berthelot, 75231 Paris Cedex 05, France

David J. Nutt Psychopharmacology Unit, University of Bristol, School of Medical Sciences, University Walk, Bristol BS8 1TD, UK

Martine Orosco Neurobiologie des Régulations, C.N.R.S. URA 1860, Collège de France, 11 place Marcelin-Berthelot, 75231 Paris Cedex 05, France

M. Qian Department of Clinical Neuroscience and Family Medicine, Division of Applied Neuroendocrinology, Karolinska Institute, Novum S-141 57 Huddinge, Sweden

G. A. Qureshi Department of Clinical Neuroscience and Family Medicine, Division of Applied Neuroendocrinology, Karolinska Institute, Novum S-141 57 Huddinge, Sweden

Rosario Samanin Istituto di Ricerche Farmacologiche 'Mario Negri', Via Eritrea 62, 20157 Milan, Italy

Kenny J. Simansky Department of Pharmacology, Medical College of Pennsylvania and Hahnemann University, 3200 Henry Avenue, Philadelphia, PA 19129, USA

Per Södersten Department of Clinical Neuroscience and Family Medicine, Division of Applied Neuroendocrinology, Karolinska Institute, Novum S-141 57 Huddinge, Sweden

Elizabeth M. Somerville School of Biology, University of Sussex, Brighton BN1 9QG, UK

B. Glenn Stanley   Departments of Psychology and Neuroscience, University of California, Riverside, CA 92521, USA

Philip Terry   School of Psychology, University of Birmingham, Edgbaston, Birmingham B15 2TT, UK

Franco J. Vaccarino   Departments of Psychology and Psychiatry, University of Toronto, 100 St George Street, Toronto, Ontario M5S 1A1, Canada

Preface

The study of neural mechanisms of ingestive behaviour has long been one of the most intensively investigated areas within behavioural neuroscience. Beginning three or four decades ago, drug studies were introduced largely with the intention of developing clinically useful anti-obesity compounds. From this largely applied start, interest rapidly developed in the use of drug studies to identify neurotransmitters that might be involved in the control of ingestive responses. More recently, there has been a shift in focus towards neurotransmitter receptors, when it became clear that there are multiple subtypes of receptors for each identified neurotransmitter. Investigators were then faced with the task of sorting through the many varieties of receptor subtypes to try to identify those with a specific connection to the control of ingestive behaviour. Consequently the field has grown rapidly, and has become quite complex. The present volume is designed to guide students and investigators through a number of different neurotransmitter systems and provide them with the latest information on the identities of receptor subtypes most relevant in the study of ingestive behaviour.

The volume opens with several chapters dealing with cholecystokinin (CCK) and 5-hydroxytryptamine (5-HT; serotonin), a neuropeptide and monoamine, respectively. Both may be involved in the process of satiety, leading to the termination of feeding. Issues of critical receptor subtypes and interactions with other factors (dopamine, insulin) are dealt with fully. Next, there are five chapters dealing with opioid peptides, widely thought to be involved in the stimulation of feeding. Once again, receptor subtype involvement in ingestive behaviour is carefully analysed, interaction with dopamine is discussed, and the topic of sensitization is introduced.

Dopamine and noradrenergic mechanisms are reviewed before relatively novel factors such as glutamate and neuropeptide Y are considered extensively. In the two final chapters, we contribute reviews of benzodiazepine receptors in relation to the interesting topic of palatability and the question of neurochemical interactions in relation to ingestive behaviour. If not completely comprehensive, the assembled chapters provide access to most of the major current research themes in the study of ingestive behaviour, where the use of drugs is a unifying research method.

We acknowledge the valuable contributions of the authors, who have provided up-to-the-minute reviews of some of the most exciting new develop-

ments in the study of ingestive behaviour. In Durham, Suzanne Higgs and
Paula Beuster have rendered much assistance, for which we are most grateful.
We thank our publisher for the efficient handling of all stages of the book's
production.

This is a unique volume. It is the first to deal explicitly with drug receptor
subtypes in relation to ingestive behaviour, and, as such, will prove to be
enormously useful to all engaged in the study of ingestive behaviour. We hope
that it will encourage much more effort in tackling the complex issues of
relating neurochemical transmission to the neural and behavioural controls of
feeding.

STEVEN J. COOPER
Durham

PETER G. CLIFTON
Sussex

1

Receptor Subtype and Affinity State Underlying the Satiety Actions of Cholecystokinin (CCK)

TIMOTHY H. MORAN

Department of Psychiatry and Behavioral Sciences, Johns Hopkins University School of Medicine, 720 Rutland Avenue/Ross 618, Baltimore, MD 21205-2196, USA

1 Introduction

Cholecystokinin (CCK) is a peptide found in significant quantities in both the upper gastrointestinal tract and the brain. In the periphery CCK serves a variety of functions involved in regulating the digestive process (Raybould and Lloyd, 1994). CCK is found in secretory cells (Buchan *et al.*, 1978) and in intrinsic neural fibres in the upper intestine (Schultzberg *et al.*, 1980). Its release stimulates pancreatic secretion, gallbladder contraction and the inhibition of gastric emptying. In the brain CCK functions as a neurotransmitter, and roles for CCK in modulating mesolimbic dopaminergic activity (Crawley, 1994), in opiate analgesia (Baber *et al.*, 1989) and in panic states (Harro *et al.*, 1993) have been documented.

CCK exists in a variety of forms in the periphery and the brain. In the gastrointestinal tract, the major biological form of CCK is CCK-58, with smaller fragments (CCK-33, CCK-25, CCK-18, CCK-8 and CCK-7) produced by cleavage (Reeve *et al.*, 1994). The primary form of CCK found in the brain is CCK-8, which represents the *C*-terminal octapeptide of the larger molecule (Dockray, 1976).

2 CCK receptor subtypes

Two CCK receptor subtypes have been identified. Heterogeneity of CCK receptors was first demonstrated in the original radioligand binding studies carried out on tissue homogenates from pancreas and brain. Innis and Snyder

DRUG RECEPTOR SUBTYPES AND INGESTIVE BEHAVIOUR
ISBN 0-12-187620-9

(1980) demonstrated that the pharmacological profile of CCK binding to these two tissues was different. Unsulfated CCK and various CCK fragments, including pentagastrin (CCK-5) and CCK-4, had the ability to inhibit the binding of ^{125}I-labelled CCK-33 to brain homogenates with much greater potency than to pancreatic homogenates. This pharmacological difference between pancreatic and brain CCK receptors has been widely replicated and has served as the basis for the identification of localized populations of the two receptor subtypes. Both types of CCK receptors were subsequently demonstrated to be present in the brain, and the nomenclature of CCK_A (A for the alimentary receptor) and CCK_B (B for the brain receptor) has been adopted (Moran et al., 1986; Hill et al., 1987). CCK_A receptors have a high affinity for CCK peptides that have a sulfated tyrosine seven amino acids from the carboxy terminus. CCK_B receptors have a high affinity for both sulfated and unsulfated forms of CCK and gastrin. As will be discussed in detail, agonists and antagonists that differentiate between the two receptor subtypes are available. The genes for the two CCK receptor subtypes have been identified and cloned (Wank et al., 1992a,b). There is a significant degree of homology between the deduced amino acid sequences of the two receptor proteins and both are members of the seven transmembrane guanine nucleotide-binding regulatory protein coupled superfamily of receptors. CCK_A receptors found in the brain have been demonstrated to be identical to peripheral CCK_A receptors (Wank et al., 1992b) and the CCK_B receptor is identical to the gastrin receptor (Wank et al., 1994). In the gastrointestinal tract CCK_A receptors are found in the pancreas (Innis and Snyder, 1980), gallbladder (Cox et al., 1990) and the circular muscle layer of the pyloric sphincter (Smith et al., 1984).

In rat brain, autoradiographic binding studies have demonstrated localized populations of CCK_A receptors in the nucleus of the solitary tract, the area postrema, the interpeduncular nucleus, the habenulum and the dorsal medial hypothalamus (Moran et al., 1986; Hill et al., 1987). Functional studies have indicated that CCK_A receptors are also present in the medial raphe, the nucleus accumbens and at other brain sites (Boden and Woodruff, 1994; Crawley, 1994). CCK_A receptors are also present in vagal afferent fibres (Moran et al., 1990). CCK_B–gastrin receptors are present in the gastrointestinal tract and, as stated, are the dominant receptor subtype found in brain. CCK_B receptors are also present in the spinal cord and in vagal afferents (Mercer and Lawrence, 1992; Corp et al., 1993). The distribution of the two CCK receptor subtypes is somewhat species specific. For example, while the rat cerebellum is devoid of CCK receptors, guinea-pig and primate cerebellum contain high densities of CCK_B receptors (Zarbin et al., 1983; Hill et al., 1990). Also, in contrast to the case in the rat, CCK_A receptors are the primary subtype found in primate spinal cord (Hill et al., 1990).

3   Satiety actions of CCK

The actions of CCK in food intake were first demonstrated in 1973 when Gibbs and co-workers (1973a) demonstrated that peripheral administration of an impure extract of porcine CCK reduced food intake. Since that time, the phenomenology of CCK's inhibitory actions on food intake have been well documented and the satiety actions of the peptide extended to a variety of species, including humans (Gibbs *et al.*, 1976; Anika *et al.*, 1981; Kissileff *et al.*, 1981). The actions of CCK are behaviourally specific in that CCK affects food but not water intake (Gibbs *et al.*, 1973a) and the pattern by which CCK reduces food intake is consistent with a satiety interpretation: CCK reduces meal size and meal duration, and results in an earlier appearance of a behavioural sequence of satiety (Antin *et al.*, 1975). CCK's effects on food intake are dose related (Fig. 1), and in sham feeding, where consumed liquid nutrients drain from the stomach without causing gastric distension or access-ing postgastric sites, CCK interrupts ongoing intake (Gibbs *et al.*, 1973b) and does so in a manner similar to that of intestinally infused nutrients (Liebling *et al.*, 1975). CCK has also been demonstrated to inhibit food intake following central administration in a variety of species including rats, sheep and baboons (Schick *et al.*, 1986; Della-Fera and Baile, 1979; Figlewicz *et al.*, 1989).

Antagonist experiments have demonstrated that inhibition of food intake is a physiological function of endogenous CCK since administration of CCK antagonists results in increased food intake in a variety of paradigms (Dourish *et al.*, 1989b; Reidelberger and O'Rourke, 1989; Silver *et al.*, 1989; Moran *et*

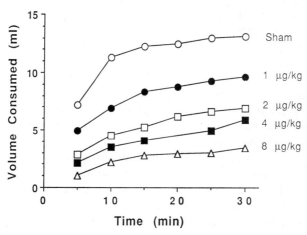

Fig. 1   Dose-related inhibition of glucose intake (0.5 kcal/ml) produced by intraperitoneal injection of CCK-8.

al., 1992, 1993). The mode and site of action for CCK satiety are still under active investigation but there is accumulating evidence that CCK affects food intake through a neurocrine or paracrine mechanism involving activation of vagal afferent fibres (for a complete discussion see Ritter *et al.*, 1994).

3.1   Receptor subtype mediating and satiety actions of exogenous CCK

Early structure–activity studies examining the inhibition of food intake by various forms of CCK clearly indicate that sulfated CCK (CCK-8, CCK-33) was 100–1000-fold more potent than unsulfated CCK, gastrin or various unsulfated CCK fragments (Gibbs *et al.*, 1973a; Lorenz *et al.*, 1979). This profile was consistent with an action of CCK at CCK_A receptors for inhibiting food intake. This conclusion has been supported in more recent studies using synthesized specific CCK_A and CCK_B receptor agonists. Asin and colleagues (1992a,b) have demonstrated that peripheral administration of a CCK-based tetrapeptide (A71623), which has greater than 1000-fold specificity for CCK_A receptors, inhibited food intake in a dose-dependent manner in a variety of paradigms. This compound was more potent than CCK in 60-min tests, even though its affinity for CCK_A receptors was ten-fold lower than that of CCK. This increased potency appears to be secondary to its increased duration of action (Asin *et al.*, 1992a). In contrast, peripheral administration of a CCK tetrapeptide analogue with high affinity ($IC_{50} = 0.7$ nmol/l and high specificity (9000-fold) for CCK_B receptors (A63387) did not affect food intake across a wide dose range (Asin *et al.*, 1992b).

Experiments examining the ability of CCK antagonists with varying degrees of specificity for the two CCK receptor subtypes to block the feeding inhibitory actions of exogenous CCK have produced a similar conclusion. As demonstrated in Table 1, a variety of CCK antagonists with relative affinities for the two CCK receptor subtypes is available. The ability of many of these compounds to block the feeding inhibitory actions of exogenous CCK have been assessed. The clearest data have been obtained with the specific CCK_A antagonist devazepide (L-364718, MK-329) and the specific CCK_B antagonist L-365260 (Dourish *et al.*, 1989a; Reidelberger *et al.*, 1991; Moran *et al.*, 1992).

As demonstrated in Fig. 2, devazepide dose-dependently reversed the feeding inhibitory actions of 4 μg/kg CCK on glucose ingestion over 30 min following a 6-h daytime deprivation. In contrast, the specific CCK_B antagonist L-356260 failed to reverse the feeding inhibitory actions of CCK in this paradigm. These results are again consistent with mediation of the feeding inhibitory actions of exogenous CCK at CCK_A receptors. Similar results using a variety of feeding paradigms have been found with these antagonists by other investigators (Schneider *et al.*, 1988; Dourish *et al.*, 1989a; Reidelberger and O'Rourke, 1989). The reversal of the feeding inhibitory actions of CCK by devazepide has been shown to be competitive. Following administration of devazepide, the dose–response curve relating food intake to increasing doses

Table 1 Relative affinity of CCK agonists and antagonists for CCK_A and CCK_B receptors

	IC_{50} (nmol/l)	
	CCK_A	CCK_B
CCK agonists		
CCK-8	0.1	0.3
CCK-8US	600	2.6
CCK-4	5330	2.6
A-71623	3.7	4400
A-63387	6300	0.7
CCK antagonists		
Proglumide	6 300 000	11 000 000
Lorglumide (CR-1409)	7.1	500
Devazepide (L-364 718 MK-329)	0.2	31
L-365 260	240	5.2
CI-988	4300	1.7
Cam 1481	2.8	260

Data compiled from Freidinger (1992), Hill et al. (1992) and Asin et al. (1992b).

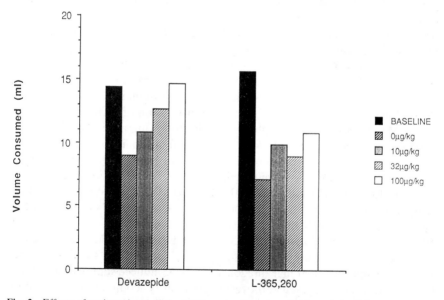

Fig. 2 Effects of various doses of the CCK_A antagonist devazepide and the CCK_B antagonist L-365 260 on the suppression of glucose intake (0.5 kcal/ml) produced by 4 μg/kg CCK-8. In the baseline condition neither CCK nor antagonist was administered. At 0, 10, 32 and 100 μg/kg doses, feeding was preceded by intraperitoneal injection of CCK-8. (From Moran et al. (1992), with permission.)

of CCK is right-shifted, and this shift is linear (Reidelberger and O'Rourke, 1989).

Together, these results with CCK agonists and antagonists indicate that exogenously administered CCK inhibits food intake through its interactions with CCK_A receptors.

3.2 Receptor affinity state mediating the satiety actions of exogenous CCK

CCK_A receptors exist in more than one affinity state. CCK's ability to stimulate pancreatic amylase secretion in the rat conforms to an inverted U-shaped dose–response curve. The upstroke of this curve reflects CCK's occupation of high-affinity CCK_A receptors stimulating amylase release, while the downstroke represents occupation of low-affinity CCK_B receptors producing an inhibition of amylase release (Jensen et al., 1982; Sankaran et al., 1982). Use of a C-terminal heptapeptide CCK analogue (BOC-Tyr(SO_3)-Nle-Gly-Trp-Nle-Asp-2-phenylethyl ester) (CCK-JMV-180) provides a functional discrimination of these two sites (Galas et al., 1988; Matozaki et al., 1989). CCK-JMV-180 is an agonist at the high-affinity site, in that it mimics the actions of CCK and stimulates amylase secretion at low concentrations. However, in contrast to CCK, at higher concentrations CCK-JMV-180 does not inhibit amylase release. In fact, CCK-JMV-180 is able to block the inhibitory actions of high concentrations of CCK on amylase release. Thus, CCK-JMV-180 has the unique profile of being an agonist at CCK_A high-affinity sites but an antagonist at CCK_A low-affinity sites in rats (Galas et al., 1988; Stark et al., 1989).

We and others (Asin and Bednarz, 1992; Weatherford et al., 1993) have used this compound to investigate whether various actions of CCK in the rat are mediated through its interactions with high- or low-affinity CCK_A receptors. As demonstrated in Fig. 3, peripheral administration of increasing doses of CCK-JMV-180 did not affect glucose intake following a 5-h daytime deprivation. Similar negative results were obtained on the ability of CCK-JMV-180 to affect intake of a complete liquid diet or of powdered chow following overnight deprivation (Asin and Bednarz, 1992; Weatherford et al., 1993). Thus, for food intake, CCK-JMV-180 did not act as a CCK agonist. These data suggest that the feeding inhibitory actions of CCK are unlikely to be mediated by its interactions with high-affinity CCK_A receptors. In contrast, when administered in combination with CCK-8, CCK-JMV-180 dose dependently attenuated CCK-8-induced suppression of food intake (Fig. 4). Thus, CCK-JMV-180 acted as a functional antagonist for CCK-induced suppression of food intake. These data suggest that the feeding inhibitory actions of CCK appear to be mediated through activation of low-affinity CCK_A receptors, the site at which CCK-JMV-180 is an antagonist.

These results have a number of implications. Actions of CCK in the inhibition of food intake at low-affinity CCK_A sites imply that the mode of

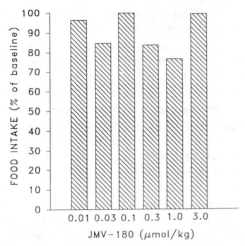

Fig. 3 Effect of intraperitoneal CCK-JMV-180 alone on glucose intake (0.5 kcal/ml) in rats following a 5-h daytime deprivation. CCK-JMV-180 did not affect intake at any dose tested. Data are expressed as a percentage of baseline glucose intake.

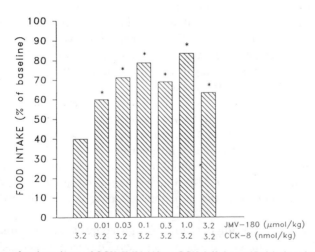

Fig. 4 Effect of various doses of CCK-JMV-180 on CCK-8 (3.2 nmol/kg) induced suppression of glucose intake in rats. CCK satiety (far left bar) was reversed by CCK-JMV-180 in a dose-related manner, with a minimum effective dose of 0.01 μmol/kg. * Indicates significant difference from intake after CCK-8 in the absence of CCK-JMV-180. (Reprinted from Weatherford *et al.* (1993), with permission.)

action for CCK in feeding is different from that of CCK in stimulating pancreatic secretion. Reidelberger and Solomon (1986) have compared the potency of CCK in stimulating pancreatic amylase release and in inhibiting food intake. Their results demonstrated that the dose of CCK required to affect food intake minimally was greater than that needed to produce maximal pancreatic amylase secretion. The stimulation of pancreatic amylase secretion has been demonstrated to be an endocrine action of CCK. Since postprandial plasma CCK levels do not exceed those that produce maximal pancreatic secretion, an endocrine action of CCK in the inhibition of food intake was thought unlikely. Actions of CCK at low-affinity CCK_A receptors in satiety require local levels in excess of those found in plasma. Therefore, the mode of action of CCK in satiety is likely to be paracrine or neurocrine. In support of this view, we have demonstrated that CCK_A receptors mediating vagal afferent responses to CCK are also low-affinity CCK sites, since CCK-JMV-180 does not result in vagal activation but, similar to devazepide, can block vagal afferent responses to CCK-8 (Schwartz et al., 1994). Similarly, CCK_A receptors mediating pyloric contraction in response to CCK or CCK-induced inhibition of gastric emptying in the rat are also low-affinity sites (Moran et al., 1994).

3.3   Receptor subtype mediating the satiety actions of endogenous CCK

Using the non-specific CCK antagonist proglumide, Shillabeer and Davison (1984) provided the first demonstration of a role for endogenous CCK in satiety. Administration of proglumide to rats that had consumed a preload resulted in greater subsequent food intake. The magnitude of the increase was related to the size of the preload consumed. Following a large preload, subsequent intake would be small in the absence of the CCK antagonist. Proglumide blocked the feeding inhibitory action of these large preloads, resulting in greater subsequent intake.

As more potent and specific CCK antagonists became available, the demonstration of a role for endogenous CCK in satiety became commonplace and the pharmacological specificity of this action was assessed. Reidelberger and O'Rourke (1989) demonstrated that intraperitoneal administration of devazepide 2.5 h into the dark cycle resulted in a dose-related increase in liquid or solid food intake at 2-, 3- or 24-h time-points following administration. For both liquid and solid food, the minimally effective dose of devazepide was $100\,\mu g/kg$.

Using a prefeeding paradigm following a 17-h deprivation, Dourish and co-workers (1989b) examined the relative abilities of devazepide and L-365 260 to affect subsequent intake. In agreement with the results of Reidelberger and O'Rourke (1989), administration of devazepide significantly increased the frequency and duration of feeding in a 60-min test session and delayed the onset of resting. In this testing situation, food intake following vehicle administration was minimal. Intake was significantly increased at a dose of 100 ng/kg and was maximal at a dose of 100 μg/kg. Administration of the specific CCK$_B$ receptor antagonist L-365 260 produced similar results, but with increased potency and efficacy, i.e. L-365 260 increased feeding frequency, decreased resting frequency and increased food consumption with a threshold of 1 ng/kg and a maximal response at 10 μg/kg. While the maximal food intake obtained with devazepide was slightly more than 4 g in the 60-min test, the maximum with L-365 260 was greater than 7 g. These data were interpreted to indicate a role for endogenous CCK in the control of food intake and an action of endogenous CCK in feeding at CCK$_B$ receptors. The difference in potency between L-365 260 and devazepide was consistent with their relative affinity for CCK$_B$ receptors and had no relationship to the affinity of these antagonists for CCK$_A$ receptors. Since exogenous CCK acts through an interaction with CCK$_A$ receptor sites, these data further suggested that endogenous and exogenous CCK were acting at different receptor subtypes in the inhibition of food intake—questioning the physiological significance of the feeding inhibitory actions of exogenous CCK.

Subsequent experiments by a variety of laboratories using other testing paradigms comparing the ability of devazepide and L-365 260 to affect food intake did not replicate these results. For example, we examined the ability of various doses of devazepide and L-365 260 to affect glucose intake in rats following a 6-h daytime deprivation. This is the same paradigm in which we examined the actions of these antagonists against exogenously administered CCK. As shown in Fig. 5, devazepide at doses of 32 and 100 μg/kg significantly increased glucose consumption at all time points during the 60-min test session. In contrast, doses of L-365 260 ranging from 3.2 to 320 μg/kg had no significant effect on glucose consumption. This dose range spans the doses found effective by Dourish and colleagues (1989b).

Similar results to ours were also reported by Reidelberger and co-workers (1991). Utilizing the paradigm in which antagonists were administered 2 h into the dark cycle, they demonstrated that devazepide increased intake with a threshold of 10 μg/kg and a maximal effect at 100 μg/kg. In contrast, no dose of L-365 260 from 100 ng/kg to 10 mg/kg affected intake. Using a prefeeding paradigm, Corwin and co-workers (1991) also demonstrated increases in test meal intake in response to devazepide in rats but, again, no increases in intake in response to L-365 260. We have also attempted to replicate directly the testing conditions of Dourish et al. (1989b). Naive rats were deprived of food for 17 h and given access to chow for a period of 40 min. Food was removed and rats were injected with 10 μg/kg devazepide, L-365 260 or vehicle. This was the dose of L-365 260 that produced a maximal effect in the experiment of Dourish and co-workers (1989b). Thirty minutes later food was returned and intake was measured over the subsequent 60 min. As shown in Fig. 6, the 10 μg/kg dose of devazepide significantly increased intake above levels following vehicle injection. In contrast, this dose of L-365 260 had no significant effect on intake.

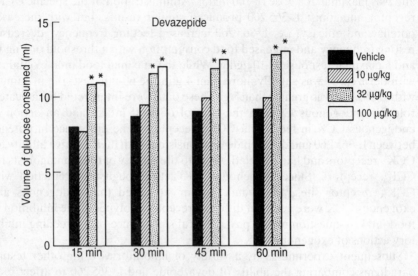

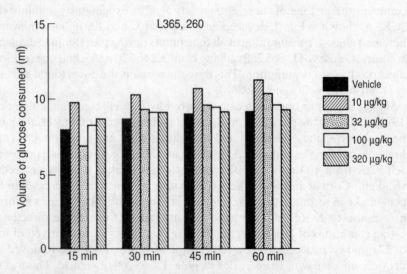

Fig. 5 Effects of various doses of the CCK_A antagonist devazepide (top panel) and the CCK_B antagonist L-365 260 on glucose intake in the absence of exogenous CCK. * Indicates significant difference from intake after vehicle administration at the same time-point. (Reprinted from Moran *et al.* (1992), with permission.)

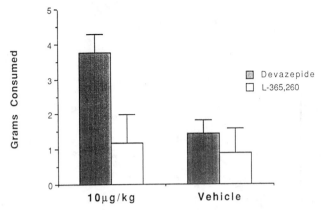

Fig. 6   Effects of devazepide and L-365 260 on 60-min chow intake in rats following a 40-min prefeed. Intake was increased from vehicle levels following devazepide but not following L-365 260.

Thus, the original results reported by Dourish and colleagues (1989b) have not been replicated.

Similar data on the ability of CCK antagonists to affect food intake have been obtained in other species. Weatherford and colleagues (1992) examined the relative ability of devazepide and L-365 260 to affect consumption of a 20% sucrose solution in mildly food-deprived mice. Devazepide administration resulted in dose-related increases in 90-min sucrose ingestion. The minimally effective dose was 31.5 μg/kg, which produced a 23% increase. The maximal effect was obtained with a dose of 315 μg/kg which increased intake by 63%. In contrast, L-365 260 in doses of up to 315 μg/kg had no effect on sucrose intake. These results again support the view that the satiety actions of endogenous CCK are mediated through CCK's interactions with CCK_A receptors.

We have also examined the relative abilities of devazepide and L-365 260 to affect food intake in rhesus monkeys (*Macaca mulatta*) (Moran *et al.*, 1993). Monkeys had chronic indwelling intragastric cannulas and were adapted to a schedule of having 4 h per day access to food. Food pellets (1 g) were obtained in response to lever pulls and intake was computer monitored through the 4-h feed period. Thirty minutes before food access, monkeys received 5 ml intragastric infusions containing 3.2–320 μg/kg devazepide or L-365 260. As demonstrated in Fig. 7. devazepide administration resulted in a dose-related increase in intake throughout the 4-h period. The threshold for a significant increase was 32 μg/kg and a maximal increase occurred at 100 μg/kg. In contrast to devazepide, L-365 260 had no significant effect on food intake at

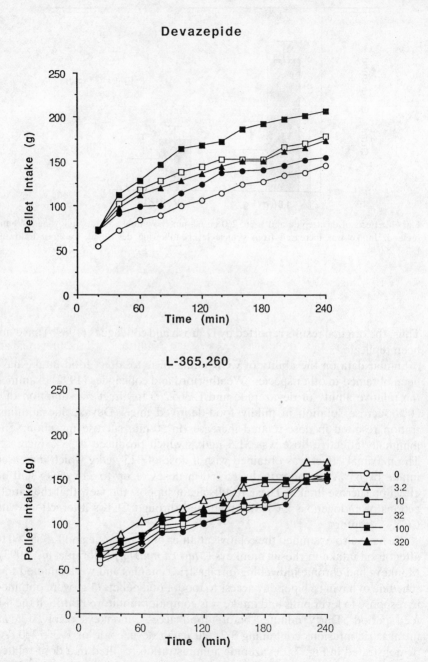

Fig. 7 Effect of various doses of devazepide (top panel) and L-365 260 (bottom panel) on 4-h chow intake in rhesus monkeys. Intake was increased in a dose-dependent fashion by devazepide but not by L-365 260. (Reprinted from Moran *et al.* (1993), with permission.)

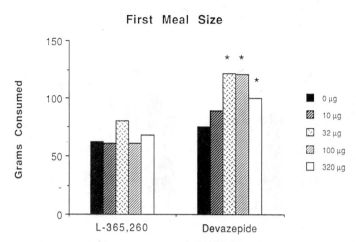

Fig. 8 Effect of various doses of L-365 260 (left panel) and devazepide (right panel) on first meal size in rhesus monkeys. * Indicates significant difference from $0\,\mu g/kg$ condition. First meal size was increased by devazepide but not by L-365 260. (From Moran *et al.* (1993), with permission.)

any dose. An analysis of meal parameters indicated that the major effect of devazepide was to produce a dose-related increase in the size of the first meal (Fig. 8). There was also a significant increase in the duration of the first meal at doses of 32 and $100\,\mu g/kg$ (Fig. 9). The interval between the first and the second meal was decreased at the $100\,\mu g/kg$ dose and the satiety ratio (intermeal interval divided by the first meal size was significantly decreased at 32, 100 and $320\,\mu g/kg$ (Fig. 10). No effects on meal patterns were obtained following L-365 260 administration.

The overall pattern of changes in food intake produced in response to devazepide administration is consistent with a satiety role for endogenous CCK acting through CCK_A receptors. Devazepide administration and the resulting blockade of CCK_A receptors decreased the satiating value of the consumed food, resulting in a larger initial meal and a shortened time period for animals to initiate a second meal.

4 Summary

Two CCK receptor subtypes have been pharmacologically differentiated, their relative distributions mapped both centrally and peripherally, and the receptors purified and sequenced. CCK agonists and antagonists with relative degrees of specificity for the two receptor subtypes have been used to address the identification of the receptor subtype underlying the satiety actions of both exogenously administered and endogenously released CCK.

The role for CCK_A receptors in the mediation of the satiety actions of exogenously administered CCK is unequivocal. CCK_A-specific receptor

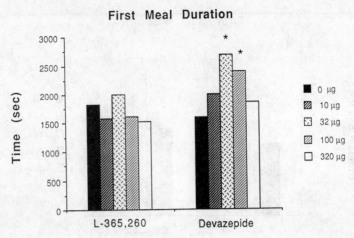

Fig. 9 Effect of various doses of L-365 260 (left panel) and devazepide (right panel) on first meal duration in rhesus monkeys. * Indicates significant difference from 0 μg/kg condition. First meal duration was increased by devazepide but not by L-365 260. (From Moran *et al.* (1991), with permission.)

agonists inhibit food intake while CCK_B-specific agonists only affect intake with significantly lower potency. Administration of CCK_A receptor antagonists blocks the feeding inhibitory actions of exogenously administered CCK, while CCK_B antagonists do not.

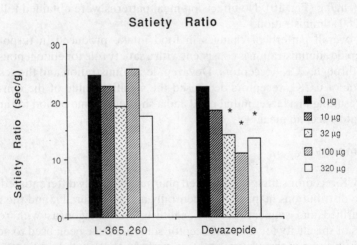

Fig. 10 Effect of various doses of L-365 260 (left panel) and devazepide (right panel) on satiety ratio (intermeal interval divided by first meal size) in rhesus monkeys. * Indicates significant difference from 0 μg/kg condition. Satiety ratio was increased by devazepide but not by L-365 260. (From Moran *et al.* (1993), with permission.)

The satiety actions of exogenously administered CCK are mediated through low-affinity CCK_A receptors. Administration of CCK-JMV-180, an agonist at CCK_A high-affinity sites and an antagonist at CCK_A low-affinity sites, had no effect on food intake when administered alone but blocked the satiety actions of endogenously administered CCK.

A physiological role for endogenous CCK in satiety has been demonstrated. Administration of CCK receptor antagonists increases food intake in a variety of experimental settings and in a variety of species. These actions appear to be mediated through CCK_A receptors since, in all cases but one, increases in food intake are obtained following administration of CCK_A but not of CCK_B receptor antagonists. The pattern of feeding changes in response to administration of CCK_A receptor antagonists is consistent with a specific role for endogenous CCK in satiety, in that meal size and duration are increased while the subsequent satiety ratio is decreased.

Acknowledgements

This work was supported by NIH grant DK19302.

References

Anika, S. M., Houpt, T. R. and Houpt, K. A. (1981). Cholecystokinin and satiety in pigs. *Am. J. Physiol.* **240**, R310–R318.

Antin, J., Gibbs, J., Holt, J., Young, R. C. and Smith, G. P. (1975). Cholecystokinin elicits the complete behavior sequence of satiety in rats. *J. Comp. Physiol. Psychol.* **89**, 784–790.

Asin, K. E. and Bednarz, L. (1982). Differential effects of CCK-JMV-180 on food intake in rats and mice. *Pharmacol. Biochem. Behav.* **42**, 291–295.

Asin, K. E., Bednarz, L., Nikkel, A. L., Gore, P. A., Jr., Montana, W. E., Cullen, M. J., Shiosaki, K., Craig, R. and Nadzan, A. M. (1992a). Behavioral effects of A-71623, a highly selective CCK-A agonist tetrapeptide. *Am. J. Physiol.* **263**, R125–R135.

Asin, K. E., Gore, P. A., Jr., Bednarz, L., Holladay, M. and Nadzan, A. M. (1992b). Effects of selective CCK receptor agonists on food intake after central or peripheral administration in rats. *Brain Res.* **517**, 169–174.

Baber, N. S., Dourish, C. T. and Hill, D. R. (1989). The role of CCK, caerulein and CCK antagonists in nociception. *Pain* **39**, 307–328.

Boden, P. and Woodruff, G. N. (1994). Ionic mechanisms underlying cholecystokinin action in the rat brain. *Ann. N. Y. Acad. Sci.* **713**, 129–137.

Buchan, A., Polak, J., Solcia, E., Capella, C., Hudson, D. and Pearse, A. (1978). Electron immunohistochemical evidence for the human intestinal I cell as the source of CCK. *Gut* **19**, 403–407.

Corp, E. S., McQuade, J., Moran, T. H. and Smith, G. P. (1993). Characterization of type A and type B CCK receptor binding sites in vagus nerve. *Brain Res.* **623**, 161–166.

Corwin, R. L., Gibbs, J. and Smith, G. P. (1991). Increased food intake after type A but not type B cholecystokinin receptor blockade. *Physiol. Behav.* **50**, 255–258.

Cox, K. L., von Schrenck, T., Moran, T. H., Gardner, J. D. and Jensen, R. T. (1990).

Characterization of cholecystokinin receptors in the sphincter of Oddi. *Am. J. Physiol.* **259**, G873–G881.

Crawley, J. N. (1994). Cholecystokinin modulates dopamine mediated behaviors: differential actions in medial posterior *versus* anterior nucleus accumbens. *Ann. N. Y. Acad. Sci.* **713**, 138–142.

Della-Fera, M. A. and Baile, C. A. (1979). Cholecystokinin octapeptide — continuous picomole injections into the cerebral ventricles of sheep suppress feeding. *Science* **206**, 471–473.

Dockray, G. J. (1976). Immunohistochemical evidence of cholecystokinin like peptides in brain. *Nature* **264**, 568–570.

Dourish, C. T., Ruckert, A. C., Tattersall, F. D. and Iversen, S. D. (1989a). Evidence that decreased feeding induced by systemic injection of cholecystokinin is mediated by CCK-A receptors. *Eur. J. Pharmacol.* **173**, 233–234.

Dourish, C. T., Rycroft, W. and Iversen, S. D. (1989b). Postponement of satiety by blockade of brain cholecystokinin (CCK-B) receptors. *Science* **245**, 1509–1511.

Figlewicz, D. P., Sipols, A. J., Porte, D. and Woods, S. C. (1989). Intraventricular CCK inhibits food intake and gastric emptying in the baboon. *Am. J. Physiol.* **256**, R1313–R1317.

Freidinger, R. M. (1992). Synthesis of non-peptide CCK antagonists. In *Multiple Cholecystokinin Receptors in the CNS* (C. T. Dourish, S. J. Cooper, S. D. Iversen and L. L. Iversen, eds), pp. 8–27. Oxford University Press, Oxford.

Galas, M.-C., Lignon, M.-F., Rodriguez, M., Mendre, C., Fulcrand, P., Laur, J. and Martinez, J. (1988). Structure–activity relationship studies on cholecystokinin: analogues with partial agonist activity. *Am. J. Physiol.* **254**, G176–G182.

Gibbs, J., Young, R. C. and Smith, G. P. (1973a). Cholecystokinin decreases food intake in rats. *J. Comp. Physiol. Psychol.* **84**, 488–495.

Gibbs, J., Young, R. C. and Smith G. P. (1973b). Cholecystokinin elicits satiety in rats with open gastric fistulas. *Nature* **245**, 323–325.

Gibbs, J., Falasco, J. D. and McHugh, P. R. (1976). Cholecystokinin decreases food intake in rhesus monkeys. *Am. J. Physiol.* **230**, 15–18.

Harro, J., Vasar, E. and Bradwejn, J. (1993). CCK in animal and human research in anxiety. *Trends Pharmacol. Sci.* **14**, 244–249.

Hill, D. R., Campbell, N. J., Shaw, T. M. and Woodruff, G. N. (1987). Autoradiographic localization and biochemical characterization of peripheral type CCK receptors in the rat CNS using highly selective nonpeptide CCK antagonists. *J. Neurosci.* **7**, 2967–1976.

Hill, D. R., Shaw, T. M., Graham, W. and Woodruff, G. N. (1990). Autoradiographical detection of cholecystokinin (CCK-A) receptors in primate brain using [^{125}I]-Bolton Hunter CCK8 and [^{3}H]-MK-329. *J. Neurosci.* **10**, 1070–1081.

Hill, D. R., Singh, L., Boden, P., Pinnock, G. N. and Hughes, J. (1992) Detection of CCK receptor subtypes in mammalian brain using highly selective non-peptide antagonists. In *Multiple Cholecystokinin Receptors in the CNS* (C. T. Dourish, S. J. Cooper, S. D. Iversen and L. L. Iversen, eds), pp. 57–76. Oxford University Press, Oxford.

Innis, R. B. and Snyder, S. H. (1980). Distinct cholecystokinin receptors in brain and pancreas. *Proc. Natl. Acad. Sci.* **77**, 6917–6921.

Jensen, R. T., Lemp, G. F. and Gardner, J. D. (1982). Interactions of COOH-terminal fragments of cholecystokinin with receptors on dispersed acini from guinea pig pancreas. *J. Biol. Chem.* **257**, 5554–5559.

Kissileff, H. R., Pi-Sunyer, X., Thornton, J. and Smith G. P. (1981). *C*-terminal octapeptide of cholecystokinin decreases food intake in man. *Am. J. Clin. Nutr.* **34**, 154–160.

Liebling, D. S., Eisner, J. D., Gibbs, J. and Smith, G. P. (1975). Intestinal satiety in rats. *J. Comp. Physiol. Psychol.* **89**, 955–965.

Lorenz, D. N., Kreielsheimer, G. and Smith, G. P. (1979). Effects of cholecystokinin, gastrin, secretin and GIP on sham feeding in the rat. *Physiol. Behav.* **23**, 1065–1072.

Matozaki, T., Martinez, J. and Williams, J. A. (1989). A new CCK analogue differentiates two functionally distinct CCK receptors in rat and mouse pancreatic acini. *Am. J. Physiol.* **257**, G594–G600.

Mercer, J. G. and Lawrence, C. B. (1992). Selectivity of cholecystokinin receptor antagonists, MK-329 and L-365 260, for axonally transported CCK binding sites in the rat vagus nerve. *Neurosci. Lett.* **137**, 229–231.

Moran, T. H., Robinson, P. H., Goldrich, M. S. and McHugh, P. R. (1986). Two brain cholecystokinin receptors: implications for behavioral actions. *Brain Res.* **362**, 175–179.

Moran, T. H., Norgren, R., Crosby, R. J. and McHugh, P. R. (1990). Central and peripheral vagal transport of cholecystokinin binding sites occurs in afferent fibers. *Brain Res.* **526**, 95–102.

Moran, T. H., Ameglio, P. J., Schwartz, G. J. and McHugh, P. R. (1992). Blockade of type A, not type B, CCK receptors attenuates the satiety action of exogenous and endogenous CCK. *Am. J. Physiol.* **262**, R46–R50.

Moran, T. H., Ameglio, P. J., Peyton, H. J., Schwartz, G. J. and McHugh, P. R. (1993). Blockade of type A, but not type B, CCK receptors postpones satiety in rhesus monkeys. *Am. J. Physiol.* **265**, R620–R624.

Moran, T. H., Kornbluh, R., Moore, K. and Schwartz, G. J. (1994). Cholecystokinin inhibits gastric emptying and contracts the pyloric sphincter in rats by interacting with low affinity CCK receptor sites. *Regul. Pept.* **52**, 165–172.

Raybould, H. E. and Lloyd, K. C. (1994). Integration of postprandial function in the proximal gastrointestinal tract: role of CCK and sensory pathways. *Ann. N. Y. Acad. Sci.* **713**, 143–156.

Reeve, J. R., Eysselein, V. E., Ho, F. J., Chew, P., Vigna, S. R., Liddle, R. A. and Evans, C. (1994). Natural and synthetic CCK-58. *Ann. N. Y. Acad. Sci.* **713**, 11–21.

Reidelberger, R. D. and O'Rourke, M. F. (1989). Potent cholecystokinin antagonist L-364 718 stimulates food intake in rats. *Am. J. Physiol.* **257**, R1512–R1518.

Reidelberger, R. D. and Solomon, T. E. (1986). Comparative effects of CCK-8 on feeding, sham feeding, and exocrine pancreatic secretion in rats. *Am. J. Physiol.* **251**, R97–R105.

Reidelberger, R. D., Varga, G. and Solomon, T. E. (1991). Effects of selective cholecystokinin antagonists L364 718 and L365 260 on food intake in rats. *Peptides* **12**, 1215–1221.

Ritter, R. C., Brenner, L. A. and Tamura, C. S. (1994). Endogenous CCK and peripheral neural substrates of intestinal satiety. *Ann. N. Y. Acad. Sci.* **713**, 255–267.

Sankaran, H., Goldfine, I. D., Bailey, A., Licko, V. and Williams, J. A. (1982). Relationship of cholecystokinin receptor binding to regulation of biological functions in pancreatic acini. *Am. J. Physiol.* **242**, G250–G257.

Schick, R. R., Yaksh, T. L. and Go, W. (1986). Intracerebroventricular injections of cholecystokinin octapeptide suppresses feeding in rats: pharmacological characterization of this action. *Regul. Pept.* **14**, 277–291.

Schneider, L. H., Murphy, R. B., Gibbs, J. and Smith, G. P. (1988). Comparative potencies of CCK antagonists for the reversal of the satiating effect of cholecystokinin. In *Cholecystokinin Antagonists* (R. Y. Wang and R. Schoenfeld, eds), pp. 263–284. Alan Liss, New York.

Schultzberg, M. T., Hokfelt, T., Nilsson, G., Terenius, L., Rehfeld, J. F., Brown, M., Rlde, R., Goldstein, M. and Said, S. (1980). Distribution of peptide and catecholamine containing neurons in the gastrointestinal tract of the rat and guinea-pig: immunohistochemical studies with antisera to substance P, vasoactive intestinal peptide, enkephalin, somatostatin, gastrin/cholecystokinin, neurotensin, and dopamine B-hydroxylase. *Neuroscience* **5**, 689–744.

Schwartz, G. J., McHugh, P. R. and Moran, T. H. (1994). Pharmacological dissociation of responses to CCK and gastric loads in rat mechanosensitive vagal afferents. *Am. J. Physiol.* **267**, R303–R308.

Shillabeer, G. and Davison, J. S. (1984). The cholecystokinin antagonist, proglumide, increases food intake in the rat. *Regul. Pept.* **48**, 640–641.

Silver, A. J., Flood, J. F., Song, A. M. and Morley, J. E. (1989). Evidence for a physiological role for CCK in the regulation of food intake in mice. *Am. J. Physiol.* **256**, R646–R652.

Smith, G. T., Moran, T. H., Coyle, J. T., Kuhar, T. L., O'Donahue, T. L. and McHugh, P. R. (1984). Anatomical localization of cholecystokinin receptors to the pyloric sphincter. *Am. J. Physiol.* **246**, R127–R130.

Stark, H. A., Sharp, C. M., Sutliff, V. E., Martinez, R. T. and Gardner, J. D. (1989). A peptide that distinguishes high-affinity cholecystokinin receptors from low-affinity cholecystokinin receptors. *Biochim. Biophys. Acta* **1010**, 145–150.

Wank, S. A., Harkins, R., Jensen, R. T., Shapira, H., de Weerth, A. and Slattery, T. (1992a). Purification, molecular cloning and functional expression of the cholecystokinin receptor from rat pancreas. *Proc. Natl. Acad. Sci.* **89**, 3125–3129.

Wank, S. A., Pisegna, J. R. and de Weerth, A. (1992b). Brain and gastrointestinal cholecystokinin receptor family: structure and functional expression. *Proc. Natl. Acad. Sci.* **89**, 8691–8695.

Wank, S. A., Pisegna, J. R. and de Weerth, A. (1994). Cholecystokinin receptor family. *Ann. N. Y. Acad. Sci.* **713**, 49–66.

Weatherford, S. C., Chiruzzo, F. Y. and Laughton, W. B. (1992). Satiety induced by endogenous and exogenous cholecystokinin is mediated by CCK-A receptors in mice. *Am. J. Physiol.* **262**, R575–R578.

Weatherford, S. C., Laughton, W. B., Salabarria, J., Danho, W., Tilley, J. W., Netterville, L. A., Schwartz, G. J. and Moran, T. H. (1993). CCK satiety is differentially mediated by high- and low-affinity CCK receptors in mice and rats. *Am. J. Physiol.* **264**, R244–R249.

Zarbin, M. A., Innis, R. B., Wamsley, J. K., Snyder, S. K. and Kuhar, M. J. (1983). Autoradiographic localization of cholecystokinin receptors in rodent brain. *J. Neurosci.* **3**, 877–906.

2

Cholecystokinin–Dopamine Interactions in Satiety

P. SÖDERSTEN[1], I. BEDNAR[1], G. A.
QURESHI[1], H. CARRER[2], M. QIAN[1],
H. MAMOUN[3], J. M. KAPLAN[4] and
A. E. JOHNSON[5]

[1] Department of Clinical Neuroscience and Family Medicine,
Division of Applied Neuroendocrinology, Karolinska Institute,
Novum S-141 57 Huddinge, Sweden
[2] Instituto de Investigación Médica, M. y M. Ferreyra, Córdoba,
Argentina
[3] Department of Renal Medicine, Karolinska Institute, S-141 86
Huddinge, Sweden
[4] Department of Psychology, University of Pennsylvania,
Philadelphia, PA 19104, USA
[5] Department of Psychiatry, Ulleråker, University of Uppsala,
S-750 17 Uppsala, Sweden

1 Introduction

1.1 Emergence of Smith's CCK-8 hypothesis of satiety

Perhaps for historical reasons, study of the neuroendocrine control of feeding behaviour concentrated on hypothalamic 'centres' for a long while (Stellar, 1954). For example, it has been known for a long time that hypothalamic damage can cause obesity (Rayer, 1823; Mohr, 1840). More recently, it was realized that, rather than interfering directly with the control of behavioural responses, hypothalamic lesions can alter peripheral mechanisms of metabolism, which produce changes in behaviour via feedback actions on the brain (Bray et al., 1990; Friedman and Stricker, 1976; Steffens et al., 1990). Peripheral messengers signalling enhanced energy and/or metabolic requirements have been considered initiators of feeding and, historically, generated lipostatic (Kennedy, 1953), glucostatic (Mayer, 1955) and aminostatic

DRUG RECEPTOR SUBTYPES AND INGESTIVE BEHAVIOUR
ISBN 0-12-187620-9

(Mellinkoff *et al.*, 1956) theories of feeding behaviour, inspired by the idea that feeding is homeostatically regulated. Although some of these peripheral signals, such as glucose (Smith and Campfield, 1993) and insulin (Schwartz *et al.*, 1992), have been studied in considerable detail, it is still uncertain exactly how feeding is initiated (Friedman, 1990). This is an important issue because knowledge of the sensory stimuli that control the initiation of a behaviour is needed for analysis of that behaviour. Partly for this reason, Smith (1982) has suggested an alternative: that we study the termination of feeding, i.e. the mechanisms of satiation. We know the stimulus, food ingestion, and the site of action, the gastrointestinal tract, which are conducive to satiety (Deutsch, 1990). Using this perspective, Smith hypothesized that release of the octapeptide of cholecystokinin (CCK-8) from the duodenum during a meal is a messenger that signals satiety (Gibbs *et al.*, 1973a,b) and, after an admirable series of experiments, now considered the hypotheses 'proven' (Smith and Gibbs, 1993).

1.2 Disproval of the CCK-8 hypothesis refuted

This is not a proper place for detailing all the arguments for and against the CCK-8 hypothesis. However, some issues may be worthy of brief discussion because there have been numerous attempts to disprove the hypothesis.

First, the suggestion that supraphysiological levels of CCK-8 are required for suppression of feeding behaviour (Deutsch, 1990) is unlikely to be true. Experiments by Lindén in this laboratory showed that suppression of feeding occurs in the presence of physiological plasma levels of CCK-8 in a variety of physiological states (Lindén and Södersten, 1990).

Second, some have argued, in extensive writing, that the action of CCK-8 on ingestive behaviour is not specific but due to the induction of aversion to the food used for testing (Deutsch, 1990). In a recent experiment in this laboratory, however, we found selective suppression of ingestive behaviour by CCK-8. Thus, rats infused intraorally with sucrose solutions through permanently implanted cannulas and presented with a rat of the opposite sex showed ingestive and sexual behaviour simultaneously (Kaplan *et al.*, 1992). When the rats were injected with CCK-8, ingestive behaviour was suppressed but sexual behaviour was unaffected (Fig. 1). This observation shows the effect of CCK-8 is behaviourally specific and undermines the suggestion that the effect of CCK-8 is caused by the induction of aversion, because rats in a state of aversion would not be expected to copulate without some sign of distress.

The idea that CCK-8 activates aversion has been suggested to have a neuroendocrine marker. Thus, injection of CCK-8 causes release of oxytocin into the peripheral circulation, as does injection of an emetic agent. Plasma levels of oxytocin were, therefore, suggested to reflect the activation of a 'a nausea pathway in the brain' (Verbalis *et al.*, 1986). This extensively published hypothesis (Olson *et al.*, 1991) is disproven by the finding that intracerebroven-

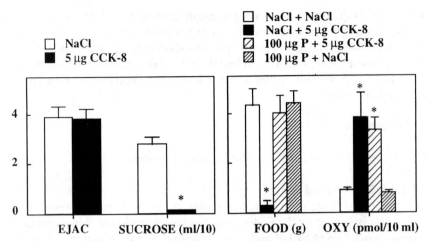

Fig. 1 Left: number of ejaculations (EJAC) and amount of sucrose ingested by male rats injected with NaCl or CCK-8. The rats were presented with a sexually receptive female and simultaneously infused with sucrose intraorally. Right: ingestion of food and release of oxytocin (OXY) in male rats treated with CCK-8 in combination with intracerebroventricular proglumide (P). The * indicates a statistically significant difference from the NaCl value. (From Lindén et al. (1989), with permission.)

tricular injection of proglumide, a non-specific CCK antagonist, reversed the inhibitory effect of CCK-8 on ingestive behaviour but did not affect the release of oxytocin (Fig. 1; Lindén et al., 1989). Clearly enough, release of oxytocin from the pituitary gland can be dissociated from inhibition of feeding.

More interesting, however, is the possibility that development of aversion during a meal is a physiological mechanism whereby the meal is terminated (Grill and Berridge, 1985). If this hypothesis proves correct, it may bridge the gap between some of the attempts at proving and disproving the CCK-8 hypothesis.

1.3 Failure of intracerebral injection of CCK-8 to suppress feeding behaviour

The finding that intracerebroventricular, but not peripheral, injection of a low dose of the non-selective CCK antagonist proglumide prevented the effect of intraperitoneal injection of CCK-8 (Fig. 1; Lindén et al., 1989) led to the suggestion that peripheral release of CCK-8 activates neural networks that control feeding and utilize CCK peptides as transmitters (Södersten et al., 1992). However, in an extensive series of experiments we failed to affect food intake in male rats by a variety of procedures of intracerebral administration of CCK-8 and CCK analogues (Lindén et al., 1990). Therefore, we suggested that CCK peptides interact with some other transmitter(s) in the brain in the control of feeding. Dopamine is a possible transmitter candidate, because it coexists with CCK peptides in neural pathways, e.g. mesolimbic neurons (Hökfelt *et al.*, 1980), from which it is released upon ingestion of food (A. G. Phillips *et al.*, 1991). Consequently, we have studied the role of dopamine in the suppressive effect of CCK-8 on feeding behaviour in a series of experiments, described in some detail below.

2 Results

2.1 Stimulation and blockade of dopamine receptors

2.1.1 Effects on food intake

Preliminary evidence that release of dopamine in the brain is important for satiety was provided by the finding that the concentration of dopamine in the cerebrospinal fluid (CSF) of male rats decreased with deprivation of food and increased in food-deprived rats 1 h after intake of food or 10 min after intraperitoneal injection of 5 μg CCK-8, the dose used in most of these experiments to inhibit food intake (Bednar *et al.*, 1991). CSF was chosen as a suitable compartment for measurement of dopamine, because turnover of dopamine in the CSF reflects turnover in the brain (Hutson *et al.*, 1984), because CSF is an extension of the extracellular fluid in which synaptic release of dopamine can be measured (Starke *et al.*, 1989) and because we had no *a priori* reason to select any specific subcortical area for measurement.

These results encouraged a study of the effect of a dopamine agonist on food intake. The combined dopamine D_1-D_2 agonist apomorphine (APO) suppressed the intake of food in a dose-dependent manner (0, 0.05, 0.1, 0.4 μg/ rat). However, so did the dopamine D_1-D_2 antagonist *cis*-flupenthixol (*cis*-FLU). Interestingly, however, it was possible to find a dose of *cis*-FLU (100 μg) that reversed the effect of APO while having no effect of its own. This dose of *cis*-FLU also antagonized the inhibitory effect of CCK-8 (Bednar *et al.*, 1991).

2.1.2 Effects on consummatory ingestive behaviour

While these results support the possibility that release of dopamine in the brain and the associated stimulation of dopamine receptors may be a mechanism whereby CCK-8 inhibits food intake, some of the results were less rewarding in that, with increasing doses, inhibition of food intake was found with the agonist as well as with the antagonist. This, however, was expected because of the well-known effects of dopamine agonists and antagonists on motor capacity. Thus, with increasing doses of an agonist, stereotyped responses such as increased motor activity, rearing, sniffing and eventually oral dyskinesias ensue, and with an antagonist inhibition of motor activity and eventually immobilization occurs (Waddington and Daly, 1993). Such behaviour will necessarily interfere with the responses used to approach food, i.e. appetitive ingestive behaviour (Craig, 1918).

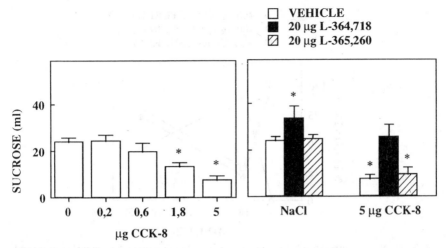

Fig. 2 Suppression of sucrose intake in male rats by CCK-8 and the effect of CCK-8 in combination with a CCK_A (L-364 718) of CCK_B (L-365 260) receptor antagonist. The sucrose was infused intraorally. The * indicates a statistically significant difference from the NaCl value. (From Bednar et al. (1992a), with permission.)

To avoid such disruptive effects we employed a test developed by Grill and Norgren (1978), which specifically measures the responses used to ingest food, i.e. consummatory ingestive behaviour (Craig, 1918), and discounts the significance of appetitive responding. In this test, a solution is delivered through permanently implanted intraoral cannulas by means of an infusion pump. In all experiments we used a 1 mol/l solution of sucrose and an infusion rate of 1 ml/min. Intake of the sucrose solution starts once the infusion starts and ends when the rat rejects the solution, either passively by letting it drip from its mouth, or actively by rubbing its chin against the floor or wall of the test arena or by trying to rid itself of the solution by forepaw chin rubbing (Grill et al., 1987). Intake of the sucrose solution stabilizes at about 20 ml within five daily tests (Kaplan et al., 1992). However, with extended testing, intake may slowly increase further.

Fig. 2 shows that CCK-8 inhibits intraoral intake of sucrose in a dose dependent fashion and that the CCK_A receptor antagonist L364 718, but not the CCK_B receptor antagonist L-365 260, reverses this effect and, by itself, stimulates intake (Bednar et al., 1992a). Ingestion of sucrose causes release of CCK-8 into the blood (Mamoun et al., 1995).

To investigate the effect of dopamine receptor stimulation on consummatory ingestive behaviour and to compare it with the effect of CCK-8, the effect of APO on stereotyped behaviour was investigated first, because it is dopamine receptor mediated (Waddington and Daly, 1993). Stereotyped behaviour appeared within 10 min of intraperitoneal administration of 400 μg APO and continued for 60 min, with 50% of the rats showing behavioural stereotypies 45

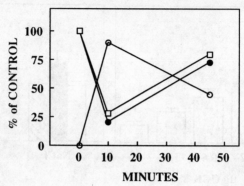

Fig. 3 Display of stereotyped behaviour and suppression of sucrose intake in male rats treated with apomorphine (APO) or CCK-8. The sucrose was infused intraorally. (From Bednar *et al.* (1992a), with permission.)

min after the injection (Fig. 3). Using this behavioural assay, maximal dopamine receptor stimulation was evident 10–35 min following injection and threshold (50%) activation occurred at 45 min. Changes in APO inhibition of consummatory ingestive behaviour paralleled changes in stereotypy, with maximum inhibition beginning after 10 min and threshold levels occurring after 45 min. Interestingly, the effect of 5 μg CCK-8 on consummatory ingestive

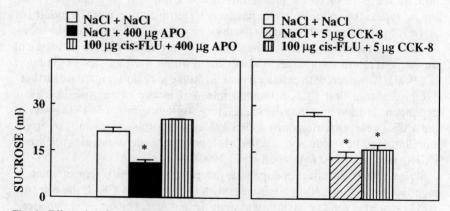

Fig. 4 Effect of *cis*-flupenthixol (*cis*-FLU) on suppression of sucrose intake in male rats treated with apomorphine (APO) or CCK-8. The sucrose was infused intraorally. The * indicates a statistically significant difference from the NaCl value. (From Bednar *et al.* (1992a), with permission.)

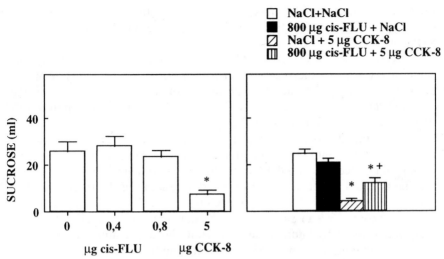

Fig. 5   Effect of *cis*-flupenthixol (*cis*-FLU) and/or CCK-8 on sucrose intake in male rats. The sucrose was infused intraorally. The * indicates a statistically significant difference from NaCl value. The + indicates a value significantly higher than for NaCl + 5 μg CCK-8. (From Bednar *et al.* (1992a), with permission.)

behaviour had a similar magnitude and time course as that of APO (Fig. 3). However, CCK-8 did not induce behavioural stereotypy (Bednar *et al.*, 1992a).

The effect of the dopamine agonist on ingestion can be dissociated from its effect on stereotyped responses. Pretreatment with 100 μg *cis*-FLU thus

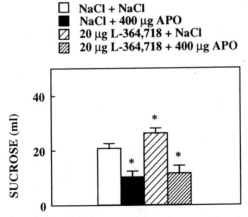

Fig. 6   Effect of apomorphine (APO) in combination with a CCK$_A$ receptor antagonist (L-364718) on sucrose intake in male rats. The sucrose was infused intraorally. The * indicates a statistically significant difference from the NaCl value. (From Bednar *et al.* (1992a), with permission.)

reversed the effect of APO on consummatory ingestive behaviour but not on stereotypy. This dose of *cis*-FLU failed to prevent the inhibitory effect of CCK-8 (Fig. 4).

Interestingly, *cis*-FLU had no effect on the intraoral intake of the sucrose solution, even when the dose was increased eight times (Fig. 5). Animals treated with this dose of cis-FLU remained motionless for over 4 h after the injection. Treatment with the high dose of *cis*-FLU in part prevented the effect of 5 μg CCK-8 (Fig. 5; Bednar *et al.*, 1992a).

These results demonstrate that rats can show ingestive and either stereotyped responses or immobility simultaneously. Therefore, the inhibitory effect of dopamine receptor stimulation on consummatory ingestive behaviour is a specific one and is not mediated by interfering non-specific responses. The results also suggest that the inhibitory effect of CCK-8 on consummatory ingestive behaviour is in part mediated by dopamine receptor stimulation. It follows that these receptors are distinct from those mediating motor stereotypes. In addition, they are possibly distinct from the CCK_A receptors which mediate the effect of CCK-8, because blockade of CCK_A receptor with L-364 718, which stimulates ingestive behaviour (Fig. 2), did not affect the inhibition induced by APO (Fig. 6).

2.1.3 Dopamine receptor blockade and reward

The normal ingestive capacity of rats rendered immobile for a prolonged period of time by treatment with 800 μg *cis*-FLU is interesting because it addresses the thoroughly studied question whether the disruptive effects of dopamine receptor blockade on behaviour is a consequence of the debilitating effect on motor capacity and/or blockade of reward (Le Moal and Simon, 1991). Ingestion of sweet solutions is rewarding (Corbin and Stellar, 1964) and reward is mediated by mesocorticolimbic dopamine neurons (Le Moal and Simon, 1991). Dopamine receptor antagonists block the rewarding aspect of food (Wise *et al.*, 1978; Weatherford *et al.*, 1990) and sweetness (Schneider *et al.*, 1990; G. Phillips *et al.*, 1991; Willner *et al.*, 1991). Such mechanisms, however, are unlikely to play a role in the present context because dopamine receptor blockade had no inhibitory effect on ingestion of the sucrose solution. Instead, it partially reversed the inhibitory effect of CCK-8, that is it actually stimulated intake. Stimulation of intake of a rewarding solution should not occur if the mechanism that mediates reward is blocked.

2.2 Stimulation and inhibition of dopamine release

Next, the effect of dopamine release in the brain was studied. Fig. 7 shows that injection of amphetamine, the model substance for eliciting release of dopamine in the brain (Segal and Kuczenski, 1992), produced a dose-dependent inhibition of the intake of pellets, a test requiring emission of appetitive and consummatory ingestive responses. However, amphetamine had no effect on

μg AMPH

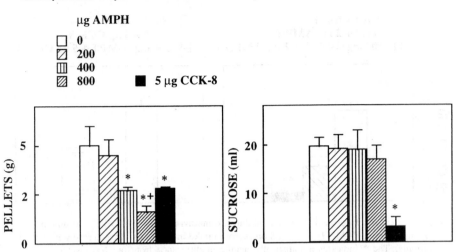

Fig. 7   Effect of amphetamine (AMPH) on intake of food pellets or sucrose in male rats. The sucrose was infused intraorally. The * indicates a statistically significant difference from the NaCl value. The + indicates a value significantly lower than for 5 μg CCK-8. (From Bednar *et al.* (1992b), with permission.)

intraoral intake of sucrose (Fig. 7; Bednar *et al.*, 1992b). These results confirm the observations of Wolgin and co-workers (1988). Interestingly, 800 μg amphetamine was more effective than CCK-8 in inhibiting the intake of pellets, but less effective in inhibiting the intake of sucrose. In fact, this dose of amphetamine had no effect on the intake of sucrose (Fig. 7), yet it induced marked behavioural stereotypy (Bednar *et al.*, 1992b). These results are in line with those of APO described above, showing that rats can display consummatory ingestive behaviour and behavioural stereotypies simultaneously.

A simple explanation for the inhibitory effect of amphetamine on food intake is, therefore, that by stimulation of motor activity as a consequence of the release of dopamine in striatal terminals amphetamine interferes with the animal's capacity to engage in appetitive responses. However, the effect of amphetamine on appetitive ingestive behaviour is transient and, with repeated injections of amphetamine, rats may learn to channel stereotyped responses into ingestive responses (Wolgin and Kinney, 1992).

Release of dopamine in the brain does not by itself affect consummatory response capacity. An extremely high dose of amphetamine (2 mg) was required for inhibition of intraoral intake of sucrose (Fig. 8; Bednar *et al.*, 1992b). However, when the release of dopamine induced by this dose of amphetamine, measured by the accumulation of 3-methoxytyramine in the striatum, was prevented with a tyrosine hydroxylase inhibitor (100 mg α-methyl-p-tyrosine, α-MPT), inhibition of intraoral intake of sucrose was enhanced (Fig. 8). The inhibitory effect of CCK-8, however, was in part reversed by α-MPT (Fig. 8).

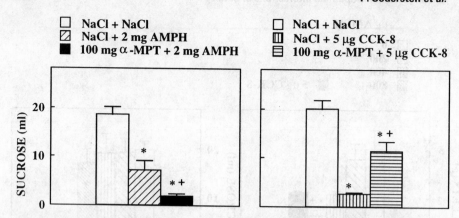

Fig. 8 Effect of a tyrosine hydroxylase inhibitor, α-methyl-p-tyrosine (α-MPT), in combination with amphetamine (AMPH) or CCK-8 on sucrose intake in male rats. The sucrose was infused intraorally. The * indicates a statistically significant difference from the NaCl value. The + indicates: left, a value significantly lower than NaCl + 2 µg AMPH; right, a value significantly higher than NaCl + 5 µg CCK-8. (From Bednar *et al.* (1992b), with permission.)

The results suggest that the inhibitory effect of a high dose of amphetamine on consummatory ingestive behaviour is not due to release of dopamine (see discussion by Bednar *et al.*, 1992b). The results also suggest that, although release of dopamine in the brain has no effect on consummatory ingestive behaviour in itself, it is part of the mechanism whereby CCK-8 inhibits this behaviour. Admittedly, however, this hypothesis rests on indirect pharmacological evidence because we found no evidence that injection of CCK-8 provokes release of dopamine in the brain in these studies (Bednar *et al.*, 1992b).

2.3 Possible sites of dopamine release

2.3.1 Effect of 6-hydroxydopamine lesion of the nucleus accumbens

Release of dopamine in the terminal region of the mesocorticolimbic dopaminergic neurons in the ventral striatum, i.e. the nucleus accumbens, occurs when rats display a variety of motivated behaviour and is a well-studied phenomenon (Le Moal and Simon, 1991). However, Fig. 9 shows that a 6-hydroxydopamine (6-OHDA) lesion of the nucleus accumbens had no effect on intraoral intake of sucrose and that rats with such lesions responded normally to injection of CCK-8. The concentration of dopamine was decreased to $15.9 \pm 3.2\%$ ($n = 12$) of that of controls ($n = 6$) in the nucleus accumbens but was unaffected in the dorsal striatum ($105.3 \pm 3.5\%$ of controls).

2.3.2 Intraoral intake in chronic decerebrate rats

In an extensive series of unpublished experiments we found no evidence that release of dopamine occurs in any forebrain structure in response to injection

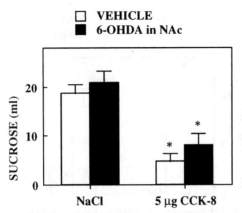

Fig. 9 Effect of CCK-8 on sucrose intake in male rats with lesions in the nucleus accumbens (NAc). 6-OHDA, 6-hydroxydopamine. The sucrose was infused intraorally. The * indicates a statistically significant difference from the NaCl value.

of CCK-8. However, this negative finding is probably due to the use of procedures with insufficient anatomical resolution (e.g. Bednar et al., 1992b), because microdialysis studies have clearly shown that CCK peptides can cause release of dopamine in the nucleus accumbens. However, the interaction between CCK and dopamine in the nucleus accumbens is exceedingly complex (Marshall et al., 1991) and as yet impossible to relate to any aspect of ingestive behaviour.

Given the negative finding with 6-OHDA lesions of the nucleus accumbens (Fig. 9), we turned to an important observation by Grill and Smith (1988). These investigators found that rats in which the forebrain had been disconnected from the brainstem at the level of the superior colliculus down to the ventral tegmental–substantia nigra region at the base of the brain are capable of responding to injection of CCK-8 by reducing their intraoral intake of sucrose. This observation directs attention to brainstem control mechanisms of ingestive behaviour. These have been extensively explored by Grill, Kaplan and collaborators (Grill and Kaplan, 1990), and it is clear that a considerable amount of regulatory competence is retained in these chronic decerebrate (CD) rats. Thus, CD rats are capable of maintaining bodyweight if given three daily intraoral intake tests (Kaplan et al., 1993). However, appetitive response capacity is absent in CD rats (Grill et al., 1987), as is the capacity to defend bodyweight when facing a challenge (Kaplan et al., 1993).

Fig. 10 shows a replication of the report by Grill and Smith (1988) that CCK-8 inhibits intraoral intake of sucrose in CD rats and that APO also suppresses intake (Kaplan and Södersten, 1994).

Interestingly, injection of APO did not stimulate display of stereotyped behaviour in the CD rats, thus supporting the suggestion that the dopamine

30 P. Södersten *et al.*

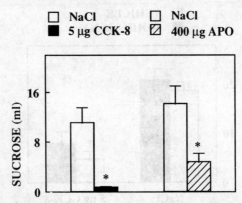

☐ NaCl   ☐ NaCl
■ 5 µg CCK-8   ▨ 400 µg APO

Fig. 10 Effects of CCK-8 or apomorphine (APO) on sucrose intake in chronic decerebrate male rats. The sucrose was infused intraorally. The * indicates a statistically significant difference from the NaCl value. (From Kaplan and Södersten (1994), with permission.)

receptors mediating ingestive behaviour can be dissociated from those mediating stereotypy (Kaplan and Södersten, 1994).

These results open the possibility that dopamine receptors in the brainstem participate in the control of consummatory ingestive behaviour. The brainstem is a rather neglected area in research on dopamine receptor localization and function, which mainly concerns nigrostriatal and mesolimbic terminal areas (Joyce *et al.*, 1993). However, dopamine receptors are present in the brainstem (Camps *et al.*, 1989; Cortés *et al.*, 1989). Obviously, these dopamine receptors deserve further investigation.

2.4 Glutamate inhibits ingestive behaviour

In all of the above-mentioned manipulations of dopaminergic mechanisms in the brain, the inhibitory effect of CCK-8 on feeding was reversed only partially. To reverse the effect completely, we depleted cerebral monoamines with reserpine. Reserpinized rats, however, showed no ingestive responses, thus making them unsuitable for studying inhibitory effects. Motor activity is activated in reserpinized rats with dopamine agonists (Carlsson *et al.*, 1957). However, ingestive behaviour is not (Bednar *et al.*, 1994). Carlsson and Carlsson (1990) reported restoration of motor activity in amine-depleted mice with the non-competitive NMDA receptor antagonist MK801, suggesting glutamate–dopamine interactions in the control of motor activity. Inspired by these findings we found that reserpine not only depleted dopamine from striatal samples but also increased the concentration of glutamate, and that ingestive responses could be reactivated in reserpinized rats by MK801 (Bednar *et al.*, 1994).

Experiments were made to investigate whether these pharmacological

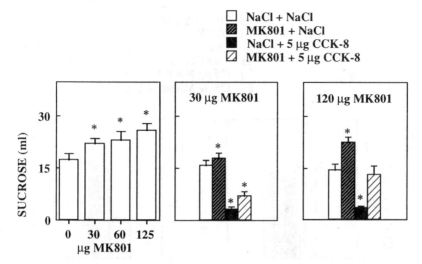

Fig. 11   Effect of an NMDA receptor antagonist (MK801) on sucrose intake in male rats. The rats were treated with MK801 in combination with CCK-8. The sucrose was infused intraorally. The * indicates a statistically significant difference from the NaCl value. (From Bednar *et al.* (1994), with permission.)

observations could be related to the mechanism of action of CCK-8. Fig. 11 shows that MK801 facilitated intraoral intake of sucrose and antagonized the effect of CCK-8 in a dose-dependent manner.

An attempt was then made to relate the effect of CCK-8 to a site in the brainstem that is of interest for ingestive behaviour. We chose to study the nucleus of the solitary tract (NTS), because of its well-known role as an interface conveying feeding-relevant information from the gastrointestinal tract to the brain (Norgren and Smith, 1988; Spector *et al.*, 1992). Fig. 12 shows that the concentration of glutamate in the NTS decreased as a consequence of food deprivation and that it increased in food-deprived rats that had ingested sucrose or had received an injection of CCK-8. Treatment with MK801 increased the concentration of glutamate in the NTS and prevented the further increase expected after injection of CCK-8. The concentration of dopamine in the NTS was unaffected by deprivation of food but increased markedly after ingestion of sucrose or injection of CCK-8 in rats deprived of food. Treatment with MK801 prevented the increase in dopamine levels seen in the NTS after injection of CCK-8 (Bednar *et al.*, 1994).

Interestingly, specific binding of MK801 was found in the caudomedial part of the NTS, where the vagal afferents mediating the effects of CCK-8 terminate (Norgren and Smith, 1988; Bednar *et al.*, 1994).

The results suggest that the inhibitory effect of CCK-8 on consummatory ingestive behaviour is, at least in part, the result of an interaction between glutamate and dopamine in the NTS.

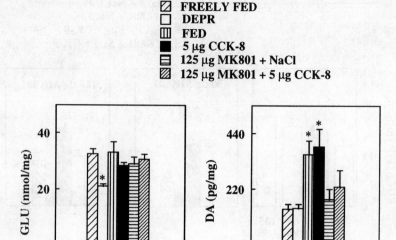

☑ FREELY FED
☐ DEPR
⊞ FED
■ 5 μg CCK-8
☰ 125 μg MK801 + NaCl
☒ 125 μg MK801 + 5 μg CCK-8

Fig. 12 Concentration of glutamate (GLU) and dopamine (DA) in the nucleus of the solitary tract of male rats treated with an NMDA receptor antagonist (MK801) in combination with CCK-8. The * indicates a statistically significant difference from the NaCl value. DEPR, Animals deprived of food. (From, Bednar *et al.* (1994), with permission.)

3 Comments

While CCK-8 is about as potent in suppressing intake in a test requiring display of appetitive ingestive responses as in one not demanding such behaviour, manipulation of dopamine function is much more effective in the former test (Bednar *et al.*, 1991, 1992a). Manoeuvres stimulating release of dopamine in the brain are in fact very potent in interfering with appetitive ingestive behaviour but ineffective in modifying consummatory ingestive behaviour (Wolgin *et al.*, 1988; Bednar *et al.*, 1992b). Interestingly, however, with repeated injections of amphetamine, for example, rats channel the stereotyped responses induced by the amphetamine, which initially compete with appetitive ingestive responses, into responses compatible with ingestion (Wolgin and Kinney, 1992). It seems possible that when facing other than feeding-relevant stimuli rats, in which ascending dopaminergic systems have been artificially aroused, might channel their behaviour in other directions (Berridge and Valenstein, 1991). Results of such experiments enforce the view that ascending dopamine systems serve no specific behavioural function but allow expression of the functions of the systems on to which they project (Le Moal and Simon, 1991).

In the present series of experiments we arrived at the hypothesis that, rather than playing a role in the initiation of ingestive behaviour, release of dopamine is involved in the mechanisms whereby CCK-8 suppresses the consummatory aspect of this behaviour. It is well known that lesioning of dopaminergic systems ascending from brainstem to forebrain eliminates ingestive behaviour (Ungerstedt, 1971; Stricker and Zigmond, 1976; Zigmond et al., 1990). However, it seems unlikely that release of dopamine in the terminal areas of these neurons, e.g. the nucleus accumbens, is of importance for the mechanism of action of CCK-8. First, a lesion in the nucleus accumbens had no effect on ingestive behaviour or on behavioural sensitivity to CCK-8. Second, consummatory (but not appetitive) response capacity as well as sensitivity to CCK-8 is retained in CD rats. In this preparation the behavioural roles of the ascending dopaminergic systems are eliminated. These findings raise the possibility that CCK-8-induced release of dopamine in the brainstem inhibits ingestive behaviour. Some support for this hypothesis is provided by the finding that the concentration of dopamine was increased in the NTS in response to feeding or injection of CCK-8 (Bednar et al., 1994). However, many facts impose restrictions on this suggestion. Thus, there is no conclusive anatomical support for the existence of dopaminergic neurons or terminals in the NTS, although this possibility has been discussed (Björklund and Lindvall, 1984). Also, a recent microdialysis study found no evidence for synaptic release of dopamine in the NTS (Yue et al., 1994). Because of the existence of noradrenergic cells in the brainstem, which are activated by CCK-8 (Luckman, 1992), it seems possible instead that dopamine serves a role as a precursor to noradrenaline, rather than as a transmitter in this brain area. However, our finding that APO suppressed consummatory ingestive behaviour in CD rats argues for a role of brainstem dopamine receptors in feeding behaviour. The possibility that dopamine acts as a transmitter in the brainstem should, therefore, be explored further.

None of the pharmacological manipulations of the dopaminergic system used in the present series of experiments prevented the inhibitory effect of CCK-8 on consummatory ingestive behaviour. Other transmitter systems, e.g. 5-hydroxytryptamine (5-HT; see Chapters 3, 4, 5 and 13) must obviously be involved. It has been suggested that 5-HT acts on the paraventricular hypothalamic nuclei to suppress carbohydrate intake (Leibowitz, 1992). This suggestion is of obvious importance in the present context because we used sucrose solutions for behavioural testing and because 5-HT is released in this brain area in response to treatment with CCK-8 (Kendrick et al., 1991). However, we found only a minor effect of inhibiting the synthesis of 5-HT on the behavioural sensitivity of CCK-8 (Esfahami et al., 1995).

Our interest in the possibility that glutamate might play a role in the mechanisms of action of CCK-8 was aroused by the observation that ingestive responses were inhibited in reserpinized rats and, correlatively, the concentration of glutamate was increased in striatal terminals. Feeding behaviour was reactivated in reserpinized rats by treatment with the NMDA receptor antagonist MK801. This finding, and the finding that MK801 facilitates the intraoral intake of sucrose and that intake of sucrose or injection of CCK-8 increases the concentration of dopamine and glutamate in the NTS, opens the possibility that an interaction between dopamine and glutamate, in the NTS in part explains the effect of CCK-8 (Bednar et al., 1994). Previous research has suggested a role for excitatory amino acids in the control of ingestive behaviour by the forebrain (see Chapter 14).

Interactive effects between dopamine and glutamate are now intensely studied using behavioural (Kelley and Delfs, 1994), microdialysis (Morari et al., 1994), electrophysiological (Zhang et al., 1994) and autoradiographic (Johnson et al., 1994) methods. These studies concentrate on mesolimbic and nigrostriatal dopaminergic systems. Our results open the possibility that interactions between dopamine and glutamate are not limited to forebrain but may also take place in the brainstem.

Acknowledgements

We thank the Swedish MRC, the Bank of Sweden Tercentenary Foundation and the Karolinska Institute for financial support, Dr L. Iversen of Merck, Sharp and Dohme for supplying MK801, L-364 718 and L-365 260, and Dr J. Hyttel for donating cis-flupenthixol. The figures were reproduced with permission from the Journal of Endocrinology Ltd, the Journal of Neuroendocrinology and Rapid Communications of Oxford Ltd.

References

Bednar, I., Forsberg, G., Lindén, A., Qureshi, G. A. and Södersten, P. (1991). Involvement of dopamine in inhibition of food intake by cholecystokinin octapeptide in male rats. J. Neuroendocrinol. 3, 491–496.

Bednar, I., Qureshi, G. A. and Södersten, P. (1992a). A comparison between the effect of cholecystokinin octapeptide and apomorphine in ingestion of intraorally administered sucrose in male rats. J. Neuroendocrinol. 4, 727–734.

Bednar, I., Qureshi, G. A. and Södersten, P. (1992b). Evidence that release of dopamine in the brain is involved in the inhibitory effect of cholecystokinin octapeptide on ingestion of intraorally administered sucrose in male rats. J. Neuroendocrinol. 4, 735–741.

Bednar, I., Qian, M., Qureshi, G. Q., Källström, L., Johnson, A. E., Carrer, H. and Södersten, P. (1994). Glutamate inhibits ingestive behaviour. J. Neuroendocrinol. 6, 403–408.

Berridge, K. C. and Valenstein, E. S. (1991). What psychological process mediates feeding evoked by electrical stimulation of the lateral hypothalamus? Behav. Neurosci. 105, 3–14.

Björklund, A. and Lindvall, O. (1984). Dopamine containing systems in the CNS. In Handbook of Chemical Neuroanatomy (A. Björklund and T. Hökfelt, eds), vol. 2, pp. 55–122. Elsevier, Amsterdam.

Bray, G. A., Fisler, J. and York, D. A. (1990). Neuroendocrine control of the development of obesity: understanding gained from studies of experimental models. Front. Neuroendocrinol. 11, 128–181.

Camps, M., Cortés, R., Gueye, B., Probst, A. and Palacios, J. M. (1989). Dopamine receptors in the human brain: autoradiographic distribution of D_2 sites. *Neuroscience* **28**, 275–290.

Carlsson, A., Lindquist, M. and Magnusson, T. (1957). 3,4-Dihydroxyphenylalanin and 5-hydroxytryptophan as reserpine antagonists. *Nature* **180**, 1200.

Carlsson, M. and Carlsson, A. (1990). Interactions between glutamatergic and monoaminergic systems within the basal ganglia—implications for schizophrenia and Parkinson's disease. *Trends NeuroSci.* **13**, 272–276.

Corbin, J. D. and Stellar, E. (1964). Palatability, food intake and obesity in normal and hyperphagic rats. *J. Comp. Physiol. Psychol.* **58**, 63–67.

Cortés, R., Gueye, B., Pazos, A. and Palacios, J. M. (1989). Dopamine receptors in human brain: autoradiographic distribution of D_1 sites. *Neuroscience* **28**, 263–273.

Craig, W. (1918). Appetites and aversions as constituents of instincts. *Biol. Bull.* **34**, 91–107.

Deutsch, J. A. (1990). Food intake, gastric factors. In *Handbook of Behavioral Neurobiology* (E. M. Stricker, ed.), vol. 10, pp. 151–182. Plenum Press, New York.

Esfahami, N., Bednar, I., Qureshi, G. A. and Södersten, P. (1995). Inhibition of serotonin synthesis attenuates inhibition of ingestive behavior by CCK-8. *Pharmacol. Biochem. Behav.* **51**, 9–12.

Friedman, M. I. (1990). Making sense out of calories. In *Handbook of Behavioral Neurobiology* (E. M. Stricker, ed.), vol. 10, pp. 513–529. Plenum Press, New York.

Friedman, M. I. and Stricker, E. M. (1976) The physiological psychology of hunger: a physiological perspective. *Psychol. Rev.* **83**, 409–431.

Gibbs, J., Young, R. C. and Smith, G. P. (1973a). Cholecystokinin decreases food intake in rats. *J. Comp. Physiol. Psychol.* **84**, 488–495.

Gibbs, J., Young, R. C. and Smith, G. P. (1973b). Cholecystokinin elicits satiety in rats with open gastric fistulas. *Nature* **245**, 243–245.

Grill, H. J. and Berridge, K. C. (1985). Taste reactivity as a measure of the neural control of palatability. *Prog. Psychobiol. Physiol. Psychol.* **11**, 1–61.

Grill, H. J. and Kaplan, J. M. (1990). Caudal brainstem participates in the distributed neural control of feeding. In *Handbook of Behavioural Neurobiology* (E. M. Stricker, ed.), vol. 10, pp. 125–149. Plenum Press, New York.

Grill, H. J. and Norgren, R. (1978). The taste reactivity test. I. Mimetic responses to gustatory stimuli in neurologically normal rats. *Brain Res.* **143**, 263–279.

Grill, H. J. and Smith, G. P. (1988). Cholecystokinin decreases sucrose intake in chronic decerebrate rats. *Am. J. Physiol.* **254**, R853–R856.

Grill H. J., Spector, A. C., Schwartz, G. J., Kaplan, J. M. and Flynn, F. W. (1987). Evaluating taste effects on ingestive behavior. In *Feeding and Drinking* (F. M. Toates and N. E. Rowlands, eds), pp. 151–188. Elsevier, Amsterdam.

Hökfelt, T., Skirboll, L. Rehfeld, J. F., Goldstein, M., Markey, K. and Dann, O. (1980). A subpopulation of mesencephalic dopamine neurons projecting to limbic areas contains a cholecystokinin-like peptide: evidence from immunohistochemistry combined with retrograde tracing. *Neuroscience* **5**, 2093–2124.

Hutson, P. H., Sarna, G. S., Kantamaniemi, B. D. and Curzon, G. (1984). Concurrent determination of brain dopamine and 5-hydroxytryptamine turnover in individual freely moving rats using repeated sampling of cerebrospinal fluid. *J. Neurochem.* **43**, 151–159.

Johnson, A. E., Liminga, U., Lindén, A., Lindefors, N., Gunne, L. M. and Wiesel, F.-A. (1994). Chronic treatment with a classical neuroleptic alters excitatory amino acid and GABAergic neurotransmission of the rat brain. *Neuroscience* **63**, 1003–1040.

Joyce, J. N., Goldsmith, S. and Murray, A. (1993). Neuroanatomical localization of D_1 *versus* D_2 receptors: similar organization in the basal ganglia of the rat, cat and human and disparate organization in the cortex and limbic system. In $D_1 : D_2$

Dopamine Receptor Interactions (J. Waddington, ed.), pp. 23–49. Academic Press, London.

Kaplan, J. M. and Södersten, P. (1994). Apomorphine suppresses ingestive behaviour in chronic decerebrate rats. *NeuroReport* **5**, 1839–1840.

Kaplan, J. M., Bednar, I. and Södersten, P. (1992). Simultaneous display of sexual and ingestive behaviour by rats. *J. Neuroendocrinol.* **4**, 381–392.

Kaplan, J. M., Seeley, R. J. and Grill, H. J. (1993). Daily caloric regulation in intact and chronic decerebrate rats. *Behav. Neurosci.* **107**, 876–881.

Kelley, A. E. and Delfs, J. M. (1994). Excitatory amino acid receptors mediate the orofacial stereotypy elicited by dopaminergic stimulation of the ventrolateral striatum. *Neuroscience* **60**, 85–95.

Kendrick, K., Leng, G. and Higushi, T. (1991). Noradrenaline, dopamine and serotonin release in the paraventricular and supraoptic nuclei of the rat in response to intravenous cholecystokinin injections. *J. Neuroendocrinol.* **3**, 139–144.

Kennedy, G. C. (1953). The role of depot of fat in the hypothalamic control of food intake in the rat. *Proc. R. Soc. Lond. Ser. B* **140**, 578–592.

Leibowitz, S. F. (1992). Neurochemical–neuroendocrine systems in the brain controlling macronutrient intake and metabolism. *Trends NeuroSci.* **15**, 491–497.

Le Moal, M. and Simon, H. (1991). Mesocorticolimbic dopaminergic network: functional and regulatory roles. *Physiol. Rev.* **71**, 155–234.

Lindén, A. and Södersten, P. (1990). Relationship between the concentration of cholecystokinin-like immunoreactivity in plasma and food intake in male rats. *Physiol. Behav.* **48**, 859–863.

Lindén, A., Uvnäs-Moberg, K., Forsberg, G., Bednar, I. and Södersten, P. (1989). Plasma concentrations of cholecystokinin octapeptide and food intake in male rats treated with cholecystokinin octapeptide. *J. Endocrinol.* **121**, 59–65.

Lindén, A., Uvnäs-Moberg, K., Forsberg, G., Bednar, I. and Södersten, P. (1990). Involvement of cholecystokinin in food intake. I. Concentrations of cholecystokinin-like immunoreactivity in the cerebrospinal fluid of male rats. *J. Neuroendocrinol.* **2**, 783–789.

Luckman, S. M. (1992). Fos-like immunoreactivity in the brain stem of the rat following peripheral administration of cholecystokinin. *J. Neuroendocrinol.* **4**, 149–152.

Mamoun, H., Anderstam, B., Bergström, J., Qureshi, G. A. and Södersten, P. (1995). Diet independent suppression of ingestive behavior by cholecystokinin octapeptide and amino acids. *Am. J. Physiol.* **268** (*Regulatory Integrated Comp. Physiol.* **37**), R520–R527.

Marshall, F. H., Barnes, S., Hughes, J., Woodruff, G. N. and Hunter, J. C. (1991). Cholecystokinin modulates the release of dopamine from the anterior and posterior nucleus accumbens by two different mechanisms. *J. Neurochem.* **56**, 917–922.

Mayer, J. (1955). Regulation of energy intake and the body weight: the glucostatic theory and the lipostatic hypothesis. *Ann. N. Y. Acad. Sci.* **63**, 15–43.

Mellinkoff, S. M., Frankland, M., Boyle, D. and Greipel, M. (1956). Relationship between serum amino acid concentration and fluctuation in appetite. *J. Appl. Physiol.* **8**, 535–538.

Mohr, B. (1840). Hypertrophie der Hypophysis cerebri und dadurch bedingter Druck auf die Hirngrundflache, insebesondere auf die Sehnerven, das Chiasm derselben und den linksseitigen Hirnschenkel. *Wochenschr. Ges. Heilk.* **6**, 565–571.

Morari, M., O'Connor, W. T., Ungerstedt, U. and Fuxe, K. (1994). Dopamine D_1 and D_2 receptor antagonism differentially modulates stimulation of striatal neurotransmitter levels by N-methyl-D-aspartate acid. *Eur. J. Pharmacol.* **256**, 23–30.

Norgren, R. and Smith, G. P. (1988). Central distribution of subdiaphragmatic vagal branches in the rat. *J. Comp. Neurol.* **273**, 207–223.

Olson, B. R., Drutarosky, M. D., Stricker, E. M. and Verbalis, J. G. (1991). Brain oxytocin receptor antagonism blunts the effects of anorexigenic treatments in rats: evidence for central oxytocin inhibition of food intake. *Endocrinology* **129**, 785–791.

Phillips, A. G., Pfaus, J. G. and Blaha, C. D. (1991). Dopamine and motivated behaviour: insights provided by *in vivo* analyses. In *The Mesolimbic Dopamine System: From Motivation to Action* (P. Willner and J. Scheel-Krüger, eds), pp. 199–224. John Wiley, Chichester.

Phillips, G., Willner, P. and Muscat, R. (1991). Reward-dependent suppression or facilitation of consummatory behaviour by raclopride. *Psychopharmacology* **105**, 355–360.

Rayer, P. F. O. (1823). Observations dur les maladies de l'appendice sussphenoidal (glande pituitaire) du cerveau. *Arch. Gen. Med.* **3**, 350–367.

Schneider, L. H., Davis, J. D., Watson, C. A. and Smith, G. P. (1990). Similar effect of raclopride and reduced sucrose concentration on the microstructure of sucrose sham feeding. *Eur. J. Pharmacol.* **186**, 61–70.

Schwartz, M. W., Fieglewicz, D. P., Baskin, D. G., Woods, S. C. and Porte, D., Jr. (1992). Insulin in the brain: a hormonal regulator of energy balance. *Endocr. Rev.* **13**, 387–414.

Segal, D. S. and Kuczenski, R. (1992). Amphetamine-induced DA response corresponding to behavioral sensitization produced by repeated amphetamine pretreatment. *Brain Res.* **571**, 330–337.

Smith, F. J. and Campfield, L. A. (1993). Meal initiation occurs after experimental induction of transient declines in blood glucose. *Am. J. Physiol.* **265**, R1423–R1429.

Smith, G. P. (1982). Satiety and the problem of motivation. In *The Physiological Mechanisms of Motivation* (D. W. Pfaff, ed.), pp. 133–144. Springer, New York.

Smith, G. P. and Gibbs, J. (1993). Satiating effect of cholecystokinin. *Ann. N. Y. Acad. Sci.* **713**, 236–241.

Södersten, P., Forsberg, G., Bednar, I., Lindén, A. and Qureshi, G. A. (1992). Cholecystokinin in the control of ingestive behaviour. In *The Peptidergic Neuron* (J. Joose, R. M. Buijs and F. J. H. Tilders, eds), pp. 335–343. Elsevier, Amsterdam.

Spector, A. C., Norgren, R. and Grill, H. J. (1992). Parabrachial gustatory lesions impair taste aversion learning in rats. *Behav. Neurosci.* **106**, 147–161.

Starke, K., Göthert, M. and Kilbringer, H. (1989). Modulation of neurotransmitter release by presynaptic autoreceptors. *Physiol. Rev.* **89**, 864–989.

Steffens, A. B., Strubbe, J. H., Balkan, B. and Scheurink, A. J. W. (1990). Neuroendocrine mechanisms involved in the regulation of body weight, food intake, and metabolism. *Neurosci. Biobehav. Rev.* **14**, 305–313.

Stellar, E. (1954). The physiology of motivation. *Psychol. Rev.* **61**, 305–331.

Stricker, E. M. and Zigmond, M. J. (1976). Recovery of function after damage to central catecholamine-containing neurons: a neurochemical model for the lateral hypothalamic syndrome. *Prog. Psychobiol. Physiol. Psychol.* **6**, 121–188.

Ungerstedt, U. (1971). Adipsia and aphagia after 6-hydroxydopamine induced degeneration of the nigro-striatal dopamine system. *Acta Physiol. Scand.* Suppl. **361**, 95–122.

Verbalis, J. G., McCann, M. J., McHale, C. M. and Stricker, E. M. (1986). Oxytocin secretion in response to cholecystokinin and food intake: differentiation of nausea from satiety. *Science* **232**, 1417–1419.

Waddington, J. L. and Daly, S. A. (1993). Regulation of unconditioned motor behaviour by D_1:D_2 interactions. In D_1:D_2 *Dopamine Receptor Interactions. Neuroscience and Neuropharmacology* (J. Waddington, ed.), pp. 52–78. Academic Press, New York.

Weatherford, S. C., Greenberg, D., Gibbs, J. and Smith, G. P. (1990). The potency of

D-1 and D-2 receptor antagonists is inversely related to the reward value of sham-fed corn oil and sucrose in rats. *Pharmacol. Biochem. Behav.* **37**, 317–323.

Willner, P., Phillips, G. and Muscat, R. (1991). Suppression of rewarded behaviour by neuroleptic drugs: can't or won't, and why? In *The Mesolimbic Dopamine System: From Motivation to Action* (P. Willner and J. Scheel-Krüger, eds), pp. 251–271. John Wiley, Chichester.

Wise, R. A., Spindler, J., De Wit, H. and Gerber, G. J. (1978). Neuroleptic-induced 'anhedonia' in rats: pimozide blocks the reward quality of food. *Science* **201**, 262–264.

Wolgin, D. L. and Kinney, G. G. (1992). Effect of prior sensitization of stereotypy on the development of tolerance to amphetamine-induced hypophagia. *J. Pharmacol. Exp. Ther.* **262**, 1232–1241.

Wolgin, D. L., Oslan, I. A. and Thompson, G. B. (1988). Effects of 'anorexia' on appetitive and consummatory behavior. *Behav. Neurosci.* **102**, 329–334.

Yue, J.-L., Okamura, H., Goshima, Y., Nakamura, S., Geffard, M. and Misu, Y. (1994). Baroreceptor–aortic nerve-mediated release of endogenous L-3,4-dihydroxyphenylalanine and its tonic depressor function in the nucleus tractus solitarii of rats. *Neuroscience* **62**, 145–161.

Zhang, J., Chiodo, L. A. and Freeman, A. S. (1994). Influence of excitatory receptor subtypes on the electrophysiological activity of dopaminergic and non-dopaminergic neurons in rat substantia nigra. *J. Pharmacol. Exp. Ther.* **269**, 313–321.

Zigmond, M. J., Abercrombie, E. D., Berger, T. W., Grace, A. A. and Stricker, E. M. (1990). Compensations after lesions of central dopaminergic neurons: some clinical and basic implications. *Trends NeuroSci.* **13**, 290–296.

3

Role of 5-Hydroxytryptamine Receptor Subtypes in Satiety and Animal Models of Eating Disorders

ROSARIO SAMANIN and GIULIANO GRIGNASCHI

Istituto di Ricerche Farmacologiche 'Mario Negri', Via Eritrea 62, 20157 Milan, Italy

1 Introduction

The evidence that brain 5-hydroxytryptamine (5-HT; serotonin) is involved in the control of feeding derives mainly from findings that agents which enhance central serotonergic transmission reduce feeding in animals and humans (Samanin *et al.*, 1972, 1977a,b, 1979, 1980; Blundell, 1984; Garattini *et al.*, 1987; Samanin and Garattini 1989, 1990). More recent studies using direct manipulations of 5-HT at central synapses have confirmed that brain 5-HT has an inhibitory role in the control of feeding. Thus, injections of 5-HT at various hypothalamic loci reduce feeding in rats (Leibowitz *et al.*, 1990), while stimulation of 5-HT$_{1A}$ autoreceptors in the raphe region produces the opposite effect (Bendotti and Samanin, 1986; Hutson *et al.*, 1986).

Recent discovery and characterization of multiple 5-HT receptor types and subtypes has made available new tools for exploring the role of 5-HT in feeding control in greater depth (Hoyer *et al.*, 1994). This review is a progress report on current research into the effects of specific agonists and antagonists at 5-HT receptor subtypes in various models proposed to provide useful information on satiety and eating disorders. In view of other contributions to the volume, our review is based primarily on work from our laboratory, although other studies with particular relevance for interpreting our results are mentioned when appropriate.

DRUG RECEPTOR SUBTYPES AND INGESTIVE BEHAVIOUR
ISBN 0-12-187620-9

2   Role of 5-HT receptors in the mechanisms specifically controlling satiety

We have conducted a number of studies measuring performance in a food-rewarded runway in order to analyse different components of the feeding process. The results suggest that D-fenfluramine, which potently and specifically enhances the release of 5-HT from nerve terminals and inhibits its reuptake into neurons (Garattini et al., 1975), over the dose range 0.6–2.0 mg/kg reduces motivation to start eating and accelerates the process of satiation (Thurlby and Samanin, 1981; Thurlby et al., 1983). The effect of D-fenfluramine (2.5 mg/kg) in the runway test was prevented by the non-selective receptor antagonist metergoline but not by xylamidine or by ritanserin, a potent $5\text{-HT}_{2A/2C}$ receptor antagonist (Neill et al., 1990). These findings suggested that 5-HT_1 receptors mediate the ability of D-fenfluramine to enhance satiation in rats.

Studying the feeding-suppressant effect of D-fenfluramine in food-deprived (Samanin et al., 1989) and free-feeding (Neill and Cooper, 1989) rats treated with antagonists at various 5-HT receptor types gave rise to a similar suggestion. In these studies high doses of ritanserin attenuated the effect of D-fenfluramine, but interference with the drug's metabolism and distribution may account for this (Samanin et al., 1989).

Using a procedure for continuously monitoring feeding patterns in slightly food-restricted rats, we found that D-fenfluramine (1.5 mg/kg) reduced meal size, meal duration and the rate of eating with no effect on meal frequency (Grignaschi et al., 1992). As previously suggested by Blundell and co-workers (1976) for fenfluramine, we interpreted these findings to indicate that D-fenfluramine specifically enhances the state of satiety in rats (Grignaschi et al., 1992). In a subsequent study, we found that (±)-cyanopindolol, an antagonist with high affinity for 5-HT_{1A} and 5-HT_{1B} receptors, specifically blocked the effect of D-fenfluramine on meal size (Grignaschi and Samanin, 1992). Since stimulation of 5-HT_{1A} receptors increases food intake (Dourish et al., 1985; Bendotti and Samanin, 1987), the results with (±)-cyanopindolol suggest that the 5-HT_{1B} receptor mediates D-fenfluramine's ability to increase the satiating effect of food. Of interest in this study was the finding that ritanserin antagonized the effect of D-fenfluramine on the rate of eating but did not modify the effect on meal size (Grignaschi and Samanin, 1992). These results clearly show that the ability of D-fenfluramine to slow eating can be separated from its effect on meal size.

Studies with 5-methoxy-3(1,2,3,6-tetrahydro-4-pyridinyl)-1H-indole (RU-24969), an agonist at 5-HT_{1A} and 5-HT_{1B} receptors, suggest that stimulation of 5-HT_{1B} receptors causes anorexia in rats. This compound dose-dependently reduced food intake in free-feeding (Dourish et al., 1986; Bendotti and Samanin, 1987) and food-deprived (Bendotti and Samanin, 1987) rats, and this effect was prevented by (±)-cyanopindolol but not by spiperone, which blocks 5-HT_{1A} and 5-HT_{2A} receptors (Kennett *et al.*, 1987).

One problem with RU-24969 is that it markedly increases the locomotor activity of rats (Green *et al.*, 1984). This seems to be mediated by an increase in mesolimbic dopamine transmission since RU-24969 significantly increases the synthesis of dopamine in the nucleus accumbens (Carli *et al.*, 1988) and its effect on locomotion, although not that on feeding, is blocked by dopamine receptor antagonists (Bendotti and Samanin, 1987; Kennett *et al.*, 1987). Although RU-24969-induced hypophagia and hyperlocomotion could be separated, the effect on motor behaviour makes it difficult to prove that it induces satiety in rats.

In a recent study using the post-prandial satiety sequence in rats, RU-24969 did not produce a behavioural profile that resembled satiety induced by food pre-load (Kitchener and Dourish, 1994), whereas in other experiments it reduced milk intake and the time spent in feeding without causing any interruption of feeding (Simansky and Vaidya, 1990). Since 5-HT infusion in the paraventricular nucleus (PVN) of the hypothalamus causes changes in meal patterns suggesting the introduction of satiety (Shor-Posner *et al.*, 1986), changes in feeding caused by RU-24969 infused into this region suggest that stimulation of central 5-HT_{1B} receptors causes satiety. Hutson and colleagues (1988) found that RU-24969 injected in the PVN caused hypophagia without hyperlocomotion, while Fletcher *et al.* (1992) found no effect. A marked reduction of food intake was also found on injecting 3-(1,2,5,6-tetrahydropyrid-4-yl)pyrrolo[3,2-b]pyrid-5-one (CP 93 129), a potent and selective agonist at 5-HT_{1B} receptors, in the PVN (Macor *et al.*, 1990).

We have re-examined the effects of RU-24969 and CP 93 129 administered in the PVN, either alone and with (−)-propranolol, a β-adrenoceptor antagonist that blocks 5-HT_{1A} and 5-HT_{1B} receptors (Hoyer, 1988). We found that 7 nmol RU-24969 significantly reduced the food intake of rats and that the effect was prevented by a local injection of 20 nmol (−)-propranolol (Fig. 1A,B). As also reported by Macor *et al.* (1990), 16 μg CP 93 129 injected into the PVN markedly reduced food intake and (−)-propranolol significantly reduced this effect (Table 1). Although further studies using more sensitive measures, such as those obtained by feeding-pattern analysis, may better clarify the feeding-suppressant effect of centrally administered RU-24969 and CP 93 129, the present findings suggest that stimulation of 5-HT_{1B} receptors in the PVN is one mechanism by which satiety is induced in rats.

Although rodent and human 5-HT_{1B} receptors show more than 90% identity of their gene amino acid sequence (Adham *et al.*, 1992), they bind with different affinity to serotonergic agonists and antagonists (Adham *et al.*, 1992; Oksenberg *et al.*, 1992). This must be considered in studies aimed at clarifying the role of 5-HT_{1B} receptors on human feeding.

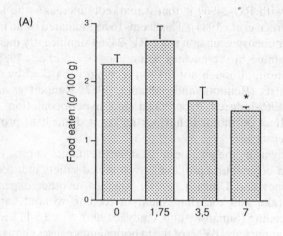

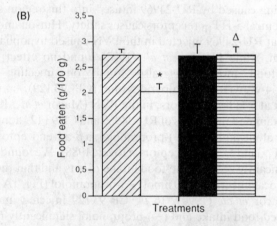

Fig. 1 (A) Effect of various doses of RU-24969 injected into the PVN on eating of food-deprived rats. Cannula implantation into the PVN was as described previously (Grignaschi *et al.*, 1993b). The animals were deprived of food 20 h before the test. RU-24969 was injected into the PVN immediately before the test. Food intake, corrected for spillage, was measured for 1 h and expressed as g per 100 g bodyweight. Each value is the mean ± SEM of at least five animals per group. *$P < 0.05$ *vs* controls (Dunnett's test). (B) Effect of (−)-propranolol on RU-24969-induced hypophagia in food-deprived rats. The experimental procedure was as described previously (see above). (−)-Propranolol (20 nmol per 0.5 μl) and RU-24969 (7 nmol per 0.5 μl) were injected into the PVN respectively 10 min and immediately before the test. Values are the mean ± SEM of seven animals per group. ▨, Saline + saline; □, saline + RU-24969; ■, (−)-propranolol + saline; ▤, (−)-propranolol + RU-24969. *$P < 0.05$ *vs* saline + saline (Tukey's test). Δ$P < 0.05$ Fint(1,27) = 4.7 (two-way analysis of variance).

Table 1 Effect of (−)-propranolol injected into the PVN on the hypophagia caused by CP 93 129 injected into the same area

	Dose (μg/0.5 μl)	Vehicle	CP 93 129 (16 μg/μl)
		Food eaten (g/30 min)	
Saline	—	3.8 ± 0.4	$0.3 \pm 0.2^*$
(−)-Propranolol	2.5	4.1 ± 0.2	$2.0 \pm 0.2^{*\dagger}$

Cannula implantation into the PVN was as described previously (Grignaschi et al., 1993b). The animals were deprived of food for 24 h before the test. (−)-Propranolol and CP 93 129 were injected into the PVN respectively 5 min and immediately before the test. Food intake corrected for spillage was measured for 30 min. Each value is the mean $\pm$ SEM of at least five animals per group.
$^*P<0.01$ vs respective controls (Tukey's test).
$\dagger^{\Delta}P<0.01$ Fint(1,17) = 10.1 (two-way analysis of variance).

2.1 5-HT–cholecystokinin interactions

The recently documented interaction between 5-HT and cholecystokinin (CCK), a peptide proposed as a link between satiety signals originating in the periphery and central mechanisms controlling feeding behaviour, may provide another means of clarifying which 5-HT receptors are involved in satiety (Stallone et al., 1989; Cooper et al., 1990; Grignaschi et al., 1993a). Stallone and colleagues (1989) found that metergoline antagonized the reduction in food intake caused by CCK-8 in slightly food-deprived rats. On the other hand, devazepide, a CCK_A receptor antagonist, blocked the effect of D-fenfluramine on sweet-mash consumption by non-deprived rats (Cooper et al., 1990). By continuously monitoring feeding patterns we confirmed that meal size is specifically controlled by the 5-HT–CCK interaction (Grignaschi et al., 1993a), suggesting that 5-HT and CCK cooperate in enhancing the satiating effect of food in rats. Clifton and Cooper (1992) reported similar results on the devazepide–D-fenfluramine interaction.

Since CCK-8 excites some 5-HT-containing cells in the raphe nuclei (Boden et al., 1991), we suggested that part of its satiating effect may be due to its ability to activate 5-HT neurons in this region. Since fenfluramine uses 5-HT neurons originating in the raphe nuclei to reduce eating (Samanin et al., 1972), 5-HT_{1B} receptors that mediate the effect of D-fenfluramine might be involved in the effect of CCK-8 on meal size. This, however, does not appear to be the case since, as shown in Table 2, a dose of (−)-propranolol previously reported to block the feeding-suppressant effect of 5-HT_{1B} receptor agonists (Kennett and Curzon, 1988) did not modify the effect of 4 μg/kg CCK-8 on meal size. Ritanserin, a potent antagonist at 5-HT_{2A} and 5-HT_{2C} receptors, also had no effect.

Poeschla and co-workers (1993) suggested that 5-HT_{2C} receptors mediate the

Table 2   Effect of ritanserin and (−)-propranolol on the reduction of meal size caused by cholecystokinin (CCK-8) in slightly deprived rats

		First meal (g)	
	Dose (mg/kg)	Saline	CCK-8 (4 μg/kg)
Vehicle	—	4.6 ± 0.4	2.7 ± 0.5*
(−)-Propranolol	16	4.2 ± 0.4	2.6 ± 0.3†
Vehicle	—	5.4 ± 0.9	2.4 ± 0.6†
Ritanserin	1.0	4.6 ± 0.3	2.9 ± 0.8

The apparatus, experimental procedure and analysis were as described previously (Grignaschi *et al.*, 1993a). (−)-Propranolol, ritanserin and CCK-8 were injected intraperitoneally 45, 45 and 15 min, respectively, before the test. Each value is the mean ± SEM of at least six animals per group.
* $P < 0.01$, † $P < 0.05$ *vs* controls (Tukey's test).
†$^{\Delta}P > 0.05$ Fint(1,25) = 0.3 ((−)-propranolol), Fint(1,30) = 0.9 (ritanserin) (two-way analysis of variance).

effect of CCK-8 since mianserin, a 5-HT$_{2A}$ and 5-HT$_{2C}$ receptor antagonist, attenuated the effect of 4 μg/kg CCK-8 on food consumption, while ketanserin, with its higher affinity for 5-HT$_{2A}$ receptors, had no such effect. Since ritanserin did not modify the effect of CCK in our experiment, the role of 5-HT$_{2C}$ receptors in the effect of CCK-8 requires further investigation. More selective 5-HT$_{2C}$ receptor antagonists are needed.

Although research into role of 5-HT$_{2C}$ receptors has been hampered by the lack of potent and selective antagonists, studies using mCPP (1–3(chlorophenyl)piperazine), an agonist at 5-HT$_{1B}$ and 5-HT$_{2C}$ receptors (Hoyer, 1988), combined with antagonists having different affinities for 5-HT$_2$ receptor subtypes, suggest that 5-HT$_{2C}$ receptors are involved in feeding control, although 5-HT$_{1B}$ receptor antagonists such as (±)-cyanopindolol and (−)-propranolol also reduced the effect of mCPP (Kennett and Curzon, 1988; Kennett and Curzon, 1991). Recent studies on the microstructure of feeding (Clifton *et al.*, 1993) or using the postprandial satiety sequence (Simansky and Vaidya, 1990; Kitchener and Dourish, 1994), suggest that mCPP specifically accelerates the appearance of satiety. Unfortunately, these studies made no attempt to modify the effect of mCPP with appropriate receptor antagonists, leaving open the question of whether 5-HT$_{1B}$, 5-HT$_{2C}$ or both receptors are involved.

3   Role of 5-HT$_{2A}$ receptors in anorexia induced by restraint stress

There is biochemical and pharmacological evidence of similarities between hypophagia caused by restraint stress and anorexia nervosa. Both are associated with an increased release of corticotropin-releasing factor (CRF) (Hotta *et al.*, 1986; Haas and George, 1988) and are attenuated by non-selective 5-HT receptor antagonists (Halmi *et al.*, 1983; Shimizu *et al.*, 1989). 5-HT-containing neurons make synaptic contact with CRF-containing cells in the PVN (Lipositis *et al.*, 1987) and there is evidence that 5-HT stimulates CRF secretion in the hypothalamus, mainly through 5-HT_{2A} receptors (Calogero *et al.*, 1989). A causal relationship between CRF secretion and hypophagia induced by restraint is suggested by the finding that a peptide antagonist completely prevented the reduction of food intake caused by restraint (Shibasaki *et al.*, 1988). The potential utility of restraint stress in anorexia nervosa prompted us to study the role of 5-HT receptor subtypes in this model.

Restraint stress-induced hypophagia was prevented by systemically administered ritanserin and ketanserin but not by ($\pm$)-cyanopindolol (Grignaschi *et al.*, 1993b). Two injections of cinanserin in the PVN also completely reversed the effect of stress on food intake. The fact that ketanserin and cinanserin have a higher affinity for 5-HT_{2A} than for 5-HT_{2C} receptors (Hoyer, 1988) makes it likely that the former receptors are involved.

A corollary of our findings with restraint stress is that, by increased 5-HT release, 5-HT_{2A} receptors and secretion of CRF in the PVN are stimulated. It was recently reported that restraint stress raised the level of CRF messenger RNA (mRNA) in the PVN, but the effect was not changed by pretreatment with parachlorophenylalanine, which caused 95% depletion of hypothalamic 5-HT (Harbuz *et al.*, 1993). Although it is not clear to what extent CRF mRNA levels are a sensitive measure of peptide release, these findings argue against 5-HT being involved in stress-induced activation of CRF.

To gain further information we studied hypophagia caused by restraint stress in animals treated with various doses of 8-hydroxy-2-(di-*n*-propylamino)-tetralin (8-OH-DPAT), a 5-HT_{1A} receptor agonist which markedly reduces the release of 5-HT in various brain regions (Hjorth and Sharp, 1991), and diazepam, which reportedly prevents the restraint stress-induced release of brain 5-HT (Shimizu *et al.*, 1992). As shown in Fig. 2, the highest dose of 8-OH-DPAT significantly attenuated the effect of stress on food intake, while diazepam was ineffective. Diazepam's lack of effect is surprising in view of its attenuating effect of stress-induced release of 5-HT. Since 5-HT fibres in the PVN arise in various cell groups in the pons-midbrain (Moore *et al.*, 1978; Sawchenko *et al.*, 1983), one possible explanation is that a 5-HT cell group not controlled by benzodiazepine sites is responsible for stress-induced anorexia in the presence of diazepam. Detailed anatomical and biochemical studies will be necessary to clarify this.

Previous studies have suggested that stimulation of 5-HT_{2A} receptors in the PVN causes anorexia in rats. Quipazine was first found to reduce rats' food intake by a 5-HT-dependent mechanism (Samanin *et al.*, 1977b) and it was subsequently suggested that 5-HT_{2A} receptors were involved in its feeding-suppressant effect (Hewson *et al.*, 1988). However, the specificity of quipazine's effect on feeding is questionable since we recently found that 'anorectic'

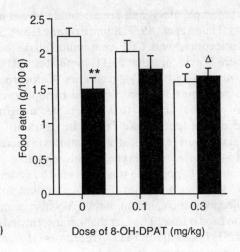

(A)   Dose of 8-OH-DPAT (mg/kg)

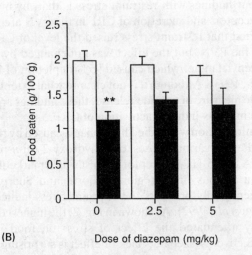

(B)   Dose of diazepam (mg/kg)

Fig. 2 (A) Effect of various doses of 8-OH-DPAT on the reduction of food intake caused by 1 h restraint stress. The experimental procedure was as described previously (Grignaschi *et al.*, 1993b). Food intake, corrected for spillage, was measured for 1 h and expressed as g per 100 g bodyweight. 8-OH-DPAT was injected subcutaneously 30 min before the stress. Values are the mean ± SEM of at least eight animals per group. □, no stress; ■, stress. **$P < .01$ *vs* no stress (Tukey's test); °$P < 0.05$ *vs* no stress + saline (Tukey's test). $^{\Delta}P < 0.05$ Fint(2,55) = 4.5 (two-way analysis of variance). (B) Effect of various doses of diazepam on the reduction of food intake caused by 2 h immobilization in rats. After 22 h of food deprivation, the animals were immobilized for 2 h by taping their paws to the plexiglas bar. The rats were then placed in the test cages with a weighed amount of food pellets in a perspex Petri dish placed on the floor and food intake, corrected for spillage, was measured for 1 h and expressed as g per 100 g bodyweight. Diazepam was injected intraperitoneally 20 min before the stress. Values are the mean ± SEM of at least eight animals per group. □, no stress; ■, stress. **$P < 0.01$ *vs* no stress (Tukey's test). $P > 0.05$ Fint(2,53) = 1.8 (two-way analysis of variance).

doses of quipazine, like lysergic acid diethylamide, impaired the visual discrimination accuracy of rats with no effect on food-motivated behavioural measures, whereas the reverse was true for D-fenfluramine and mCPP (Carli and Samanin, 1992).

Associational disturbances and/or disruption of motor behaviour may be responsible for the hypophagic effect of systematically administered 1-(2,5-dimethoxy-4-iodophenyl)-2-amino-propane (DOI), a 5-HT_{2A} and 5-HT_{2C} receptor agonist (Simansky and Vaidya, 1990; Kitchener and Dourish, 1994). We reasoned that intracerebral injections of DOI might better clarify the role of 5-HT_{2A} receptors in feeding. We therefore measured food intake by rats that had received various concentrations of DOI in the PVN. As shown in Fig. 3, we found that 20 and 40 nmol per 0.5 μl significantly reduced the amount eaten by food-deprived rats without causing any apparent changes in motor behaviour. The effect of 20 nmol DOI was completely prevented by a local injection of 30 nmol mianserin, an antagonist at 5-HT_{2A} and 5-HT_{2C} receptors (Hoyer, 1988) and by 25 nmol spiperone, a potent 5-HT_{2A} receptor antagonist with relatively low affinity for 5-HT_{2C} sites (Hoyer, 1988).

Our studies clearly suggest that stimulation of 5-HT_{2A} receptors is one mechanism by which restraint stress causes anorexia. In view of some analogies with this model, it would be interesting to assess whether 5-HT_{2A} receptor antagonists are useful in the treatment of anorexia nervosa. Further studies with more sophisticated measures of feeding behaviour are necessary to clarify the significance of hypophagia caused by direct stimulation of 5-HT_{2A} receptors in the PVN, but, as we will see in the next section, we found an interesting interaction between these receptors and feeding caused by neuropeptide Y (NPY) in the PVN.

4   Role of 5-HT receptor subtypes in neuropeptide Y-induced hyperphagia

The findings described above indicate that different 5-HT receptors are involved in the process of satiation and pathological anorexia as assessed by restraint stress. It is therefore reasonable to examine whether the same is true for pathological conditions involving excessive food consumption.

Although NPY is probably involved in the control of natural eating behaviour (Stanley et al., 1992; Shibasaki et al., 1993), we chose to study in some detail the role of 5-HT receptor subtypes in controlling NPY-induced hyperphagia for several reasons. Intracerebral injection of NPY has a potent and long-lasting orexigenic effect, which overrides physiological satiety signals (Morley et al., 1987; Paez and Myers, 1990). Experimental hyperphagia in diabetic rats and in some forms of genetic obesity are associated with increased hypothalamic levels of NPY and NPY gene expression (Williams et al., 1989; Sanacora et al., 1990), and concentrations of peptide YY, a peptide structurally

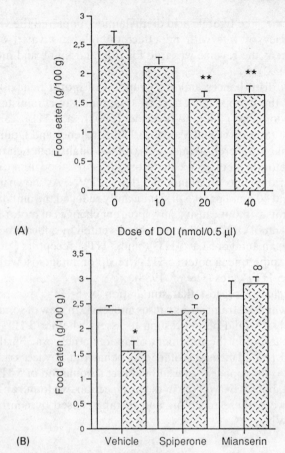

(A)   Dose of DOI (nmol/0.5 µl)

(B)   Vehicle   Spiperone   Mianserin

Fig. 3 (A) Effect of various doses of DOI injected into the PVN on eating of food-deprived rats. The experimental procedure was as described previously (see legend to Fig. 1A). DOI was injected into the PVN immediately before the test. Each value is the mean ± SEM of at least five animals per group. **$P < 0.01$ vs controls (Dunnett's test). (B) Effect of spiperone and mianserin on DOI-induced hypophagia in food-deprived rats. The experimental procedure was as described previously (see legend to Fig. 1A). Spiperone (25 nmol per 0.5 µl) and mianserin (30 nmol per 0.5 µl) were injected into the PVN 10 min before the test. DOI (20 nmol per 0.5 µl) was injected into the PVN immediately before the test. Values are the mean ± SEM of at least five animals per group. □, Saline. ▨, DOI. *$P < 0.05$ vs vehicle + saline; °$P < 0.05$, °°$P < 0.01$ vs vehicle + DOI (Tukey's test). $P < 0.01$ Fint(2,31) = 5.7 (two-way analysis of variance).

related to NPY, also with potent orexigenic effect, are high in the cerebrospinal fluid of bulimic patients (Berrettini et al., 1988).

NPY increases the motivation to eat by a mechanism different from that elicited by hunger, as shown by the fact that NPY and food deprivation produce different behavioural profiles (Levine et al., 1991) and the discriminative stimulus of food deprivation does not generalize to NPY (Jewett et al., 1991).

Table 3 Effect of various 5-HT receptor antagonists on D-fenfluramine-induced inhibition of NPY hyperphagia in rats

		Food eaten (g/100 g)	
Treatment	Dose	Saline	D-fenfluramine (0.63 mg/kg)
Vehicle	—	1.44 ± 0.20	$0.35 \pm 0.12^*$
Metergoline	2.0	1.19 ± 0.14	0.94 ± 0.04^a
Vehicle	—	1.12 ± 0.11	$0.32 \pm 0.14^*$
($\pm$)-Cyanopindolol	8.0	1.08 ± 0.13	1.14 ± 0.08^b
Vehicle	—	1.18 ± 0.15	$0.34 \pm 0.12^*$
Mesulergine	0.3	1.30 ± 0.17	0.64 ± 0.16^c
Vehicle	—	1.32 ± 0.18	$0.47 \pm 0.13^*$
Ketanserin	5.0	1.06 ± 0.10	0.49 ± 0.16^d

The experimental procedure was as described previously by Bendotti et al. (1987). Metergoline, ketanserin and D-fenfluramine were injected intraperitoneally 3 h, 45 min and 15 min, respectively, before the test. ($\pm$)-Cyanopindolol and mesulergine were injected subcutaneously 45 min before testing. All the animals received 235 pmol NPY in 0.5 μl distilled water in the PVN immediately before the test. After NPY injection, food intake corrected for spillage was measured for 1 h and expressed as g per 100 g bodyweight. Food intake of vehicle-treated rats was: 0.08 ± 0.05 g per 100 g. Values are the mean $\pm$ SEM of at least five rats per group.
$^*P < 0.01$ vs. respective controls (Tukey's test).
$^aP < 0.01$ Fint(1,21) = 8.2; $^bP < 0.01$ Fint(1,21) = 12.3; $^cP > 0.05$ Fint(1,27) = 0.3; $^dP > 0.05$ Fint(1,30) = 0.9 (two-way analysis of variance).

As regards the 5-HT–NPY relation, it is interesting that increased concentrations (Kakigi and Maeda, 1992) and synthesis (Bendotti et al., 1993) of NPY were found on depleting 5-HT in the rat brain. Particularly intriguing is the interaction between NPY and CRF in the PVN (Heinrichs et al., 1993). Some years ago we found that D-fenfluramine was particularly potent in blocking the hyperphagia caused by NPY administered into the PVN (Bendotti et al., 1987). We therefore planned a series of experiments aimed at clarifying the 5-HT receptor subtypes controlling NPY-induced hyperphagia. In a first experiment, we studied the effect of 0.63 mg/kg D-fenfluramine on eating induced by 235 pmol per 0.5 μl NPY administered into the PVN in rats treated with antagonists having different affinities for various 5-HT receptor subtypes.

The results are shown in Table 3. Metergoline (2 mg/kg) and ($\pm$)-cyanopindolol (8 mg/kg) did not modify NPY hyperphagia but completely prevented the effect of D-fenfluramine. NPY-induced eating and the effect of D-fenfluramine were not changed in rats treated with mesulergine (0.3 mg/kg) and ketanserin (5 mg/kg).

As discussed above, these findings suggest that 5-HT$_{1B}$ receptors mediate

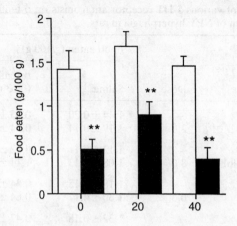

Dose of (-)-propranolol (nmol/0.5 μl)

Fig. 4 Effect of (−)-propranolol injected into the PVN on D-fenfluramine-induced inhibition of NPY hyperphagia in rats. The experimental procedure was as described previously (Bendotti *et al.*, 1987). All the animals received 235 pmol per 0.5 μl NPY in the PVN immediately before the test. (−)-Propranolol was injected bilaterally into the PVN 20 min before the test. D-fenfluramine (0.63 mg/kg) was injected intraperitoneally 15 min before the test. Food intake, corrected for spillage, was measured for 1 h and expressed as g per 100 g bodyweight. Each value is the mean ± SEM of at least nine animals per group. □, Saline; ■, D-fenfluramine. $**P < 0.01$ *vs* respective controls (Tukey's test). $P > 0.05$ Fint(2,58) = 0.2 (two-way analysis of variance).

the effect of D-fenfluramine on NPY overeating. Since, as we have seen, 5-HT_{1B} receptor agonists injected in the PVN reduce eating in deprived rats, we examined the effect of 0.6 mg/kg D-fenfluramine on NPY-induced eating by rats bilaterally injected in the PVN with 20 and 40 nmol per 0.5 μl of the 5-HT_{1A}/5-HT_{1B} receptor antagonist (−)-propranolol. As shown in Fig. 4, neither dose of (−)-propranolol modified the effect of D-fenfluramine, suggesting that 5-HT_{1B} receptors outside the PVN mediate it.

In another study, we examined whether direct stimulation of these receptors in the PVN attenuated the effect of NPY in the same area. Doses of RU-24969 ranging from 7 to 14 nmol per 0.5 μl had no effect on eating caused by 235 pmol per 0.5 μl NPY, whereas 10 and 20 nmol per 0.5 μl DOI significantly reduced the effect of NPY (Fig. 5A, B). Since DOI has affinity for both 5-HT_{2A} and 5-HT_{2C} receptors (Van Wijngaarden *et al.*, 1990) and previous studies (see above) suggested that 5-HT_{2A} receptors mediate its effect on food intake by deprived rats, we examined whether 5-HT_{2A} receptors also mediate the effect of DOI on NPY overeating by injecting spiperone, which has high affinity for 5-HT_{2A} but not for 5-HT_{2C} sites, into the PVN (Hoyer, 1988). The complete antagonism of DOI's effect confirmed that 5-HT_{2A} receptors are involved (Fig. 6A). In view of the fact that stimulation of 5-HT_{2A} receptors facilitates the release of CRF in the PVN (Calogero *et al.*, 1989) and this peptide blocks the

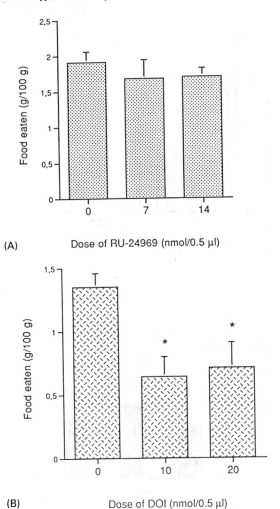

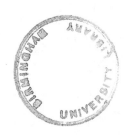

(A)   Dose of RU-24969 (nmol/0.5 µl)

(B)   Dose of DOI (nmol/0.5 µl)

Fig. 5 Effect of RU-24969 (A) and DOI (B) injected into the PVN on NPY-induced hyperphagia in rats. The experimental procedure was as described previously (Bendotti *et al.*, 1987). RU-24969 and DOI were injected into the PVN 5 min before the test. NPY (235 pmol per 0.5 µl) was injected into the PVN immediately before the test. Food intake, corrected for spillage, was measured for 1 h and expressed as g per 100 g bodyweight. Each value is a mean ± SEM of at least six animals per group. *$P < 0.05$ *vs* controls (Dunnett's test).

effect of NPY on eating (Morley *et al.*, 1987), it is likely that the effect of DOI on NPY eating was mediated by release of CRF. To prove this, we injected rats with 235 pmol per 0.5 µl NPY in the PVN and administered 10 nmol per 0.5 µl DOI together with two doses of the CRF antagonist α-helical CRF_{9-41}. As shown in Fig. 6B, the antagonist significantly attenuated the effect of DOI, confirming that stimulation of 5-HT_{2A} receptors in the PVN reduces the effect

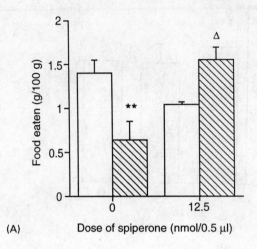

(A)   Dose of spiperone (nmol/0.5 μl)

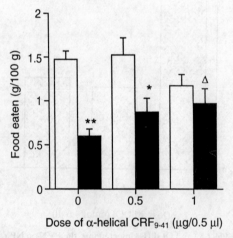

(B)   Dose of α-helical CRF₉₋₄₁ (μg/0.5 μl)

Fig. 6 (A) Effect of spiperone on DOI-induced inhibition of NPY hyperphagia in rats. The experimental procedure was as described previously (Bendotti *et al.*, 1987). Spiperone (12.5 nmol per 0.5 μl), DOI (10 nmol per 0.5 μl) and NPY (235 pmol per 0.5 μl) were injected into the PVN respectively 15 min, 5 min and immediately before the test. Food intake, corrected for spillage, was measured for 1 h and expressed as g per 100 g bodyweight. Each value is the mean ± sem of at least five animals per group. □, Saline; ▨, DOI. **$P < 0.01$ *vs* vehicle + saline (Tukey's test). ᐃ$P < 0.01$ Fint(1,19) = 18.3 (two-way analysis of variance). (B) Effect of α-helical CRF₉₋₄₁ on DOI-induced inhibition of NPY hyperphagia in rats. The experimental procedure was as described previously (Bendotti *et al.*, 1987). α-Helical CRF₉₋₄₁ (0.5–1.0 μg per 0.5 μl), DOI (10 nmol per 0.5 μl) and NPY (235 pmol per 0.5 μl) were injected into the PVN respectively 15 min, 5 min and immediately before the test. Food intake, corrected for spillage, was measured for 1 h and expressed as g per 100 g bodyweight. Each value is the mean ± sem of at least seven animals per group. □, Saline; ■, DOI. **$P < 0.01$, *$P < 0.05$ *vs* vehicle + saline (Tukey's test). ᐃ$P < 0.05$ Fint(2,60) = 3.4 (two-way analysis of variance).

of NPY on eating by an action of CRF. It seems, therefore, that overeating induced by NPY in the PVN is controlled by 5-HT$_{2A}$ receptors in the same area, in relation with changes in CRF release, and by 5-HT$_{1B}$ receptors outside the PVN, as suggested by the results with D-fenfluramine. While the finding that fenfluramine reduced eating in patients with bulimia nervosa (Robinson *et al.*, 1986) agrees with the proposal that NPY overeating models are important aspects of the human disease, further studies are needed with more selective agonists at the human 5-HT$_{1B}$ receptors, which we hope will soon be developed, to establish the extent to which NPY overeating is predictive of effective pharmacotherapy in humans. Although, according to the NPY model, stimulation of 5-HT$_{2A}$ receptors should also be of therapeutic utility in bulimia nervosa, the perceptual disturbances caused by stimulating these receptors in the whole brain may seriously limit its clinical verification.

5 Conclusions

Our findings suggest that stimulation of 5-HT$_{1B}$ receptors accelerates the process of satiation and blocks eating caused by NPY injection in the PVN. Stimulation of 5-HT$_{2A}$ receptors in the PVN mediates stress-induced anorexia and blocks eating caused by NPY. Both conditions may involve changes in the release of CRF.

The role of 5-HT$_{2C}$ receptors in feeding control is not clearly defined. Studies using mCPP, a non-selective 5-HT$_{1B}$/5-HT$_{2C}$ receptor agonist, in combination with antagonists having different affinities for the various receptors, suggest that stimulation of 5-HT$_{2C}$ receptors reduces food intake, but the specificity of the effect of mCPP on feeding is not clear. Recent investigation of the effect of mCPP on more sensitive measures of feeding behaviour suggest that it can enhance satiety, but the receptor involved is not known.

The spectacular progress in the discovery of 5-HT receptor types and subtypes (14 up to now) highlights limitations in our knowledge of the organization of these systems in the brain. Further progress in 5-HT receptor pharmacology is necessary to clarify how each 5-HT receptor type and subtype is involved in feeding. Although we have no certainty that the mechanisms controlling feeding in rats are similar to those governing anorexia and excessive eating in humans, our studies provide an example of how the new knowledge of some 5-HT receptors, together with advances in sensitive measures of feeding behaviour, can indicate novel strategies for modifying appetite and perhaps correcting eating disorders.

Acknowledgements

We thank Dr Jean Rivier and Dr E. Merlo Pich for generously providing the α-helical-CRF$_{9-41}$. This study was partially supported by National Research Council (CNR), Rome, Italy, Convenzione Psicofarmacologia.

References

Adham, N., Romanienko, P., Hartig, P., Weinshank, R. L. and Branchek, T. (1992). The rat 5-hydroxytryptamine$_{1B}$ receptor is the species homologue of the human 5-hydroxytryptamine$_{1Db}$ receptor. *Mol. Pharmacol.* **41**, 1–7.

Bendotti, C. and Samanin, R. (1986). 8-Hydroxy-2-(di-*n*-propylamino)tetralin (8-OH-DPAT) elicits eating in free-feeding rats by acting on central serotonin neurons. *Eur. J. Pharmacol.* **121**, 147–150.

Bendotti, C. and Samanin, R. (1987). The role of putative 5-HT$_{1A}$ and 5-HT$_{1B}$ receptors in the control of feeding in rats. *Life Sci.* **41**, 635–642.

Bendotti, C., Garattini, S. and Samanin, R. (1987). Eating caused by neuropeptide-Y injection in the paraventricular hypothalamus: response to (+)-fenfluramine and (+)-amphetamine in rats. *J. Pharm. Pharmacol.* **39**, 900–903.

Bendotti, C., Tarizzo, G., Fumagalli, F., Baldessari, S. and Samanin, R. (1993). Increased expression of preproneuropeptide Y and preprosomatostatin mRNA in striatum after selective serotoninergic lesions in rats. *Neurosci. Lett.* **160**, 197–200.

Berrettini, W. H., Kaye, W. H., Gwirtsman, H. and Allbright, A. (1988). Cerebrospinal fluid peptide YY immunoreactivity in eating disorders. *Neuropsychopharmacology* **19**, 121–124.

Blundell, J. E. (1984). Serotonin and appetite. *Neuropharmacology* **23**, 1537–1551.

Blundell, J. E., Latham, C. J. and Leshem, M. B. (1976). Differences between the anorexic actions of amphetamine and fenfluramine; possible effects on hunger and satiety. *J. Pharm. Pharmacol.* **28**, 471–477.

Boden, P. R., Woodruff, G. N. and Pinnock, R. D. (1991). Pharmacology of a cholecystokinin receptor on 5-hydroxytryptamine neurones in the dorsal raphe of the rat brain. *Br. J. Pharmacol.* **102**, 635–638.

Calogero, A. E., Bernardini, R., Margioris, A. N., Bagdy, G., Gallucci, W. T., Munson, P. J., Tamarkin, L., Tomai, T. P., Brady, L., Gold, P. W. and Chrousos, G. P. (1989). Effects of serotonergic agonists and antagonists on corticotropin-releasing hormone secretion by explanted rat hypothalami. *Peptides* **10**, 189–200.

Carli, M. and Samanin, R. (1992). Serotonin$_2$ receptor agonists and serotonergic anorectic drugs affect rats' performance differently in a five-choice serial reaction time task. *Psychopharmacology* **106**, 228–234.

Carli, M., Invernizzi, R., Cervo, L. and Samanin, R. (1988). Neurochemical and behavioural studies with RU 24969 in the rat. *Psychopharmacology* **94**, 359–364.

Clifton, P. G. and Cooper S. J. (1992). CCK–5-HT interactions influence meal size in free-feeding rat. In *Multiple Cholecystokinin Receptors in the CNS* (C. T. Dourish, S. J. Cooper, S. D. Iversen and L. L. Iversen, eds), pp. 286–289, Oxford Science Publications, Oxford.

Clifton, P. G., Barnfield, A. M. and Curzon, G. (1993). Effects of food deprivation and mCPP treatment on the microstructure of ingestive behaviour of male and female rats. *J. Psychopharmacol.* **7**, 257–264.

Cooper, S. J., Dourish, C. T. and Barber, D. J. (1990). Reversal of the anorectic effect of (+)-fenfluramine in the rat by the selective cholecystokinin receptor antagonist MK-329. *Br. J. Pharmacol.* **99**, 65–70.

Dourish, C. T., Hutson, P. H. and Curzon, G. (1985). Low doses of the putative serotonin agonist 8-hydroxy-2-(di-*n*-propylamino) tetralin (8-OH-DPAT) elicit feeding. *Psychopharmacology* **86**, 197–204.

Dourish, C. T., Hutson, P. H., Kennett, G. A. and Curzon, G. (1986). 8-OH-DPAT-induced hyperphagia: its neural basis and possible therapeutic relevance. *Appetite* **7** (supplement), 127–140.

Fletcher, P. J., Ming, Z. H., Zack, M. H. and Coscina, D. V. (1992). A comparison of the effects of the 5-HT$_1$ agonists TFMPP and RU 24969 on feeding following peripheral or medial hypothalamic injection. *Brain Res.* **580**, 265–272.

Garattini, S., Buczko, W., Jori, A. and Samanin, R. (1975). The mechanism of action of fenfluramine. *Postgrad. Med. J.* **51 (supplement 1)**, 27–35.

Garattini, S., Mennini, T. and Samanin, R. (1987). From fenfluramine racemate to D-fenfluramine: specificity and potency of the effects on the serotoninergic system and food intake. *Ann. N. Y. Acad. Sci.* **409**, 156–166.

Green, A. R., Guy, A. P. and Gardner, C. R. (1984). The behavioural effects of RU-24969, a suggested 5-HT, receptor agonist in rodents and the effect on the behaviour of treatment with antidepressants. *Neuropharmacology* **23**, 655–661.

Grignaschi, G. and Samanin, R. (1992). Role of 5-HT receptors in the effect of D-fenfluramine on feeding patterns in the rat. *Eur. J. Pharmacol.* **212**, 287–289.

Grignaschi, G., Neill, J. C., Petrini, A., Garattini, S. and Samanin, R. (1992). Feeding pattern studies suggest that D-fenfluramine and sertraline specifically enhance the state of satiety in rats. *Eur. J. Pharmacol.* **211**, 137–142.

Grignaschi, G., Mantelli, B., Fracasso, C., Anelli, M., Caccia, S. and Samanin, R. (1993a). Reciprocal interaction of 5-hydroxytryptamine and cholecystokinin in the control of feeding patterns in rats. *Br. J. Pharmacol.* **109**, 491–494.

Grignaschi, G., Mantelli, B. and Samanin, R. (1993b). The hypophagic effect of restraint stress in rats can be mediated by 5-HT$_2$ receptors in the paraventricular nucleus of the hypothalamus. *Neurosci. Lett.* **152**, 103–106.

Haas, D. A. and George, S. R. (1988). Single or repeated mild stress increases synthesis and release of hypothalamic corticotropin-releasing factor. *Brain Res.* **461**, 230–237.

Halmi, K. A., Eckert, E. and Falk, J. R. (1983). Cyproheptadine, an antidepressant and weight inducing drug for anorexia nervosa. *Psychopharmacol. Bull.* **19**, 103–105.

Harbuz, M. S., Chalmers, J., De Souza, L. and Lightman, S. L. (1993). Stress-induced activation of CRF and c-*fos* mRNAs in the paraventricular nucleus are not affected by serotonin depletion. *Brain Res.* **609**, 167–173.

Heinrichs, S. C., Menzaghi, F., Merlo Pich, E., Hauger, R. L. and Koob, G. F. (1993). Corticotropin-releasing factor in the paraventricular nucleus modulates feeding induced by neuropeptide Y. *Brain Res.* **611**, 18–24.

Hewson, G., Leighton, G. E., Hill, R. G. and Hughes, J. (1988). Quipazine reduces food intake in the rat by activation of 5-HT$_2$ receptors. *Br. J. Pharmacol.* **95**, 598–604.

Hjorth, S. and Sharp, T. (1991). Effect of the 5-HT$_{1A}$ receptor agonist 8-OH-DPAT on the release of 5-HT in dorsal and median raphe-innervated rat brain regions as measured by *in vivo* microdialysis. *Life Sci.* **48**, 1779–1786.

Hotta, M., Shibasaki, T., Masuda, A., Imaki, T., Demura, H., Ling, N. and Shizume, K. (1986). The response of plasma adrenocorticotropin and cortisol to corticotropin-releasing hormone (CRH) and cerebrospinal fluid immunoreactive CRH in anorexia nervosa patients. *J. Clin. Endocrinol. Metab.* **62**, 319–324.

Hoyer, D. (1988). Functional correlates of serotonin in 5-HT$_1$ recognition sites. *J. Recept. Res.* **8**, 59–81.

Hoyer, D., Clarke, D. E., Fozard, J. R., Hartig, P. R., Martin, G. R., Mylecharane, E. J., Saxena, P. R. and Humphrey, P. A. (1994). VII. International Union of Pharmacology classification of receptors for 5-hydroxytryptamine (serotonin). *Pharmacol. Rev.* **46**, 157–203.

Hutson, P. H., Dourish, C. T. and Curzon, G. (1986). Neurochemical and behavioural evidence for mediation of the hyperphagic action of 8-OH-DPAT by 5-HT cell body autoreceptors. *Eur. J. Pharmacol.* **129**, 347–352.

Hutson, P. H., Donohoe, T. P. and Curzon, G. (1988). Infusion of the

5-hydroxytryptamine agonist RU24969 and TFMPP into the paraventricular nucleus of the hypothalamus causes hypophagia. *Psychopharmacology* **95**, 550–552.

Jewett, D. C., Schaal, D. W., Cleary, J., Thompson, T. and Levine, A. S. (1991). The discriminative stimulus effects of neuropeptide Y. *Brain Res.* **561**, 165–168.

Kakigi, T. and Maeda, K. (1992). Effect of serotonergic agents on regional concentrations of somatostatin- and neuropeptide Y-like immunoreactivities in rat brain. *Brain Res.* **599**, 45–50.

Kennett, G. A. and Curzon, G. (1988). Evidence that hypophagia induced by mCPP and TFMPP requires 5-HT_{1C} and 5-HT_{1B} receptors; hypophagia induced by RU 24969 only requires 5-HT_{1B} receptors. *Psychopharmacology* **96**, 93–100.

Kennett, G. A., and Curzon, G. (1991). Potencies of antagonists indicate that 5-HT_{1C} receptors mediate 1-3(chlorophenyl) piperazine-induced hypophagia. *Br. J. Pharmacol.* **103**, 2016–2020.

Kennett, G. A., Dourish, C. T. and Curzon, G. (1987) 5-HT_{1B} agonists induce anorexia at a postsynaptic site. *Eur. J. Pharmacol.* **141**, 429–435.

Kitchener, S. J. and Dourish, C. T. (1994). An examination of the behavioural specificity of hypophagia induced by 5-HT_{1B}, 5-HT_{1C} and 5-HT_2 receptor agonists using the post-prandial satiety sequence in rats. *Psychopharmacology* **113**, 369–377.

Leibowitz, S. F., Weiss, G. F. and Suh, J. S. (1990). Medial hypothalamic nuclei mediate serotonin's inhibitory effect on feeding behavior. *Pharmacol. Biochem. Behav.* **37**, 735–742.

Levine, A. S., Kuskowski, M. A., Grace, M. and Billington, C. J. (1991). Food deprivation-induced *vs.* drug-induced feeding: a behavioural evaluation. *Am. J. Physiol.* **260**, R546–R552.

Lipositis, Z. S., Phelix, C. and Paull, W. K. (1987). Synaptic interaction of serotonergic axons and corticotropin releasing factor (CRF) synthesizing neurons in the hypothalamic paraventricular nucleus of the rat. A light and electron microscopic immunocytochemical study. *Histochemistry* **86**, 541–549.

Macor, E. J., Burkhart, C. A., Heym, J. H., Ives, J. L., Lebel, L. A., Newman, M. E., Nielsen, J. A., Ryan, K., Schulz, D. W., Torgersen, L. K. and Koe, B. K. (1990). 3-(1,2,5,6-Tetrahydropyrid-4-yl)pyrrolo[3,2-b]pyrid-5-one: a potent and selective serotonin (5-HT_{1B}) agonist and rotationally restricted phenolic analogue of 5-methoxy-3-(1,2,5,6-tetrahydropyrid-4-yl) indole. *J. Med. Chem.* **33**, 2087–2093.

Moore, R. Y., Halaris, A. E. and Jones, B. E. (1978). Serotonin neurons of the midbrain raphe: ascending projections. *J. Comp. Neurol.* **180**, 417–438.

Morley, J. E., Levine, A. S., Gosnell, B. A., Kneip, J. and Grace, M. (1987). Effect of neuropeptide Y on ingestive behaviors in the rat. *Am. J. Physiol.* **252**, R599–R609.

Neill, J. C. and Cooper, S. J. (1989). Evidence that D-fenfluramine anorexia is mediated by 5-HT_1 receptors. *Psychopharmacology* **97**, 213–218.

Neill, J. C., Bendotti, C. and Samanin, R. (1990). Studies on the role of 5-HT receptors in satiation and the effect of D-fenfluramine in the runway test. *Eur. J. Pharmacol.* **190**, 105–112.

Oksenberg, D., Marsters, S. A., O'Dowd, B. F., Jin, H., Havlik, S., Peroutka, S. J. and Ashkenazi, A. (1992). A single amino-acid difference confers major pharmacological variation between human and rodent 5-HT_{1B} receptors. *Nature* **360**, 161–163.

Paez, X. and Myers, R. D. (1990). Non-satiable feeding induced by multiple perfusions of neuropeptide Y (NPY) in medial hypothalamus of the rat. *FASEB J.* **4**, 882.

Poeschla, B., Gibbs, J., Simansky, K. J., Greenberg, D. and Smith, G. P. (1993). Cholecystokinin-induced satiety depends on activation of 5-HT_{1C} receptors. *Am. J. Physiol.* **264**, R62–R64.

Robinson, P. H., Checkley, S. A. and Russell, G. F. M. (1986). Suppression of eating by fenfluramine in patients with bulimia nervosa. *Br. J. Psychiatry* **146**, 169–176.

Samanin, R. and Garattini, S. (1989). Serotonin and the pharmacology of eating disorders. *Ann. N. Y. Acad. Sci.* **575**, 194–208.

Samanin, R. and Garattini, S. (1990). The pharmacology of serotoninergic drugs affecting appetite. In *Nutrition and the Brain* (R. J. Wurtman and J. J. Wurtman, eds), vol. 8, pp. 163–192. Raven Press, New York.

Samanin, R., Ghezzi, D., Valzelli, L. and Garattini, S. (1972). The effects of selective lesioning of brain serotonin or catecholamine containing neurons on the anorectic activity of fenfluramine and amphetamine. *Eur. J. Pharmacol.* **19**, 318–322.

Samanin, R., Bendotti, C., Candelaresi, G. and Garattini, S. (1977a). Specificity of serotoninergic involvement in the decrease of food intake induced quipazine in the rat. *Life Sci.* **21**, 1259–1265.

Samanin, R., Bendotti, C., Miranda, F. and Garattini, S. (1977b). Decrease of food intake by quipazine in the rat: relation to serotonergic receptor stimulation. *J. Pharm. Pharmacol.* **29**, 53–54.

Samanin, R., Mennini, T., Ferraris, A., Bendotti, C., Borsini, F. and Garattini, S. (1979). *m*-Chlorophenylpiperazine: a central serotonin agonist causing powerful anorexia in rats. *Naunyn Schmiedebergs Arch. Pharmacol.* **308**, 159–163.

Samanin, R., Caccia, S., Bendotti, C., Borsini, F., Borroni, E., Invernizzi, R., Pataccini, R. and Mennini, T. (1980). Further studies on the mechanism of serotonin-dependent anorexia in rats. *Psychopharmacology* **68**, 99–104.

Samanin, R., Mennini, T., Bendotti, C., Caccia, S. and Garattini, S. (1989). Evidence that central 5-HT$_2$ receptors do not play an important role in the anorectic activity of D-fenfluramine in the rat. *Neuropharmacology* **5**, 465–469.

Sanacora, G., Kershaw, M., Finkelstein, J. A. and White, J. D. (1990). Increased hypothalamic content of preproneuropeptide Y messenger ribonucleic acid in genetically obese Zucker rats and its regulation by food deprivation. *Endocrinology* **127**, 730–737.

Sawchenko, P. E., Swanson, L. W., Steinbush, H. W. M. and Verhofstad, A. A. J. (1983). The distribution of cells of origin of serotoninergic inputs to the paraventricular and supraoptic nuclei of the rat. *Brain Res.* **277**, 355–360.

Shibasaki, T., Yamauchi, N., Kato, Y., Masuda, A., Imaki, T., Hotta, M., Demura, H., Oono, H., Ling, N. and Shizume, K. (1988). Involvement of corticotropin-releasing factor in restraint stress-induced anorexia and reversion of the anorexia by somatostatin in the rat. *Life Sci.* **43**, 1103–1110.

Shibasaki, T., Oda, T., Imaki, T., Ling, N. and Demura, H. (1993). Injection of anti-neuropeptide Y g-globuline into the hypothalamic paraventricular nucleus decreases food intake in rats. *Brain Res.* **601**, 313–316.

Shimizu, N., Oomura, Y. and Kai, Y. (1989). Stress-induced anorexia in rats mediated by serotonergic mechanisms in the hypothalamus. *Physiol. Behav.* **46**, 835–841.

Shimizu, N., Take, S., Hori, T. and Oomura, Y. (1992). *In vivo* measurement of hypothalamic serotonin release by intracerebral microdialysis: significant enhancement by immobilization stress in rats. *Brain Res. Bull.* **28**, 727–734.

Shor-Posner, G., Grinker, J. A., Marinescu, C., Brown, O. and Leibowitz, S. F. (1986). Hypothalamic serotonin in the control of meal patterns and macronutrient selection. *Brain Res. Bull.* **17**, 663–671.

Simansky, K. J. and Vaidya, A. H. (1990). Behavioural mechanisms for the anorectic action of the serotonin (5-HT) uptake inhibitor sertraline in rats: comparison with directly acting 5-HT agonists. *Brain Res. Bull.* **25**, 953–960.

Stallone, D., Nicholaidis, S. and Gibbs, J. (1989). Cholecystokinin-induced anorexia depends on serotoninergic function. *Am. J. Physiol.* **256**, R1138–R1141.

Stanley, B. G., Magdalin, W., Seirafi, A., Nguyen, M. M. and Leibowitz, S. F. (1992).

Evidence for neuropeptide Y mediation of eating produced by food deprivation and for a variant of the Y_1 receptor mediating this peptide's effect. *Peptides* **13**, 581–587.

Thurlby, P. L. and Samanin, R. (1981). Effects of anorectic drugs and prior feeding on food-rewarded behaviour. *Pharmacol. Biochem. Behav.* **14**, 799–804.

Thurlby, P. L., Grimm., V. E. and Samanin, R. (1983). Feeding and satiation observed in the runway: the effects of D-amphetamine and D-fenfluramine compared. *Pharmacol. Biochem. Behav.* **18**, 841–846.

Van Wijngaarden, I., Tulp, M.Th.M. and Soudijn, W. (1990). The concept of selectivity in 5-HT receptor research. *Eur. J. Pharmacol.* **188**, 301–312.

Williams, G., Gill, J. S., Lee, Y. C., Cardoso, H. M., Okpere, B. E. and Bloom, S. R. (1989). Increased neuropeptide Y concentrations in specific hypothalamic regions of streptozocin-induced diabetic rats. *Diabetes* **38**, 321–327.

4

5-HT Receptor Subtypes Influencing Feeding and Drinking: Focus on the Periphery

KENNY J. SIMANSKY

Department of Pharmacology, Medical College of Pennsylvania and Hahnemann University, 3200 Henry Avenue, Philadelphia, PA 19129, USA

1 Introduction

During the past few decades, a vast body of data accumulated implicating the indoleamine serotonin (5-hydroxytryptamine; 5-HT) in the inhibitory control of feeding. Evidence relating 5-HT to ingestion came primarily from pharmacological demonstrations that enhancing postsynaptic serotonergic activity reduced the amount of food eaten, whereas decreasing serotonergic neurotransmission increased intake. For the most part, investigations of these phenomena have focused on mechanisms in the central nervous system. In some studies, for example, selectively manipulating 5-HT function in the brain altered either feeding itself or ingestive actions of systemically administered serotonergic drugs. In comparison, the peripherally acting 5-HT antagonist xylamidine (Copp *et al.*, 1967) generally failed to inhibit the anorectic effects of 5-HT agonists which could penetrate the blood–brain barrier (see discussions by other contributors in this volume and in reviews elsewhere, e.g. Blundell, 1977; Carruba *et al.*, 1986; Samanin and Garattini, 1989; Cooper, 1992; Leibowitz, 1993; Simansky, 1995).

Other data, however, have questioned the universal importance of central 5-HT in regulating food intake. For example, destruction of serotonergic neurons in the brain inhibited the anorectic effects of presumably indirectly acting 5-HT agonists under certain conditions (Samanin *et al.*, 1972; Davies *et al.*, 1983; Lucki *et al.*, 1988) but not uniformly (Davies *et al.*, 1983; Carlton and Rowland, 1984; Grignaschi and Samanin, 1992). It is possible that the failures were due to inadequate depletion of 5-HT in critical terminal fields or, in the case of fenfluramine (Davies *et al.*, 1983; Carlton and Rowland, 1984), to direct

DRUG RECEPTOR SUBTYPES AND INGESTIVE BEHAVIOUR
ISBN 0-12-187620-9

actions of its metabolite at 5-HT$_{2C}$ receptors (Gibson *et al.*, 1993). None the less, in one study xylamidine antagonized fenfluramine's actions to reduce food intake and to delay clearance of gastric contents (Baker *et al.*, 1988). Raphe lesions did not attenuate either of these effects in non-deprived rats (Davies *et al.*, 1983). Thus, the results suggested that peripheral serotonergic mechanisms might also serve to modulate feeding, and that this function might involve actions in the gastrointestinal system (Davies *et al.*, 1983; Booth *et al.*, 1986).

The largest stores of 5-HT are, in fact, in the gastrointestinal system, where this indoleamine acts as a neurotransmitter in enteric neurons and as a paracrine or endocrine substance released from enterochromaffin cells (see reviews by Gershon *et al.*, 1990; Sanger, 1992). Enterochromaffin cells are present within the mucosa from the stomach to the colon. Under vagal and sympathetic control (see Sanger, 1992), these bipolar cells release 5-HT either luminally or into the blood, except in the stomach where their apices fail to reach the lumen (Rubin and Schwartz, 1979). A variety of stimuli release 5-HT intraluminally (e.g. Bulbring and Crema, 1959; O'Hara *et al.*, 1959; Kellum *et al.*, 1983) and humorally (e.g. Drapanas *et al.*, 1962; Kellum and Jaffe, 1976) and concentrations of circulating 5-HT increase postprandially in humans (Jaffe *et al.*, 1978; Richter *et al.*, 1986). Most 5-HT that reaches the blood supply draining the gut is eventually sequestered by platelets or degraded. None the less, the localization of this indoleamine within the gastrointestinal system, its actions to modulate the activity of smooth muscles and enteric neurons, and its access to the blood make serotonin a prominent candidate for mediating a peripheral inhibitory control of feeding.

Pharmacological evidence has emerged that is consistent with a role for peripheral 5-HT in curtailing feeding. This review describes those data and evaluates the mechanisms involved. Particular consideration is given to the subtypes of 5-HT receptors responsible for the decreased food intake produced by peripheral serotonergic stimulation. Systemically administered 5-HT also increases water intake. Accordingly, the mechanisms for this dipsogenic effect are discussed and compared with 5-HT's actions in feeding.

2 Peripheral 5-HT and feeding

Investigations of the role of peripheral 5-HT in feeding have relied on evidence that this indoleamine penetrates poorly across the blood–brain barrier (e.g. Garattini *et al.*, 1961; Oldendorf, 1971). Thus, the effects of parenterally administered 5-HT, as an exogenous drug, on food intake are assumed to probe serotonergic functions outside the central nervous system and in circumventricular organs in the brain, in ingestion.

In the first such study, Soulairac and Soulairac (1960) observed that subcutaneous administration of 3 mg/kg serotonin creatinine sulfate to non-deprived male rats decreased their 24-h intake of standard laboratory chow while their concurrent ingestion of glucose was unaltered. Bray and York

(1972) subsequently demonstrated that 5-HT reduced short-term (2 h) consumption of ground chow by food-deprived obese Zucker rats and their lean controls. Furthermore, 5-HT decreased food intake in rats made obese by central lesions in the ventromedial hypothalamus. In contrast, the anorectic action of 5-HT (in food-deprived female rats) was inhibited by the peripheral serotonergic antagonist xylamidine (Clineschmidt *et al.*, 1978).

The above results provided the experimental framework that exogenous 5-HT reduces food intake in a number of models in rats via a primary site of action at peripheral serotonergic receptors. In 1981, Pollock and Rowland broadened the scope of this inquiry. They showed that intraperitoneal injection of 5-HT in rats after 24-h food deprivation decreased their intake of pellets in a dose-related manner, that the monoamine oxidase type A inhibitor clorgyline potentiated this action of 5-HT, and that a dose of 5-HT that reduced intake by approximately 60% did not impair locomotor or sensorimotor function or act as the unconditional stimulus in a conditioned taste aversion paradigm. Their results implied that systemically administered 5-HT did not require biotransformation for activity and reduced food intake in a behaviourally selective manner. Thus, this study set the occasion for carefully describing and analysing the bases for peripheral serotonergic anorexia.

2.1   Behavioural analysis

2.1.1   Characterization
As is evident from Table 1, both intraperitoneal and subcutaneous injection of 5-HT in rats have been shown to reduce food intake across a range of deprivation conditions and with liquid, solid and semisolid test diets of varying palatabilities. Common dose ranges, pretreatment intervals of 0–15 min and measurement periods of 0.5–3.0 h have typically been effective with both routes of administration. The major anorectic action of 5-HT occurs within the first 30–60 min after injection and generally without compensatory overeating in subsequent intervals (Fletcher and Burton, 1984; Montgomery *et al.*, 1986; Edwards and Stevens, 1989). Tolerance did not develop in male rats that were injected once daily before a 4-h feeding period over the course of 8 (Rowland *et al.*, 1982) or 30 (Edwards and Stevens, 1994) days. When rats were offered a diet with separate sources of carbohydrate, fat and protein, 5-HT reduced total caloric intake by preferentially decreasing the consumption of fat (Kanarek and Dushkin, 1988). Thus, the macronutrient composition, taste or texture of the test food may influence the actions of 5-HT. The inhibitory effect of exogenous 5-HT on feeding seems to arise early in development because this indoleamine reduces the duration of nipple attachment in 20- and 30-day-old food-deprived pups (Bateman *et al.*, 1990).

Some apparent disparities with the uniformity of the data exist. For example, Kanarek and Dushkin (1988) found that 2.0 mg/kg 5-HT actually increased the amount of ground chow eaten during the first 3 h of the dark period. In a

Table 1 Studies of the effects of peripheral 5-HT on food intake

Deprivation conditions (h)	Route	Dose (mg/kg)	Test diet	Change in food intake	References
Non-deprived	i.p.	2.0–4.0	Macronutrients	Decreased	Kanarek and Dushkin (1988)
	s.c.	1.0–4.0	Pellets, saccharin solution, sucrose solution, milk	Decreased	Soulairac and Soulairac (1960); Montgomery and Burton (1986a,b); Montgomery et al. (1986); Fletcher and Yu (1989)
Non-deprived (+ INS + 2-DG)	s.c.	2.5–10.0	Pellets	Decreased	Carruba et al. (1986)
Non-deprived (dark period)	i.p.	2.0–4.0	Ground chow	Increased	Kanarek and Dushkin (1988)
			Macronutrients	Decreased	Kanarek and Dushkin (1988)
Non-deprived (rabbits)	s.c.	2.0	Pellets	Decreased	Montgomery et al. (1986)
	Hepatic-portal vein	0.05–0.15	Pellets	Decreased	Rezek and Novin (1975)
Short deprivation (3–4 h)	i.p.	1.5–3.9	Sweetened mash, sucrose solution	Decreased	Neill and Cooper (1989a); Eberle-Wang and Simansky (1992); Eberle-Wang et al. (1993)
	s.c.	1.25–5.0	Pellets	Decreased	Edwards and Stevens (1989)

Condition	Route	Dose	Food type	Effect	References
Long deprivation (17–24 h)	i.p.	0.5–6.0	Ground chow, pellets, sweetened mash, sweetened milk, macronutrients	Decreased	Bray and York (1972); Pollock and Rowland (1981); Rowland et al. (1982); Fletcher (1987); Massi and Marini (1987); Kanarek and Dushkin (1988); Eberle-Wang and Simansky (1992); Simansky et al. (1992); Eberle-Wang et al. (1993); Adipudi and Simansky (1995); Francis et al. (1995)
	s.c.	0.5–5.0	Pellets	Decreased	Lehr and Goldman (1973); Clineschmidt et al. (1978); Fletcher and Burton (1984, 1985, 1986a,b); Carruba et al. (1986); Montgomery et al. (1986); Edwards and Stevens (1991, 1994)
Long deprivation (dark period)	i.p.	2.0–6.0	Ground chow, macronutrients	Decreased	Kanarek and Dushkin (1988)
Long deprivation (ovariectomized rats)	s.c.	5.0	Pellets	No change	Edwards and Stevens (1994)

Doses are in the weights of the salt. Tests were conducted during the light period of the light–dark cycle unless stated otherwise. INS, insulin-stimulated feeding; 2-DG, feeding stimulated by 2-deoxy-D-glucose; i.p., intraperitoneal; s.c., subcutaneous.

different study, however, this same dose reduced pelleted chow intake at the beginning of nocturnal feeding (Montgomery *et al.*, 1986). Furthermore, as noted previously, Kanarek and Dushkin (1988) reported that 5-HT did not increase, but instead decreased, total caloric intake of a macronutrient diet in non-deprived rats. Moreover, when they tested rats after an 18-h deprivation, 5-HT produced dose-related decreases in each type of diet. The increased feeding consumption of ground chow in the dark might hint at significant influences of the stimulus properties of the diet or other test conditions on the actions of 5-HT. The interaction of 5-HT with macronutrient composition, however, would appear to be a more compelling issue to pursue.

Potential sex-based differences pose a more serious concern for understanding the actions of peripheral 5-HT. Edwards and Stevens (1994) assessed the acute and chronic effects of 5.0 mg/kg 5-HT subcutaneously on food intake and bodyweight for 30 days in normal male and female Wistar rats, in obese Zucker male rats, in ovariectomized female Wistars and in male Wistars fed a palatable cafeteria diet. The first four groups were restricted to 4 h of chow daily, whereas the cafeteria group fed freely. 5-HT reduced food intake in lean and obese Zucker males but not in ovariectomized females. 5-HT did produce an anorectic effect during the first hour of the first test day in normal females (also in Clineschmidt *et al.*, 1978), but overall food intake was unaltered on this or subsequent days. In comparison, 5-HT uniformly suppressed the gradual weight gain seen in saline-injected controls in all groups. Food intake was not reported for the cafeteria-fed rats but their weight gain was also inhibited.

Edwards and Stevens (1994) concluded that reduced food intake due to 5-HT contributed at least partly to the suppression of bodyweight in males but that metabolic or other mechanisms were responsible for this action in females. Certainly, this study suggests a role for processes other than those that control feeding in peripheral serotonergic modulation of bodyweight. None the less, it is premature to exclude the possibility that higher doses of 5-HT would reliably decrease food intake in females. If so, it would be critical to determine whether such higher doses inhibited feeding in a behaviourally specific manner.

2.1.2 Specificity

A variety of evidence demonstrates that the reduction of food intake by acute peripheral administration of 5-HT comes from a primary action of the indoleamine on feeding rather than from behavioural toxicity. A dose (2.0 mg/kg) of 5-HT that reduced food intake by 60–70% in food-deprived rats failed to act as an unconditional stimulus in a one-bottle conditioned taste aversion paradigm in one study (Pollock and Rowland, 1981) and produced only a nominal transient aversion in a two-bottle test in a second experiment (Fletcher and Burton, 1984). As cited above, Pollock and Rowland (1981) showed that this dose of 5-HT also failed to alter sensorimotor performance or locomotion in non-deprived rats. Simansky *et al.* (1992) analysed exploratory behaviour in rats that were maintained with the same diet and deprived for the same overnight interval as employed for feeding tests. In that study, 1.6 mg/kg intraperitoneally (ED_{50} for anorexia) did not change the latency to touch a novel object in an open field, the number of contacts made with the object or the time course for this investigatory response, or the frequencies or time courses for rearing and square crossings. Fletcher (1987) reported that 1.0–2.0 mg/kg subcutaneous 5-HT did not alter initial running speeds during a meal in a runway task.

Together, these results argued against 5-HT reducing food intake because it produced malaise, sedation or gross motor impairment. This inference was also supported by evidence that 5-HT decreased gastric sham feeding of liquid diets but not sham drinking of water that was sustained at the same rate (Neill and Cooper, 1989a; Simansky et al., 1992). Furthermore, when non-fistulated rats were given access to a sweet fluid and to water during normal ingestion, 5-HT preferentially decreased consumption of the sweetened solution (Montgomery and Burton, 1986a,b). In contrast, when saline and water were offered in a two-bottle test, peripheral 5-HT increased consumption of water and saline. Thus, 5-HT appeared selectively to inhibit intake of substances identified as food-like (Montgomery and Burton, 1986a) (although 5-HT increased water intake without decreasing saccharin consumption when rats were water deprived before testing (Cooper and Barber, 1994; see section 3.1 below)).

The dipsogenic action raised the possibility that anorexia occurred because 5-HT stimulated drinking at the expense of feeding. The effects of various behavioural manipulations and the different time courses for anorexia and the later-onset drinking, however, indicated that 5-HT produced a primary action on feeding (Montgomery et al., 1986). Studies in which propranolol, an angiotensin-converting enzyme inhibitor, and abdominal vagotomy each prevented drinking but not anorexia in response to serotonergic stimulation established the independence of these two ingestive actions (Montgomery and Burton, 1986b; Montgomery et al., 1986; Simansky, 1991; Eberle-Wang et al., 1993; see also section 3).

2.1.3   Behavioural mechanisms
Several paradigms have been used to analyse the behavioural mechanisms by which peripheral 5-HT reduces food intake in rats. Fletcher (1987) measured the motor performance and food intake of food-deprived rats during 15 trials in a runway task. 5-HT decreased running speed only after some pellets were consumed. The decay in food intake over trials paralleled that for running.

These data implied that peripheral 5-HT interacted with stimuli from ingested food, from feeding or with their combination to enhance the rate of satiation. Using a time-sampling method (Antin et al., 1975), Edwards and Stevens (1991) observed that, after 5-HT, rats progressed more rapidly from eating pellets, to non-feeding activities such as exploration, to resting without altering the normal sequence of these periprandial (i.e. meal-related) behaviours. Simansky et al. (1992) demonstrated a similar accelerated transition in

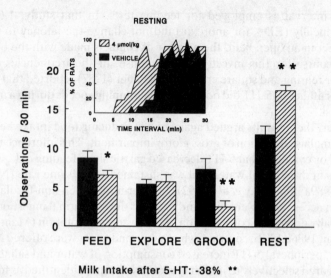

Milk Intake after 5-HT: -38% ★★

Fig. 1 Peripheral 5-HT accelerates satiation in rats. Effect of 4.0 μmol/kg 5-HT intraperitoneally on the incidence of four categories of periprandial behaviour (mean ± SE) as determined by time-sampling observations (one per min) during a 30-min test. Rats (n = 11) were provided with sweetened milk after 17 h food deprivation and were tested under each condition (vehicle and 5-HT). Injections were given 6 min before the start of the test. Inset panel shows that 5-HT reduced the time until rats began resting during the test period. 5-HT also decreased the size of the meal from 12.5 ± 1.0 to 7.8 ± 0.7 ml ($P < 0.01$). $*P < 0.05$, $**P < 0.01$ vs mean after vehicle. (Reprinted by permission of the publisher from Simansky et al. (1992), *Pharmacol. Biochem. Behav.* **43**, 847–854. Copyright 1992 by Elsevier Science Inc.)

the satiety sequence in rats consuming sweetened milk (Fig. 1). When rats were sham-fed with open gastric cannulas, however, 5-HT decreased intake of milk in a dose-related fashion without producing behavioural satiety (Simansky et al., 1992).

Overall, the results suggested that peripheral serotonergic stimulation exerts two dissociable behavioural actions: 5-HT reduces food intake and speeds the onset of satiety. Clearly, this indoleamine must interact with stimuli from the stomach (such as distension) or from postgastric sites in order to enhance satiation. In contrast, 5-HT does not require this stimulus background to diminish the amount of food eaten. Instead, the inhibition of intake may require taste input or other oropharyngeal information. In normal feeding, 5-HT reduces food intake by decreasing the size and duration of bouts without altering their frequency or eating rate (Fletcher and Burton, 1986b). It remains to be determined whether 5-HT limits sham intake by inhibiting the local rate of licking or by otherwise changing the distribution of these motor responses (see Davis et al., 1993).

2.2 Pharmacological analysis

The demonstration that systemically administered 5-HT inhibits feeding implicates peripheral serotonergic mechanisms in controlling food intake but fails to elucidate the subtypes of receptor(s) involved. It is of historical interest that Gaddum and Picarelli (1957) established the first nomenclature for multiple serotonergic receptors based on work in the gut. Serotonergic contractions were antagonized by morphine acting at M sites on neurons and by dibenzyline (phenoxybenzamine) at D sites on smooth muscle. M receptors were also blocked by cocaine, which formed the structural basis for later development of tropine-based 5-HT_3 antagonists such as MDL 72222 and tropisetron (formerly ICS 205-930) (see Fozard, 1989). D receptors were also blocked by various ergots, which led to the later emergence of methysergide as a tool for antagonizing this site.

It is now known that morphine acted indirectly to block neuronal actions of 5-HT by inhibiting the release of acetylcholine from enteric nerves and that dibenzyline lacked specificity for defining a subtype on smooth muscle (Gershon et al., 1990). None-the-less, this receptor distinction proved useful when later radioligand binding studies revealed two 5-HT sites in the brain (Peroutka and Snyder, 1979). Using additional functional data from peripheral models, Bradley and colleagues (1986) subsumed these four sites (M, D, 5-HT_1, 5-HT_2) under three classes within a new major nomenclature. This classification system defined three sets of 5-HT receptors in terms of their ability to be stimulated selectively by structural analogues of serotonin and antagonized by certain antagonists (Fig. 2). 5-HT_2 receptors have generally been considered to correspond to D sites and 5-HT_3 to M sites, although details of each of these points have been argued.

Evidence from operational (i.e. functional and ligand binding), transductional (i.e. intracellular signalling) and structural (molecular biological) studies has now revealed seven classes of 5-HT receptors, including a number that have subtypes (Hoyer et al., 1994). In the periphery, direct actions of endogenous 5-HT at its receptors produce important, sometimes profound, changes in cardiovascular, gastrointestinal and other autonomic functions. Because of the likely relevance to the physiology of feeding, Table 2 lists some prominent features of neurocrine and paracrine responses that have been linked to serotonergic receptors in the gastrointestinal systems of various mammalian species. The pharmacological distinctions among the first three major classes of receptors that were described by Bradley et al. (1986) have been maintained; comparisons across subtypes within these classes often remain problematic (see Hoyer et al., 1994). The profiles of 5-HT_3, 5-HT_4 and 5-HT_{1P} receptors overlap in some cases. For example, tropisetron blocks 5-HT_3 sites and (at much higher concentrations) antagonizes 5-HT_4 sites. In comparison, though, a number of compounds that appear to be pure potent antagonists at 5-HT_3 receptors display intrinsic activity as agonists at 5-HT_4 sites.

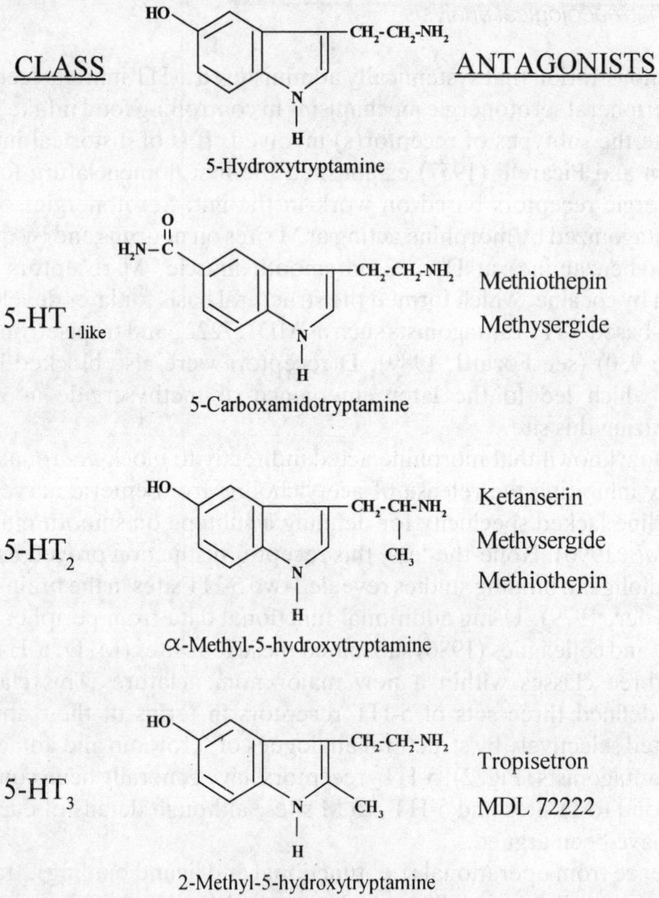

CLASS

5-Hydroxytryptamine

ANTAGONISTS

5-HT₁-like

5-Carboxamidotryptamine

Methiothepin
Methysergide

5-HT₂

α-Methyl-5-hydroxytryptamine

Ketanserin
Methysergide
Methiothepin

5-HT₃

2-Methyl-5-hydroxytryptamine

Tropisetron
MDL 72222

Fig. 2 Prototypical compounds in 5-HT receptor nomenclature of Bradley *et al.* (1986). 5-Carboxamidotryptamine (5-CT), α-methyl-5-hydroxytryptamine (α-methyl-5-HT) and 2-methyl-5-hydroxytryptamine (2-methyl-5-HT) are the agonists for 5-HT$_{1-Like}$, 5-HT$_2$ and 5-HT$_3$ receptors, respectively. Distinguishing antagonists are shown on the right.

2.2.1 Studies using 5-HT antagonists

Across various testing conditions, methysergide has prevented the reduction of food intake produced by systemically administered 5-HT (Fletcher and Burton, 1984, 1985, 1986a; Kanarek and Dushkin, 1988). Given methysergide's pharmacological profile, such observations appeared to implicate subtypes of 5-HT$_1$ or 5-HT$_2$ receptors, or both classes, in mediating peripheral serotonergic anorexia and to exclude other sites.

To discriminate between 5-HT$_1$ and 5-HT$_2$ sites, Massi and Marini (1987) tested the ability of ritanserin (0.01–1.0 mg/kg subcutaneously) to block anorexia produced by 5-HT (6.0 mg/kg intraperitoneally) in rats trained to eat

Table 2 5-HT receptor subtypes involved in gastrointestinal function

Receptor subtype	Role in gastrointestinal function	comment
5-HT$_{1A}$	Inhibits enteric neuronal activity	(**AG**) 5-CT and 8-OH-DPAT; (**P**) methysergide; (**ANT**) propranolol; WAY 100635
5-HT$_{1-Like}$	Gut relaxation (e.g. ileum; see footnote) Increased intragastric pressure	(**AG**) 5-CT > 5-HT; (**ANT**) methysergide, metergoline (**AG**) 5-HT > 5-CT; (**ANT**) methysergide
5-HT$_{2A/2C}$	Gut contraction (e.g. pylorus); vasoconstriction (mesenteric and hepatic portal vasculature); intestinal secretion	(**AG**) α-Me-5-HT, DOI; (**ANT**) ketanserin, ritanserin, methysergide, xylamidine, SB 200646A (5-HT$_{2C}$)
5-HT$_{2B}$	Contracts fundus of the stomach in rats; peripheral and central in humans (close homology and pharmacology to rat)	(**AG**) rat, 5-HT = α-Me-5-HT > 5-CT; (**ANT**) methysergide, ritanserin, SB 200646A, not ketanserin in rats
5-HT$_3$	Rapid neuronal depolarization; activates vagal afferents in gut wall; emesis; increases postprandial colonic propulsion; may slow gastric emptying in rats	(**AG**) 2-Me-5-HT, mCPBG; (**ANT**) tropisetron, MDL 72222, granisetron, ondansetron, zacopride, renzapride
5-HT$_4$	Relaxes oesophagus; stimulates gastric emptying in dogs and humans, not rats; excitatory modulation of peristalsis; increases secretion; may depolarize vagal afferents in rats; may mediate emesis	(**AG**) 5-MeOT > α-Me-5-HT > 5-CT, 2-Me-5-HT is inactive; (**P**) cisapride, renzapride, zacopride, others; (**ANT**) tropisetron, DAU 6285, SDZ 205-557
5-HT$_{1P}$	Slow depolarization of myenteric neurons; slows gastric emptying	(**AG**) 5-OH- and 6-OH-indalpine, S-zacopride, 2-Me-5-HT is weak; (**ANT**) 5-HTP-DP, renzapride

This information provides notable actions mediated by activating each subtype in the gastrointestinal system. The 1B (in rodents), 1D$_α$, 1D$_β$, 1E and 1F subtypes and the 5-HT$_{5-7}$ classes have either not been identified or not well defined in gut-related functions. The 5-HT$_{1-Like}$ receptor that relaxes ileum may actually be a 5-HT$_7$ site (Hoyer et al., 1994). Methysergide and metergoline display partial agonist activity with varying efficacy at many 1A, 1B, 1D and 1-Like receptors. Actions of the two drugs differ at some receptors. Complete pharmacological and physiological profiles can be found in Gershon et al. (1990), Sanger (1992), Ford and Clarke (1993) and Hoyer et al. (1994); see Kursar et al. (1994) for human 5-HT$_{2B}$ receptor. **AG**, agonist; **P**, partial agonist; **ANT**, antagonist.

Drug abbreviations: 5-HTP-DP, 5-hydroxytryptophyl-5-hydroxytryptophan amide; 5-MeOT, 5-methoxytryptamine; DAU 6285, endo-6-methoxy-8-methyl-8-azabicyclo[3.2.1]oct-3-yl-2,3-dihydro-2-oxo-1H-benzimidazole-1-carboxylate; DOI, 1-(2,5-dimethoxy-4-iodophenyl)-2-aminopropane; mCPBG, meta-chlorophenylbiguanide; MDL 72222, 1α, 3α, 5αH-tropan-3-yl-3,5-dichlorobenzoate; 8-OH-DPAT, 8-hydroxy-di-N-propyl aminotetralin; SB 200646A, N-(1-methyl-5-indonyl)-N'-(3-pyridyl)urea hydrochloride; SDZ 205557, 2-methoxy-4-amino-5-chlorobenzoic acid-2-(diethylamino)ethyl ester; WAY 100635, N-[2-[4-(2-methoxyphenyl)-1-piperazinyl]ethyl]-N-(2-pyridinyl)cyclohexanecarboxamide trihydrochloride.

pellets during a 6-h period in the light. Ritanserin attenuated the action of 5-HT in a dose-related manner but the asymptotic effect of the antagonist was incomplete. Together with the methysergide data, the results suggested that ritanserin-sensitive 5-HT_2 sites and ritanserin-insensitive 5-HT_1 sites were responsible for 5-HT to reduce food intake.

Ritanserin cannot distinguish among the subtypes of 5-HT_2 receptors (see Table 2; Baez et al., 1990; Hoyer et al., 1994). In contrast, ketanserin has very high binding affinity for 5-HT_{2A} sites (0.4 nmol/l, equivalent to ritanserin; Leysen, 1992), 100-fold lower affinity for 5-HT_{2C} sites, and fails to block serotonergic contractions mediated by 5-HT_{2B} receptors in the rat fundus, in vitro (Clineschmidt et al., 1985; Cohen and Fludzinski, 1987; Baxter et al., 1994). In vivo, ketanserin displays 300-fold lower potency for blocking 5-HT_{2C}-mediated hypophagia produced by m-chlorophenylpiperazine (mCPP) in rats compared with antagonizing 5-HT_{2A}-mediated stereotypy (Kennett and Curzon, 1991).

Experiments were therefore conducted comparing the abilities of ketanserin and methysergide to inhibit hypophagia produced by 5-HT in rats given access to sweetened milk after overnight food deprivation. Based on separate dose–response studies (unpublished results), rats were pretreated with a supramaximal dose of ketanserin or methysergide before 5-HT. A similar large dose of tropisetron was used to assess the contribution of 5-HT_3 and 5-HT_4 receptors (see Table 2) to serotonergic anorexia. The results in Table 3 show that methysergide completely prevented the decrease in milk consumption produced by this dose of 5-HT whereas ketanserin only partially reversed the anorexia, and tropisetron was ineffective.

Table 3 Comparison of the effects of methysergide, ketanserin and tropisetron on the anorectic action of 5-HT

		Milk intake (ml/30 min)		
Pretreatment	Treatment	Methysergide	Ketanserin	Tropisetron
Vehicle	Vehicle	17.8 ± 1.8	21.2 ± 2.1	21.0 ± 1.3
Vehicle	5-HT	5.4 ± 1.2†	6.8 ± 1.4†	2.6 ± 0.9†
Antagonist	Vehicle	19.5 ± 2.1	20.7 ± 2.2	19.8 ± 1.7
Antagonist	5-HT	18.8 ± 2.6§	12.8 ± 2.9‡	1.0 ± 0.7†

Three experiments were conducted in which four groups of 7–9 rats each were tested after 17 h food deprivation. Pretreatment was injected intraperitoneally 15 min before vehicle or 5-HT, and sweetened milk was provided 6 min later for the 30-min test. Doses of all antagonists and of 5-HT were 10 μmol/kg (approximately 3.9, 3.5, 5.4 and 2.8 mg/kg for 5-HT creatinine sulfate, methysergide maleate, ketanserin tartrate and 3-tropanyl-indole-3-carboxylate (tropisetron), respectively).

Data are expressed as mean ± SE.

$*P < 0.05$, †$P < 0.01$ vs respective vehicle + vehicle control and vs antagonist + vehicle group; ‡$P < 0.05$, §$P < 0.01$ vs respective vehicle + 5-HT group.

These data confirmed and extended Massi and Marini's (1987) findings and clearly implicated 5-HT_1 and $5\text{-HT}_{2A/2C}$ (probably 2A) receptors in the anorectic action of peripheral 5-HT. It was intriguing, then, that Edwards and Stevens (1989) also reported that the peripheral antagonist, xylamidine, only partly reversed 5-HT-induced anorexia. In binding, xylamidine displays very high and equal affinity for 2A and 2C receptors and extremely low affinity for 1A and 1B sites (Leysen, 1992). Thus, once again, it appeared that 5-HT_2 receptors and also other peripheral sites are involved in serotonergic inhibitory effects on feeding.

Some discrepancies with these data exist. For example, the ergoline metergoline failed to reverse, at all, 5-HT-induced anorexia in one study in which methysergide was effective (Fletcher and Burton, 1984), although others reported that metergoline produced total antagonism (Carruba *et al.*, 1986). In other work, xylamidine completely reversed 5-HT in real feeding (Carruba *et al.*, 1986) and in sham feeding (Neill and Cooper, 1989a). It is possible that 5-HT operates solely via 5-HT_2 receptors to inhibit sham feeding. This hypothesis can be tested by the judicious choice of antagonist drugs. The differences among laboratories in the antagonist profiles during real feeding, however, cannot yet be reconciled because the testing conditions across laboratories were reasonably similar. Under our conditions using food-deprived rats and sweetened milk, xylamidine and metergoline each produced large but incomplete reversals of 5-HT (unpublished results).

2.2.2 Studies using 5-HT analogues as agonists

The differential selectivity of structural analogues of 5-HT for serotonergic receptors (Fig. 2) offered a complementary approach for testing the roles of peripheral 5-HT_1 and 5-HT_2 mechanisms in anorexia. As can be seen in Fig. 3, the 5-HT_1 agonist 5-carboxamidotryptamine (5-CT) and the 5-HT_2 agonist α-methyl-5-hydroxytryptamine (α-Me-5-HT) each decreased milk consumption in a dose-related manner (Simansky *et al.*, 1989–1990). The curves for the two analogues were parallel and the ED_{50} for 5-CT was 100-fold lower than that for α-Me-5-HT. This was not simply a matter of 5-CT acting more potently than α-Me-5-HT at a single type of receptor, however, because ketanserin blocked only the anorectic effect of the latter indole (see also Hewson *et al.*, 1989). In contrast, methysergide prevented the anorexia produced by both analogues.

The agonist effects of these two analogues could also be distinguished on the basis of their sensitivity to xylamidine. As can be seen in Fig. 4, a dose of xylamidine as small as $0.25\ \mu$mol/kg (approximately 0.13 mg/kg of the tosylate salt) completely reversed anorexia produced by α-Me-5-HT, but a 40-fold larger dose of the antagonist failed to attenuate the action of 5-CT. In a separate study using different experimental conditions, methysergide but not ritanserin blocked 5-CT-induced anorexia (Simansky, 1991). Thus, 5-CT reduces food intake via a 5-HT_1 receptor whereas α-Me-5-HT's action is

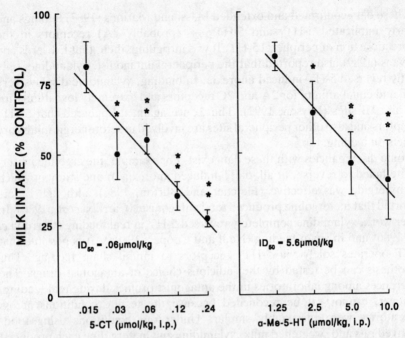

Fig. 3   Anorectic actions of 5-CT and (±)-α-methyl-5-HT. Data are expressed as the percentage of the baseline (mean ± SE). Separate groups of 7–8 rats were tested at each dose of each analogue. Rats were provided with sweetened milk after 18 h food deprivation. Baseline was 15.9 ± 1.3 ml for the 5-CT experiment and 18.7 ± 0.7 ml for the α-methyl-5-HT experiment. *$P < 0.05$, **$P < 0.01$ vs baseline. (Adapted by permission of the publisher from Simansky et al. (1989–1990), Behav. Pharmacol. 1, 241–246, Rapid Science Publishers, Oxford.)

mediated by a 5-HT$_2$ site. These effects are additive: in an experiment in which controls consumed 31.1 ± 2.0 ml milk in 30 min, 0.03 μmol/kg 5-CT reduced intake by 40%, 4.0 μmol/kg of α-Me-5-HT by 35%, and the combination of these treatments by 76%.

The precise nature of the 5-HT subtypes that mediate the actions of these analogues requires further attention. The relative importance of 5-HT$_{2A}$ vs 5-HT$_{2C}$ sites is readily amenable to analysis with a series of 5-HT$_2$ antagonists, including the 2B/2C antagonist SB 200646A (see Table 2; Kennett et al., 1994). Developing a profile for 5-CT may be less straightforward. Besides ketanserin, ritanserin and xylamidine, 16 μmol/kg (4.7 mg/kg) of (−)-propranolol failed to antagonize 5-CT-induced anorexia (Simansky, 1991). This was consistent with the failure of 5 mg/kg of the less potent and less selective racemate, (±)-propranolol, to attenuate hypophagia produced by 5-HT (Montgomery et al., 1986). In addition to its high affinity as an antagonist at β-adrenergic receptors, (−)-propranolol displays approximately micromolar affinity for 5-HT$_{1A}$, 5-HT$_{1B}$ and the 5-HT$_2$ sites but not for 5-HT$_{1D}$ or 5-HT$_{1-Like}$ receptors (e.g. see Clineschmidt et al., 1985; Hoyer, 1989; Hoyer et al., 1994). Thus, it appeared

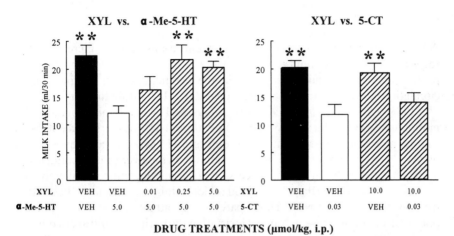

DRUG TREATMENTS (μmol/kg, i.p.)

Fig. 4 Xylamidine (XYL) prevents the anorectic action of α-methyl-5-HT but not that of 5-CT. Left panel shows the milk intake of groups of seven rats treated 60 min apart with: two intraperitoneal (i.p.) injections of vehicle (VEH); vehicle (no dose of XYL) before 5.0 μmol/kg (±)-α-methyl-5-HT; or one of three doses of XYL before α-methyl-5-HT. Right panel depicts the results of a separate experiment with groups of 11 rats each in which XYL or its vehicle was administered 60 min before 0.03 μmol/kg 5-CT or its vehicle. The analogues (0 dose pretreatment + analogue) significantly decreased milk intake in each study compared with the controls (VEH + VEH), $P < 0.01$. A dose of xylamidine as large as 10.0 μmol/kg did not affect baseline (right panel). **$P < 0.01$ vs group injected with 0 dose of XYL + analogue. (Adapted by permission of the publisher from Simansky et al. (1989–1990), Behav. Pharmacol. **1**, 241–246, Rapid Science Publishers, Oxford.)

that 5-CT did not act via the 1A or the 1B subtypes. However, Lehr and Goldman (1973) did find that a larger dose of racemic propranolol (6.2 mg/kg) antagonized 5-HT-induced anorexia. Thus, further analysis is required.

The 5-HT_{2B} sites in the fundus do not mediate the anorectic effect of 5-CT, nor are these receptors involved in the anorexia produced by α-Me-5-HT. 5-CT does contract the stomach but less potently than either 5-HT or α-Me-5-HT (see Table 2). As noted above, ketanserin blocks the anorectic effect of α-Me-5-HT but not contractions in the isolated fundus. In comparison, ritanserin does inhibit serotonergic contractions in the rat stomach but not the anorectic action of 5-CT (see above).

Besides 1A, 1B and 2B receptors, a role for 5-HT_{1D} receptors in 5-CT-induced anorexia should be considered. The serotonergic $1D_\alpha$ subtype, however, is sparse in rats and the 1B subtype is the rodent homologue of $1D_\beta$ receptors found in lagomorphs, guinea-pigs, primates and other mammals (Hoyer et al., 1994). It is also possible that an atypical, $5\text{-HT}_{1\text{-Like}}$ receptor is involved, such as that which relaxes smooth muscle in the ileum of the guinea-pig (Feniuk et al., 1983; Kalkman et al., 1986) or which increases intragastric pressure in rats (Dhasmana et al., 1992). Clearly, these are concerns for immediate study.

2.3   Sites of action

After parenteral administration, local concentrations of 5-HT increase in the region of the gut and other abdominal viscera, in the mesenteric and hepatic–portal vasculature, and conceivably in the posthepatic and postpulmonary circulation. Given the transmural movement of 5-HT within the gut (Cooke *et al.*, 1983; Larsson *et al.*, 1990), exogenous 5-HT that is not degraded by monoamine oxidase has access to mucosal afferents, serotonergic receptors on smooth muscle and possibly enteric receptors. 5-HT that escapes sequestration by platelets (see Sanger, 1992) and degradation in the liver or lung could reach targets in the hindbrain that are accessible to circulating amines—namely, the area postrema and, perhaps, a confined region within the nucleus of the solitary tract (Gross *et al.*, 1990). Thus, parenterally administered 5-HT can act potentially at numerous anatomical loci within the periphery and at circumventricular organs of the brain to produce physiological changes that influence feeding. The relevant changes could involve direct, receptor-mediated, modulation of neuronal feedback in the hindbrain or within afferent pathways to the brain. Just as likely, however, 5-HT could alter muscle tone within smooth muscle of the gut or vasculature to produce changes that secondarily modify neuronal activity.

2.3.1   Abdominal vagus nerve

The vagus nerve provides a major source of sensory information from the gut and other abdominal viscera. Some of this information appears to be critical to the normal control of the size of meals because bilateral transection of the abdominal vagus, or interrupting its afferent pathway in the medulla, prevents the satiating effects of the peptide cholecystokinin (CCK) (e.g. Smith *et al.*, 1981, 1985). Hepatic vagotomy interferes with a similar action of glucagon (Geary and Smith, 1983).

In contrast, Fletcher and Burton (1985) reported that abdominal vagotomy enhanced the anorectic effects of 5-HT. Their vagotomies, however, spared the hepatic branch of the vagus, and it was previously suggested that anorectic effects of 5-HT infused via the hepatic portal vein in non-deprived rabbits were mediated by vagal afferents from the liver (Rezek and Novin, 1975). Accordingly, we tested rats with vagotomies that transected the tenth nerve above the level at which the hepatic branch leaves the right vagal trunk (Eberle-Wang *et al.*, 1993). These rats displayed normal sensitivity to 5-HT, although, as expected, the lesions did prevent the satiety effect of CCK octapeptide (CCK-8). Furthermore, the vagotomized rats responded normally to the reductions in food intake produced by 5-CT, despite blocking the dose-related increases in water intake elicited by this 5-HT analogue in the same experiment (see Section 3.3.1).

The study by Fletcher and Burton (1985) used rats, 3 weeks after operation, that were deprived of food for 18 h and tested with pelleted chow. In our study

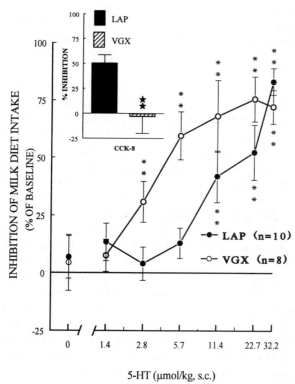

5-HT (μmol/kg, s.c.)

Fig. 5 Abdominal vagotomy dissociates the mechanisms for the satiating actions of 5-HT and cholecystokinin octapeptide (CCK-8) in rats. Rats with bilateral abdominal vagotomy (VGX) and their laparotomized controls (LAP) were given sweetened milk for 17 h daily; the first 30-min access to milk served as the test period (as in Figs 1, 3 and 4). *Main panel*: Each rat received each of the six doses of 5-HT (5-hydroxytryptamine creatinine sulfate) and the 0 dose (32.2 μmol/kg creatinine sulfate) 12 min before milk was provided. Data are expressed as the percentage decrease from average overall baseline (LAP, 13.6 ± 3.6 ml; VGX, 6.2 ± 0.8 ml, $P < 0.01$) determined on the day before the test with 5-HT or creatinine. $**P < 0.01$ *vs* creatinine treatment (two-tailed Dunnett's t test after analysis of variance). Dose–response functions differed by two-way ANOVA ($P < 0.01$ for lesion–dose interaction) and regression analysis; ED_{50} and 95% confidence limits were 11.5 (8.9–14.9) μmol/kg for LAP and 3.8 (1.7–8.1) μmol/kg for VGX; the slopes did not differ. After completing the dose–response function with 5-HT, the rats were tested with vehicle and CCK-8 (3.5 nmol/kg intraperitoneally). CCK-8 decreased intake in controls but not in vagotomized rats ($**P < 0.01$, see inset). Baseline was 15.7 ± 2.4 ml for LAP and 5.8 ± 0.6 ml for VGX ($P < 0.01$). Testing occurred 3–8 weeks after surgery.

with 5-HT (Eberle-Wang *et al.*, 1993), rats were tested with sweetened mash after 3 h of deprivation; the experiment began 11 weeks after operation. When rats were tested after a shorter postoperative recovery, and using a milk diet after 17-h deprivation, vagotomy produced supersensitivity to 5-HT but still blocked CCK-8 (Fig. 5). Thus, either the length of food deprivation or the duration of postoperative recovery, or both, appear to influence the sensitivity of rats to 5-HT after vagotomy. These factors may determine compensatory changes in neuronal or in muscle function that dictate responsiveness to serotonin. None the less, it is clear that the abdominal vagus is not necessary for peripheral 5-HT to reduce food intake in rats.

The abdominal vagus nerve is thought to mediate effects of excessive local concentrations of 5-HT in the gut to cause gastrointestinal malaise and emesis (Andrews et al., 1990). These responses involve 5-HT_3 and possibly 5-HT_4 receptors on vagal afferents in the abdominal viscera and in the hindbrain (Andrews et al., 1990; Ford and Clarke, 1993). Thus, the failure of vagotomy to alter the anorectic action of 5-HT would appear to be consistent with the failure of a high dose of the $5\text{-HT}_{3/4}$ antagonist tropisetron to block this effect. Furthermore, the results are interesting in view of the conclusion that an ED_{50} dose of 5-HT decreases food intake without causing toxicity.

These data also clearly separate the neuronal pathways by which peripheral 5-HT and CCK-8 elicit satiety. In another study, the CCK_A receptor antagonist devazepide blocked the reduction of food intake produced by CCK-8 but not that after 5-HT (Eberle-Wang and Simansky, 1992). Thus, surgical and pharmacological manipulations dissociate the mechanisms by which these two satiety agents limit feeding. It should be noted that devazepide did inhibit the anorectic effect of fenfluramine in rats that were either non-deprived or deprived for 4 h (Cooper et al., 1990a; Grignaschi et al., 1993) but not after 22 h of deprivation (Li and Rowland, 1994). Devazepide failed, however, to inhibit the anorectic action of fluoxetine in freely feeding rats (Cooper et al., 1990b). Eberle-Wang and Simansky (1992) used a 3-h deprivation period. Therefore, it appears that fenfluramine recruits central rather than peripheral CCKergic mechanisms to inhibit feeding (cf. Cooper et al., 1992). The nature of this interaction may depend on the deprivational state of the animal. Neither fluoxetine nor peripheral 5-HT, itself, recruit CCK_A mechanisms. Other evidence exists for central 5-HT mediating satiety induced by peripheral CCK (e.g. Poeschla et al., 1992).

2.3.2   Gastric emptying, the stomach and pylorus

Baker and co-workers (1988) observed that xylamidine antagonized the action of fenfluramine to increase retention of food. They therefore suggested that peripheral serotonergic mechanisms enhance satiation by slowing gastric emptying. Fletcher and Burton (1985) reported that subcutaneous administration of 2.0 mg/kg 5-HT also increased retention of food but methysergide did not block this effect. Given that methysergide did antagonize the anorectic action of 5-HT in the same study, it would appear that serotonergic effects on gastric emptying were not responsible for the ability of this indoleamine to reduce food intake. Similarly compelling data were presented recently by Francis et al. (1995), who demonstrated that 5-HT (0.1–3.0 mg/kg intraperitoneally) increased gastric emptying within the same dose range as it decreased food intake. A discussion of the issues surrounding differences among laboratories in determining effects of 5-HT on gastric kinetics can be found in this latter paper. None the less, to the present, the data argue against a role for gastric emptying in peripheral inhibition of feeding by 5-HT.

It is possible that local changes in muscle tension, *per se*, rather than effects due to altered gastric emptying are sufficient for 5-HT to provide a satiety stimulus to the brain. One such potential site is at the gastroduodenal junction, where 5-HT contracts the pylorus *in vitro* by a mechanism that is antagonized by methysergide, ketanserin and xylamidine but not by tropisetron, atropine, various adrenergic antagonists or the CCK_A antagonist devazepide (Eberle-Wang *et al.*, 1994). Thus, this $5\text{-}HT_2$-type receptor may mediate one of the components of anorexia produced by exogenous 5-HT. As already noted, it is clear that the fundic $5\text{-}HT_{2B}$ receptor is unimportant because ketanserin blocks $5\text{-}HT_2$-related anorexia but not the 2B receptor in rats. A role for increased intragastric pressure in the effects of 5-CT, operating via a $5\text{-}HT_{1\text{-}Like}$ site (Dhasmana *et al.*, 1992), has also been mentioned above. If so, then rats feeding with an open gastric cannula might not respond to this particular serotonergic signal. It is therefore significant that Neill and Cooper (1989a) reported that xylamidine completely antagonized peripheral serotonergic inhibition of sham feeding, as would be expected if $5\text{-}HT_2$ but not $5\text{-}HT_{1\text{-}Like}$ mechanisms decreased sham feeding.

2.3.3 Central nervous system

In 1972, Bray and York reported that obese rats with lesions in the ventromedial area of the hypothalamus responded normally to the anorectic effect of systemic 5-HT. Thus, this region of the forebrain was unnecessary for ultimately processing serotonergic inhibitory signals from the periphery.

The area postrema is a more interesting candidate as a target for 5-HT to decrease food intake because of its ability to monitor information from circulating amines and peptides that normally penetrate poorly across the blood–brain barrier (Borison, 1989). This circumventricular organ receives serotonergic innervation (including from vagal afferents; Sykes *et al.*, 1994) and sends 5-HT-containing projections to other regions of the hindbrain (e.g. parabrachial nucleus; Lanca and van der Kooy, 1985). More significantly for the current discussion, the area postrema contains populations, though sparse, of several 5-HT receptor subtypes (Laporte *et al.*, 1992; Thor *et al.*, 1992). Thus, it may integrate neuronal and hormonal information from 5-HT that serve functions in normal physiology and pathology. It is perhaps relevant that lesions of this region prevent conditioned taste aversions produced by the 5-HT precursor, 5-hydroxy-L-tryptophan (5-HTP) (Ossenkopp *et al.*, 1985; see also Ervin *et al.*, 1984).

Recently, we observed that ablating the area postrema blunted the anorectic response to $8.0\,\mu\text{mol/kg}$ (approximately 3.1 mg/kg intraperitoneally) but not to $2.0\,\mu\text{mol/kg}$ in rats that were fed sweet-mash after 19 h of deprivation (Adipudi and Simansky, 1995). The attenuated response to the higher dose after ablation was correlated with a decreased incidence of resting and an abnormal posture. Conversely, lesioned rats were observed eating more frequently than controls after the higher dose of 5-HT. These data suggested that, under these testing conditions, 8.0 μmol/kg inhibited feeding partly by causing behavioural toxicity. The lesions were very selective. Thus, destroying the area postrema either removed the target for this behavioural effect of 5-HT or otherwise produced secondary changes in the hindbrain that interfered with the response. It remains possible that the loss of resting reflected the disruption of a normal role for this organ in serotonergic synchronization of sleep (cf. Borison, 1989; Koella, 1974). A more likely site for 5-HT to mediate the important postprandial relationship between satiety and sleep (Danguir et al., 1979) is in the nucleus of the solitary tract (e.g. Key and Mehta, 1977). To date, low densities of 5-HT$_{1A}$, 5-HT$_{1B}$ and 5-HT$_3$ receptors have been found in the area postrema (Laporte et al., 1992; Thor et al., 1992). As none of these matches the pharmacology of the ingestive responses described for peripheral 5-HT, it remains to be determined whether 5-HT$_2$ or 5-HT$_{1-Like}$ sites exist in this region of the hindbrain.

Perhaps most significantly, this study leaves open the question of the neuronal substrates responsible for behaviourally selective effects of lower doses of 5-HT to reduce food intake and promote satiation. The half-life of a few minutes for 5-HT and the layers of protection along the circulatory path, especially in the lung (Vane, 1969), would appear to favour abdominal loci as the primary site(s) for the major actions of intraperitoneal 5-HT in feeding. Identification of the neuronal representation of the serotonergic signal, therefore, should focus on peripheral afferent pathways for relaying information to the brain.

2.4 Future directions

Significant progress has been achieved during the past 15 years in describing the effects of parenterally administered 5-HT in feeding and in analysing the mechanisms for those actions. None the less, the substantial body of evidence that has emerged merely provides the foundation for understanding the function of subtypes of serotonergic receptors, and of the native indoleamine in general, in peripheral controls of feeding and satiety. The following issues need to be addressed, although this list is certainly not exhaustive.

Role of 5-HT receptor subtypes in modulating the organization of feeding and satiety. The roles of different pharmacological mechanisms in the separate actions of peripheral 5-HT to reduce food intake and to enhance satiety can be defined by probing with structural analogues of 5-HT and their antagonists. In addition, the effects of 5-HT and its analogues on eating rate and other microstructural parameters of feeding require further analysis. Although a moderate dose of 5-HT reportedly did not change the rate of eating (Fletcher and Burton, 1986a), xylamidine antagonized the ability of 5-HTP to slow eating. This suggests that more intensive stimulation of peripheral serotonergic (5-HT$_2$) receptors inhibits rate;

Stimulus background for satiety. The critical stimulus or stimuli that enable peripheral 5-HT to accelerate satiation remains to be identified;

Characterization of receptor subtypes. The pharmacological profiles for the different serotonergic components of peripheral anorexia require more precise definition. Furthermore, the effects of activating 5-HT receptors of the 3, 4, 1P and other classes on ingestion should be explored for comparison with the data already in hand. We found that 2-methyl-5-HT reduces food intake in a behaviourally selective manner but were unable to inhibit this action with any of the classical 5-HT$_3$ antagonists (Simansky *et al.*, 1991; see also Kennett and Grewal, 1992) or with 5-HT$_{1P}$ antagonists (unpublished);

Actions of 5-HT antagonists in feeding. Methysergide has been demonstrated to disinhibit satiety under optimal conditions (e.g. Fletcher, 1988; Dourish *et al.*, 1989; Dryden *et al.*, 1993) but the role of peripheral *vs* central mechanisms in this response cannot be ascertained. In one study, xylamidine increased bout size (Fletcher and Burton, 1986a), but generally this agent has been tested in situations that are relatively insensitive for detecting drug-induced increases in food intake. Some evidence exists that blocking peripheral 5-HT$_3$ receptors increases consumption of a diet with imbalanced amino acids (Hrupka *et al.*, 1991). In other work, the 5-HT$_3$ antagonist ondansetron decreased intake of a palatable diet (van der Hoek and Cooper, 1994) although, once again, the contribution of peripheral *vs* central mechanisms is uncertain.

It is important to emphasize that the failure of xylamidine to block 5-CT's anorectic action, and the poor affinity of xylamidine for non-5-HT$_2$ receptors, seriously questions the general use of this agent to define central *vs* peripheral sites for serotonergic actions. Specifically, demonstrating that a drug action is insensitive to antagonism by xylamidine does not necessarily establish that the agent is acting centrally. Certainly, new tools are needed to explore the actions of peripheral 5-HT in feeding.

Comparison with centrally acting agonists. The structure of 5-CT, like that of 5-HT, should greatly restrict its access to the brain. By comparison, 2-Me-5-HT is known to cross the blood–brain barrier (Kilpatrick and Rogers, 1993). α-Me-5-HT also might penetrate better than 5-HT into the brain, but xylamidine completely blocked the hypophagic action of this drug. In comparison, xylamidine did not inhibit the anorectic effect of systemic administration of DOI (1-[2,5-dimethoxy-4-iodophenyl]-2-aminopropane), which definitely enters the brain and reduces food intake by stimulating 5-HT$_2$ receptors

(Schechter and Simansky, 1988). Thus, we presume that ingestive actions of parenterally injected 5-CT and α-Me-5-HT act at primary receptor targets in the periphery.

In rodents, the satiating and other inhibitory actions of serotonergic stimulation in the brain in feeding appear to be mediated by the 1B and 2C subtypes; in contrast, activating central 5-HT_{2A} receptors disrupts the continuity of feeding (see Cooper, 1992; Dourish, 1992; Simansky, 1995). 5-HT_{1B} receptors are found peripherally in rats where they control vasomotor function and act as heteroreceptors to modulate neurotransmitter release (e.g. see Hoyer *et al.*, 1994). The 1B subtype does not appear to be associated with gut function and, in fact, the significance of 2C (*vs* 2A and 2B) sites in the gut also remains arguable. Thus, the profile of central serotonergic mechanisms in feeding differs from that developing for peripheral 5-HT. Given this overall context, it will be useful to compare the relative potencies and the nature of the behavioural actions of the 5-HT analogues after central and peripheral administration.

Sites of action of peripheral 5-HT. Peripheral 5-HT reduces food intake by an extravagal pathway. This observation classifies 5-HT with the peptidergic satiety factor bombesin (Stuckey *et al.*, 1985) and distinguishes it from CCK and glucagon (Smith *et al.*, 1981, 1985; Geary and Smith, 1983). The ability of bombesin to reduce food intake is prevented by total neural disconnection of the gut from the brain in which abdominal vagotomy is combined with spinal cord transection at the sixth thoracic segment and dorsal rhizotomy at T3–6 (Stuckey *et al.*, 1985). Analogous surgical interruptions, selective and combined, of non-vagal afferent pathways will elucidate the neuronal substrates for peripheral serotonergic anorexia. Complementary information may come from more local administration of 5-HT, as noted previously for hepatic portal infusions in rabbits. It is intriguing that in that study (Rezek and Novin, 1975) portal 5-HT administration increased food intake in deprived female rabbits. This experiment warrants replication and comparison to rats.

3 Peripheral 5-HT and drinking

The myriad subtypes of 5-HT receptors mediate serotonergic responses causing vasoconstriction and vasodilatation, chronotropic and inotropic effects in the heart, and widespread modulation of endocrine systems. Physiologically (and pathophysiologically) some of these changes reflect the functions of endogenous serotonergic systems throughout the central neuraxis (McCall, 1990; Van de Kar, 1991). Many of these events, though, can be attributed to direct actions of 5-HT at receptors on vascular and cardiac muscle, to presynaptic inhibition of neurotransmitter release and to reflexes initiated by stimulating neuronal afferents in the periphery (see Sanger, 1992; Ford and Clarke, 1993; Hoyer *et al.*, 1994). Associated with the varied haemodynamic and neuroendocrine changes, parenteral administration of exogenous 5-HT causes the primary behavioural response for maintaining body fluid homoeostasis: namely, drinking.

3.1 Characterization

Thirty years ago, Zamboni (1965, 1966) reported that subcutaneous administration of 5-HT creatinine sulfate (1 and 4 mg/kg) increased consumption of an electrolyte solution containing 0.9 mmol/l NaCl and other salts. The increase was marked (2–5-fold), dose related, occurred primarily in the first 2 h after injection and was associated with a concomitant decrease in urinary excretion. The dipsogenic action of parenteral 5-HT has been replicated numerous times in male and female rats that were maintained with *ad libitum* acess to food and water before the experiment (e.g. Lehr and Goldman, 1973; Kikta *et al.*, 1981, 1983; Kraly *et al.*, 1985; Montgomery and Burton, 1986a,b; Rowland *et al.*, 1987) or after 15–18 h of food deprivation (Meyer *et al.*, 1974; Fletcher and Burton, 1984; Montgomery *et al.*, 1986).

Generally, food has been removed from the cage for the duration of the test and water has been used as the solution for drinking. 5-HT has also been shown to increase the intake of saline, citric acid and quinine in the absence of food (Montgomery and Burton, 1986a,b). When food remained in the cage, however, increases in drinking were sometimes mitigated by the higher baseline in controls due to prandial drinking (Fletcher and Burton, 1984; Montgomery *et al.*, 1986). Similarly, 5-HT did not enhance the intake of water, 0.9% NaCl or 1.8% NaCl when baselines were high due to 22-h water deprivation (Neill and Cooper, 1989b). When non-deprived rats were given a choice between water and a second solution in two-bottle tests, 5-HT increased total consumption of water and 0.9% saline without altering preference for saline, but decreased consumption and preference for 0.1% saccharin and for sucrose (Montgomery and Burton, 1986a,b). Rats selectively increased their water intake, though, without suppressing saccharin consumption when they were tested after a 20-h period of water deprivation (Cooper and Barber, 1994). In non-deprived rats, 5-HT also increased water intake without decreasing the volume of ethanol ingested during the first 2 h of the dark period (Higgins *et al.*, 1992). As mentioned above, Montgomery and Burton (1986a) suggested that 5-HT reduced the intake of 'food-like' solutions and increased drinking of 'water-like' liquids. The failure of 5-HT to decrease intake of dilute (0.1%) sodium saccharin in Cooper and Barber's study presumably demonstrated that the deprivation conditions altered the valence for generalization of flavoured liquids to water as opposed to food. The unchanged ethanol intake probably reflected the already nominal baseline that might be insensitive to inhibitory effects of drug. Notwithstanding these interpretations, it is clear that peripherally administered 5-HT causes hyperdipsia in rats across a broad range of conditions.

3.2   Pharmacological analysis

3.2.1   Studies using 5-HT antagonists and 5-HT analogues

As can be seen in Table 4, numerous pharmacological approaches have been employed to inhibit the dipsogenic action of 5-HT. Meyer et al. (1974) demonstrated that relatively non-selective blockade of $5\text{-}HT_1$ and $5\text{-}HT_2$ receptors with methysergide antagonized drinking produced by 5-HT. This finding was confirmed for methysergide (Kikta et al., 1981; Kraly et al., 1985; Montgomery et al., 1986) and extended to another ergot derivative, the $5\text{-}HT_{1/2}$ antagonist metergoline (Rowland et al., 1987). In those studies, 3 mg/ kg methysergide blocked drinking elicited by 2 mg/kg 5-HT, and 2 mg/kg metergoline blocked 3.9 mg/kg 5-HT. In contrast, however, a dose as large as 25 mg/kg of the more selective $5\text{-}HT_2$ antagonist cinanserin did not affect serotonergic dipsogenesis (Kikta et al., 1983). Cinanserin has slightly higher affinity than the ergots for $5\text{-}HT_{2A}$ sites and considerably lower affinity for 2C sites (Hoyer et al., 1994). Thus, the data implicated either $5\text{-}HT_1$ or $5\text{-}HT_{2C}$ receptors in 5-HT-induced drinking.

Administration of 5-CT but not α-Me-5-HT mimicked the dipsogenic effect of 5-HT (Simansky et al., 1989–1990; Simansky, 1991). This action of 5-CT (ED_{50} 0.04 μmol/kg subcutaneously) was antagonized by methysergide but not by ketanserin, ritanserin, mianserin (2A/2C antagonist) or MDL 72222. Thus, 5-CT presumably stimulated a $5\text{-}HT_1$ subtype to produce drinking. Neither RU 24969 (5-methoxy-3-[1,2,3,6-tetrahydropyridin-4-yl]-1H-indole) nor 8-OH-DPAT (8-hydroxy-di-N-propyl aminotetralin) increased water intake. These agents have prominent agonist actions at 1A/1B and 1A subtypes, respectively, and readily enter the brain. Thus, 5-CT-induced drinking appeared to be mediated by a $5\text{-}HT_{1\text{-Like}}$, or perhaps a $5\text{-}HT_{1D}$, receptor in the periphery.

3.2.2   Studies using other receptor antagonists and agonists

Although ($-$)-propranolol has poor if any antagonist activity at $5\text{-}HT_{1\text{-Like}}$ and $5\text{-}HT_{1D}$ sites, this agent blocked the dipsogenic but not the anorectic effect of 5-CT (Simansky, 1991). This finding agreed with previous studies in which the racemate of propranolol antagonized drinking produced by 5-HT (Lehr and Goldman, 1973; Meyer et al., 1974; Kikta et al., 1983; Montgomery et al., 1986). The blockade by propranolol is more likely related to antagonism of β-adrenergic receptors rather than $5\text{-}HT_{1A}$ or $5\text{-}HT_{1B}$ receptors. First, the agonist profile noted above seemed to eliminate 1A and 1B sites. Second, we found that the β_1-blocker atenolol was equally potent with propranolol in reversing 5-CT-induced drinking (unpublished results), and atenolol is essentially devoid of activity at 5-HT receptors (Hoyer, 1989).

Propranolol also blocked drinking elicited by the non-selective β-agonist isoproterenol, but methysergide did not (e.g. Kikta et al., 1983). These results suggested that 5-HT and isoproterenol acted at different primary receptor targets but shared a common final pathway for stimulating thirst. It was

Table 4 Manipulations that inhibit drinking elicited by peripheral serotonergic stimulation in rats

Intervention	Dipsogen	References
Pharmacological antagonists and agonists		
Serotonergic (5-HT$_1$ and 5-HT$_2$) blockade	5-HT	Meyer et al. (1974); Kikta et al. (1981); Kraly et al. (1985); Montgomery et al. (1986); Rowland et al. (1987)
	5-CT	Simansky (1991)
β-Adrenergic blockade	5-HT	Lehr and Goldman (1973); Meyer et al. (1974); Kikta et al. (1983); Montgomery et al. (1986)
	5-CT	Simansky (1991)
Dopaminergic (primarily DA$_{2\text{-Like}}$) blockade	5-HT	Lehr and Goldman (1973); Kikta et al. (1983)
Nicotinic (ganglionic) blockade	5-HT	Meyer et al. (1974)
α_2-Adrenergic stimulation	5-HT	Kikta et al. (1983)
Impaired functioning of renin–angiotensin system		
Inhibition of angiotensin-converting enzyme activity	5-HT	Kikta et al. (1983); Montgomery and Burton (1986b); Rowland et al. (1987)
Nephrectomy	5-HT	Meyer et al. (1974); Rowland et al. (1987)
Peripheral nervous system lesion		
Bilateral abdominal vagotomy	5-HT	This chapter
	5-CT	Eberle-Wang et al. (1993)
Central nervous system lesion		
Destruction of subfornical organ	5-HT	Hubbard et al. (1989)

pertinent, therefore, that the α_2-adrenergic agonist clonidine (Kikta *et al.*, 1983) and the ganglionic blocker camphidonium (Meyer *et al.*, 1974) also reduced 5-HT-induced drinking. One interpretation of these data was that exogenous 5-HT recruited sympathetic nerve activity to increase consumption of water. Other evidence implied that expression of the behaviour also depended on dopaminergic systems (Lehr and Goldman, 1973; Kikta *et al.*, 1983).

3.2.3 Role of the renin–angiotensin system

Several indications focused attention on the renin–angiotensin system as the mediator of drinking elicited by peripheral 5-HT in rats. First, subcutaneous administration of dipsogenic doses of 5-HT increased plasma renin activity and circulating concentrations of renin and angiotensin I (AI) (Meyer *et al.*, 1974; Barney *et al.*, 1981). The time course for these endocrine changes paralleled that for drinking. As with drinking, methysergide, propranolol and ganglionic blockade antagonized the increases in renin and AI (Meyer *et al.*, 1974). Second, systemic administration of the angiotensin-converting enzyme inhibitors, captopril and MK 421, to block the conversion of AI to AII, also blocked 5-HT-induced dipsogenesis (Kikta *et al.*, 1983; Montgomery and Burton, 1986b; Rowland *et al.*, 1987). Finally, bilateral nephrectomy prevented drinking that was elicited by peripheral 5-HT (Meyer *et al.*, 1974; Rowland *et al.*, 1987).

As an aside, interesting comparative data on this issue came from the finding that neither isoproterenol nor 5-HT elicited drinking in two species of hamsters despite the ability of the former agent to increase plasma renin concentrations. These animals also were unresponsive to AII and AIII. Thus, it appeared that the amines failed to produce drinking because peripheral angiotensins are ineffective as dipsogens in these species (Rowland, 1988).

Administration of 5-HT generally causes a triphasic change in blood pressure in rats that is mediated by 5-HT_3, 5-HT_2 and 5-HT_1 (probably 1-Like) receptors in succession with the final depressor stage persisting longest. In contrast, 5-CT produces only a prolonged hypotensive action (e.g. Saxena and Lawang, 1985). The sympathetic reflex activity in response to lowered blood pressure would be expected to increase renin release via β_1-adrenergic receptors in the kidney (Milavec-Krizman *et al.*, 1985). It has been suggested that systemic reductions in blood pressure may not, however, be necessary for 5-HT to stimulate drinking (Barney *et al.*, 1981). 5-CT might also increase renin release by a local action to constrict the renal vasculature, thereby decreasing glomerular blood flow. Such 5-HT_{1D} or $5\text{-HT}_{1\text{-Like}}$ receptors have been reported in the dog but not yet in rats (Cambridge *et al.*, 1991). Conversely, though, opposing actions via 5-HT_1 receptors for vasodilation may exist in rat kidney; 5-CT could also lower noradrenergic drive to the kidney by activating inhibitory presynaptic heteroreceptors on sympathetic nerves in rats (Charlton *et al.*, 1986). Thus, the net effect of 5-CT on renin release, the relationship between renin levels and 5-CT-induced drinking, and the receptor(s) at which 5-CT acts remain to be studied.

Although the data seem to converge on a role for renin secretion in the dipsogenic effect of 5-HT, the action of serotonergic agonists to increase circulating renin is not tantamount to their ability to produce drinking. Stimulation by 5-HT of 5-HT_2 receptors in the kidney causes vasoconstriction, a reduction in glomerular blood flow, and a concomitant increase in renin release (Bond et al., 1989; Takahashi et al., 1991; Endlich et al., 1993). α-Me-5-HT is one-third as potent as 5-HT and 30 times as potent as 5-CT at these 5-HT_2 sites (Bond et al., 1989) but does not increase drinking (Simansky et al., 1989–1990; also, unpublished data). Similarly, in our hands, DOI has never increased water intake but this $5\text{-HT}_{2A/2C}$ agonist raises levels of circulating renin at least partly by a xylamidine-sensitive (i.e. peripheral) mechanism (see review by Van de Kar, 1991). Indeed, besides DOI a number of directly acting 5-HT agonists increase renin secretion (see Van de Kar, 1991) without increasing water intake. These drugs include the $5\text{-HT}_{1A/1B}$ agonist RU 24969 and the $5\text{-HT}_{1B/2C}$ agonists mCPP (1-3-[chlorophenyl]-piperazine) and TFMPP (1-[3-(trifluoromethyl) phenyl] piperazine). In fact, in water-deprived rats they either decreased saline intake or decreased saline and water intake (Neill and Cooper, 1989b; Cooper and Ciccocioppo, 1993). mCPP has been shown to inhibit food-related drinking (Clifton et al., 1993). At least some of these hypodipsic effects have been attributed to a general suppression of ingestion driven by palatability, an action associated primarily with 5-HT_{2C} receptor function (e.g. Cooper and Barber, 1994).

The agents just cited readily enter the brain where they activate central receptors, probably in the hypothalamic paraventricular nucleus, to initiate processes that release renin (Rittenhouse et al., 1992; Van de Kar, 1991). It might be hypothesized that other central effects of these drugs oppose the dipsogenic stimulus that would otherwise be provided by increasing renin or by other challenges to thirst. None the less, the explanation may be more complicated because the less selective 5-HT agonists fenfluramine (e.g. Cooper and Barber, 1994) and intracerebroventricular L-5-HTP (Rowland et al., 1987) actually produced mild hyperdipsia in limited circumstances.

Other data also questioned the role of the renin–angiotensin system in 5-HT-induced drinking. For example, systemically administered L-5-HTP increased drinking in nephrectomized rats (Rowland et al., 1987). None the less, drinking produced by substantial hypotensive–hypovolaemic challenge can survive nephrectomy and work via afferent neuronal feedback to the brain— independently of AII mediation (Rettig et al., 1981). In intact rats, L-5-HTP elicits drinking without significantly altering arterial pressure (Barney et al., 1981) but in nephrectomized rats it is plausible that this precursor causes marked hypotension in the absence of renal defence mechanisms. It is possible that neuronal feedback from thoracic receptors also accounts for the failure of the AII type 1 (AT_1) receptor antagonist, losartan, to reduce water intake after peripheral 5-HT (Fregly and Rowland, 1992). None the less, nephrectomy did abolish drinking to peripheral 5-HT (see above). Furthermore, in a preliminary report, losartan did inhibit drinking elicited by 5-CT (Dourish *et al.*, 1992). Thus, the relationship between either peripheral or central serotonergic stimulation and the renin–angiotensin system in thirst requires further investigation.

3.3 Sites of action

3.3.1 Abdominal vagus nerve
In contrast with the failure of abdominal vagotomy to alter the anorectic action of either 5-CT or 5-HT (section 2.3.1), bilateral transection of the main vagal trunks along the oesophagus attenuated or blocked completely the dipsogenic effect of each of these indoleamines. In one study, we tested five subcutaneous doses of 5-CT, ranging from 0.01 to 0.16 μmol/kg, in non-deprived rats given water and sweetened mash during a 2-h period (Eberle-Wang *et al.*, 1993). In laparotomized controls, each dose of 5-CT increased 2-h water intake; the increases were dose-related, with an ED_{50} of approximately 0.04 μmol/kg. By comparison, none of the doses of 5-CT increased water intake after vagotomy. Vagotomy also markedly reduced drinking elicited by 5-HT and by AII in rats that were maintained with 7-h daily access to milk and free access to water and tested after 15 h of milk deprivation (Fig. 6). Thus, vagotomy impaired the dipsogenic response to peripheral serotonergic stimulation whether the rats were non-deprived and tested with food present or deprived (to minimize stomach contents) and tested in the absence of food.

These results are consistent with numerous other studies in which abdominal vagotomy impaired drinking to various dipsogenic stimuli including those thought to be mediated by the renin–angiotensin system (for a review see Smith, 1986). The disruption of drinking elicited by subcutaneously administered AII appears within the first 2 days after surgery (Simansky and Smith, 1983). Furthermore, the deficit is behaviourally specific because vagotomy does not alter the dipsogenic response to the same peptide given into the lateral cerebral ventricles (Rowland, 1980; Simansky and Smith, 1983). The impairment to AII occurs after selective lesions of the coeliac or gastric branches of the vagus. Different patterns of vagal denervation underlie deficits to other dipsogens (Smith, 1986). Thus, it remains to be determined whether 5-HT-related drinking depends on the integrity of the same vagal, probably afferent, branches and terminal fields as reported for AII.

3.3.2 Lesions of the subfornical organ
The subfornical organ is a circumventricular organ that functions as a sensor for circulating angiotensin in an integrated neuroendocrine system that controls extracellular thirst (Johnson, 1990). Consistent with the hypothesized role for the renin–angiotensin system in 5-HT-induced drinking, ablation of the subfor-

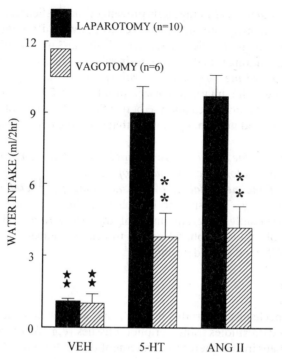

Fig. 6   Abdominal vagotomy attenuates the dipsogenic action of peripherally administered 5-HT in rats. Water intake (mean ± SE) of laparotomized and vagotomized rats after subcutaneous administration of vehicle, 11.4 μmol/kg 5-HT and 0.97 nmol/kg asp[1]-ile[5]-angiotensin II (ANG II). Rats were maintained with 7 h daily access to milk and free access to water. Tests were conducted during the 2 h before milk was provided. The experiment with 5-HT was conducted 13 weeks after surgery and that with AII 2 weeks later. Bodyweights differed at each test (e.g. laparotomy 440 ± 15 g *vs* vagotomy 368 ± 20 g at 5-HT test, $P < 0.01$) but vagotomy still reduced drinking responses when water intakes were corrected for weight ($P < 0.01$). **$P < 0.01$ *vs* laparotomized control $\star\star P < 0.01$ *vs* 5-HT and ANG II.

nical organ prevented drinking that was elicited by subcutaneous 5-HT (Hubbard *et al.*, 1989). The subfornical organ is innervated by 5-HT projections from the midbrain raphe (Lind, 1986) and it is possible that subcutaneous 5-HT influences drinking by direct actions in this site.

3.4   Future directions

A considerable amount of evidence has been presented above suggesting that serotonergic mechanisms in the periphery are interesting and important targets for investigating the physiological controls of feeding. In comparison, similar compelling arguments for 5-HT-induced drinking remain to be developed.

1 *Studies using 5-HT antagonists.* The most significant experiments would

investigate whether 5-HT antagonists prevent drinking elicited by feeding or even by other more profound challenges to body fluid homoeostasis. By analogy, in an elegant series of studies, Kraly has implicated peripheral histamine in mediating prandial drinking in rats (e.g. Kraly and Arias, 1990).

2 *Characterization of the 5-HT receptor subtype mediating peripheral seroto-nergic drinking.* The pharmacological profile of 5-CT-induced drinking requires further definition to analyse better the site(s), physiological trans-duction systems and neuronal pathways that subserve peripheral serotoner-gic drinking.

3 *Further analysis of the roles of the renin–angiotensin system, and of extrarenal mechanisms, in serotonergic stimulation of thirst.*

4 *Delineation of the neuronal pathways mediating peripheral serotonergic stimulated drinking.* The specific branches of the abdominal vagus, the relevant (presumably) afferent limbs of the pathway and the potential contribution of other peripheral nerves to drinking elicited by peripheral 5-HT and 5-CT need to be determined.

4 Conclusion

Serotonergic mechanisms for the psychotropic actions of drugs were first postulated based on studies using peripheral tissues (e.g. Woolley and Shaw, 1954). It is perhaps ironic, therefore, that attention has turned only recently to the periphery as a physiological target, rather than simply a bioassay, for understanding the role of this indoleamine in behaviour.

The data reviewed in this chapter established that peripherally administered 5-HT produces systematic, robust changes in feeding and drinking in rats. Although at an early stage, analysis of these ingestive effects has already revealed important differences in their mechanisms. First, the anorectic action is mediated by 5-HT$_1$ and by 5-HT$_2$ receptors, whereas the dipsogenic effect relies only on 5-HT$_1$ receptors. It is quite possible that separate subtypes of 5-HT$_1$ receptors are involved in the actions on feeding and drinking. Second, the neurological underpinnings of the two responses differ. For example, the drinking elicited by peripheral serotonergic stimulation depends on the inte-grity of abdominal vagal neurons, whereas vagotomy spares the anorexia. Finally, the hypothesis that exogenous 5-HT probes a physiological role for this peripheral indoleamine in feeding and satiety is still viable and invites further serious consideration. Whether exogenous 5-HT also tests a physiological function in the periphery in drinking awaits more incisive experimental analysis.

A major goal of future research must be to link specific subtypes of peripheral serotonergic receptors to satiety and to other ingestive actions of 5-HT. In the short term, such information using new pharmacological tools may identify, in the periphery, mechanisms that are unresolved for the anorectic properties of clinical agents such as 5-HT reuptake inhibitors (Garattini *et al.*, 1992). In the longer term, more precise delineation of peripheral 5-HT subtypes in ingestion may help to develop novel therapeutic agents for obesity. These drugs would act outside the brain to influence eating while minimizing deleterious effects in the cardiovascular and central nervous systems.

Acknowledgements

Preparation of this manuscript and some of the research reported were supported by USPHS grant no. MH 41987 from the National Institute of Mental Health. The author is grateful to Wayne Kachelries for preparing the figures.

References

Adipudi, V. and Simansky, K. J. (1995). Lesions of area postrema attenuate but do not prevent anorectic action of peripheral serotonin in rats. *Amer. J. Physiol.* **269**, R1314–R1320.

Andrews, P. L. R., Davis, C. J., Bingham, S., Davidson, H. I. M., Hawthorn, J. and Maskell, L. (1990). The abdominal visceral innervation and the emetic reflex: pathways, pharmacology, and plasticity. *Can. J. Physiol. Pharmacol.* **68**, 325–345.

Antin, J., Gibbs, J., Holt, J., Young, R. C. and Smith, G. P. (1975). Cholecystokinin elicits the complete behavioral sequence of satiety in rats. *J. Comp. Physiol. Psychol.* **89**, 784–790.

Baez, M., Yu, L. and Cohen, M. L. (1990). Pharmacological and molecular evidence that the contractile response to serotonin in rat stomach fundus is not mediated by activation of the 5-hydroxytryptamine$_{1C}$ receptor. *Mol. Pharmacol.* **38**, 31–37.

Baker, B. J., Duggan, J. P., Barber, D. J. and Booth, D. A. (1988). Effects of DL-fenfluramine and xylamidine on gastric emptying of maintenance diet in freely feeding rats. *Eur. J. Pharmacol.* **150**, 137–142.

Barney, C. C., Threatte, R. M., Kikta, D. C. and Fregly, M. J. (1981). Effects of serotonin and L-5-hydoxytryptophan on plasma renin activity in rats. *Pharmacol. Biochem. Behav.* **14**, 895–900.

Bateman, S. T., Lichtman, A. H. and Cramer, C. P. (1990). Peripheral serotonergic inhibition of suckling. *Pharmacol. Biochem. Behav.* **37**, 219–225.

Baxter, G. S., Murphy, O. E. and Blackburn, T. P. (1994). Further characterization of 5-hydroxytryptamine receptors (putative 5-HT$_{2B}$) in rat stomach fundus longitudinal muscle. *Br. J. Pharmacol.* **112**, 323–331.

Blundell, J. E. (1977). Is there a role for serotonin (5-hydroxytryptamine) in feeding? *Int. J. Obes.* **1**, 15–42.

Bond, R. A., Ornstein, A. G. and Clarke, D. E. (1989). Unsurmountable antagonism to 5-hydroxytryptamine in rat kidney results from pseudoirreversible inhibition rather than multiple receptors or allosteric receptor modulation. *J. Pharmacol. Exp. Ther.* **249**, 401–410.

Booth, D. A., Gibson, E. L. and Baker, B. J. (1986). Gastromotor mechanism of fenfluramine anorexia. *Appetite* **7** (supplement), 57–69.

Borison, H. L. (1989). Area postrema: chemoreceptive circumventricular organ of the medulla oblongata. *Progr. Neurobiol.* **32**, 351–390.

Bradley, P. B., Engel, G., Feniuk, W., Fozard, J. R., Humphrey, P. P. A., Middlemiss, D. N., Mylecharane, E. J., Richardson, B. P. and Saxena, P. R. (1986). Proposals for the classification and nomenclature of functional receptors for 5-hydroxytryptamine. *Neuropharmacology* 25, 563–576.

Bray, G. A. and York, D. A. (1972). Studies on food intake of genetically obese rats. *Amer. J. Physiol.* 223, 176–179.

Bulbring, E. and Crema, A. (1959). The release of 5-hydroxytryptamine in relation to pressure exerted on the intestinal mucosa. *J. Physiol. (London)* 146, 18–28.

Cambridge, D., Whiting, M. V. and Butterfield, L. J. (1991). 5-Carboxamidotryptamine induced renal vasoconstriction in the dog. In *Serotonin: Molecular Biology, Receptors and Functional Effects* (J. R. Fozard and P. R. Saxena, eds), pp. 282–299. Birkhäuser, Basel.

Carlton, J. and Rowland, N. (1984). Anorexia and brain serotonin: development of tolerance to the effects of fenfluramine and quipazine in rats with serotonin-depleting lesions. *Pharmacol. Biochem. Behav.* 20, 739–745.

Carruba, M. O., Mantegazza, P., Memo, M., Missale, C., Pizzi, M. and Spano, P. F. (1986). Peripheral and central mechanisms of action of serotonergic anorectic drugs. *Appetite* 7 (supplement), 15–38.

Charlton, K. G., Bond, R. A. and Clarke, D. E. (1986). An inhibitory prejunctional 5-HT$_1$-like receptor in the isolated perfused rat kidney. Apparent distinction from the 5-HT$_{1A}$, 5-HT$_{1B}$ and 5-HT$_{1C}$ subtypes. *Naunyn Schmiedebergs Arch. Pharmacol.* 332, 8–15.

Clifton, P. G., Barnfield, A. M. and Curzon, G. (1993). Effects of food deprivation and mCPP treatment on the microstructure of ingestive behaviour of male and female rats. *J. Psychopharmacol.* 7, 257–264.

Clineschmidt, B. V., McGuffin, J. C., Pfleuger, A. B. and Totaro, J. A. (1978). A 5-hydroxytryptamine-like mode of anorectic action for 6-chloro-2-[1-piperazinyl]-pyrazine (MK-212). *Br. J. Pharmacol.* 62, 579–589.

Clineschmidt, B. V., Reiss, D. R., Pettibone, D. J. and Robinson, J. L. (1985). Characterization of 5-hydroxytryptamine receptors in rat stomach fundus. *J. Pharmacol. Exp. Ther.* 235, 696–708.

Cohen, M. L. and Fludzinski, L. A. (1987). Contractile serotonergic receptor in rat stomach fundus. *J. Pharmacol. Exp. Ther.* 243, 264–269.

Cooke, H. J., Montakhab, M., Wade, P. R. and Wood, J. D. (1983). Transmural fluxes of 5-hydroxytryptamine in guinea pig ileum. *Am. J. Physiol.* 244, G421–G425.

Cooper, S. J. (1992). 5-HT and ingestive behaviour. In *Central Serotonin Receptors and Psychotropic Drugs* (C. A. Marsden and D. J. Heal, eds), pp. 260–291. Blackwell Scientific Publications, London.

Cooper, S. J. and Barber, D. J. (1994). Evidence for serotonergic involvement in saccharin preference in a two-choice test in rehydrating rats. *Pharmacol. Biochem. Behav.* 47, 541–546.

Cooper, S. J. and Ciccocioppo, R. (1993). Effects of selective 5-HT$_1$ receptor agonists in water-deprived rats on salt intake in two-choice tests. *Pharmacol. Biochem. Behav.* 45, 513–518.

Cooper, S. J., Dourish, C. T. and Barber, D. J. (1990a). Reversal of the anorectic effect of (+)-fenfluramine in rat by the selective cholecystokinin receptor antagonist MK-329. *Br. J. Pharmacol.* 99, 65–70.

Cooper, S. J., Dourish, C. T. and Barber, D. J. (1990b). Fluoxetine reduces food intake by a cholecystokinin-independent mechanism. *Pharmacol. Biochem. Behav.* 35, 51–54.

Cooper, S. J., Dourish, C. T. and Clifton, P. G. (1992). CCK antagonists and CCK–monoamine interactions in the control of satiety. *Am. J. Clin. Nutr.* 55, 291S–295S.

Copp, F. C., Green, A. F., Hodson, H. F., Randall, A. W. and Sim, M. F. (1967). New peripheral antagonists of 5-hydroxytryptamine. *Nature* 214, 200–201.

Danguir, J., Nicolaïdis, S. and Gerard, H. (1979). Relations between feeding and sleep patterns in the rat. *J. Comp. Physiol. Psychol.* **93**, 820–830.

Davies, R. F., Rossi, J., III, Panksepp, J., Bean, N. J. and Zolovick, A. J. (1983). Fenfluramine anorexia: a peripheral locus of action. *Physiol. Behav.* **30**, 723–730.

Davis, J. D., Smith, G. P. and Meissner, J. (1993). Postpyloric stimuli are necessary for the normal control of meal size in real feeding and sham feeding rats. *Am. J. Physiol.* **265**, R888–R895.

Dhasmana, K. M., Villalon, C. M., Zhu, Y. N., Tadipatri, S. and Saxena, P. R. (1992). Role of 5-HT$_1$-like receptors in the increase in intragastric pressure induced by 5-hydroxytryptamine in the rat. *Eur. J. Pharmacol.* **213**, 293–299.

Dourish, C. T. (1992). 5-HT receptor subtypes and feeding behaviour. In *Serotonin, CNS Receptors and Brain Function* (P. B. Bradley, S. L. Handley, S. J. Cooper, B. J. Key, N. M. Barnes and J. Coote, eds), pp. 179–202. Pergamon Press, London.

Dourish, C. T., Clark, M. L., Fletcher, A. and Iversen, S. D. (1989). Evidence that blockade of postsynaptic 5-HT$_1$ receptors elicits feeding in satiated rats. *Psychopharmacology* **97**, 54–58.

Dourish, C. T., Francis, J. and Duggan, J. A. (1992). Multiple angiotensin receptors and angiotensin/5-HT interactions in the control of drinking in rats. *Appetite* **19**, 174.

Drapanas, T., McDonald, J. C. and Stewart, J. D. (1962). Serotonin release following instillation of hypertonic glucose into the proximal intestine. *Ann. Surg.* **156**, 528–536.

Dryden, S., McCarthy, H. D., Malabu, U. H., Ware, M. and Williams, G. (1993). Increased neuropeptide Y concentrations in specific hypothalamic nuclei of the rat following treatment with methysergide: evidence NPY may mediate serotonin's effects on food intake. *Peptides* **14**, 791–796.

Eberle-Wang, K. and Simansky, K. J. (1992). The CCK-A receptor antagonist, devazepide, blocks the anorectic action of CCK but not peripheral serotonin in rats. *Pharmacol. Biochem. Behav.* **43**, 943–947.

Eberle-Wang, K., Levitt, P. and Simansky, K. J. (1993). Abdominal vagotomy dissociates the anorectic mechanisms for peripheral serotonin and cholecystokinin. *Am. J. Physiol.* **265**, R602–R608.

Eberle-Wang, K., Braun, B. T. and Simansky, K. J. (1994). Serotonin contracts the isolated rat pylorus via a 5-HT$_2$-like receptor. *Am. J. Physiol.* **266**, R284–R291.

Edwards, S. and Stevens, R. G. (1989). Effects of xylamidine on peripheral 5-hydroxytryptamine-induced anorexia. *Pharmacol. Biochem. Behav.* **34**, 717–720.

Edwards, S. and Stevens, R. (1991). Peripherally administered 5-hydroxytryptamine elicits the full behavioural sequence of satiety. *Physiol. Behav.* **50**, 1075–1077.

Edwards, S. and Stevens, R. (1994). Effects of chronic systemic administration of 5-HT on food intake and body weight in rats. *Pharmacol. Biochem. Behav.* **47**, 865–872.

Endlich, K., Kuhn, R. and Steinhausen, M. (1993). Visualization of serotonin effects on renal vessels of rats. *Kidney Int.* **43**, 314–323.

Ervin, G. N., Carter, R. B., Webster, E. L., Moore, S. I. and Cooper, B. R. (1984). Evidence that taste aversion learning induced by 1-5-hydroxytryptophan is mediated peripherally. *Pharmacol. Biochem. Behav.* **20**, 799–802.

Feniuk, W., Humphrey, P. P. A. and Watts, A. D. (1983). 5-Hydroxytryptamine-induced relaxation of isolated mammalian smooth muscle. *Eur. J. Pharmacol.* **96**, 71–78.

Fletcher, P. J. (1987). The anorectic action of peripheral 5-HT examined in the runway: evidence for an action on satiation. *Psychopharmacology* **93**, 498–501.

Fletcher, P. J. (1988). Increased food intake in satiated rats induced by the 5-HT antagonists methysergide, metergoline and ritanserin. *Psychopharmacology* **96**, 237–242.

Fletcher, P. J. and Burton, M. J. (1984). Effects of manipulations of peripheral serotonin on feeding and drinking in the rat. *Pharmacol. Biochem. Behav.* **20**, 835–840.

Fletcher, P. J. and Burton, M. J. (1985). The anorectic action of peripherally administered 5-HT is enhanced by vagotomy. *Physiol. Behav.* **34**, 861–866.

Fletcher, P. J. and Burton, M. J. (1986a). Dissociation of the anorectic actions of 5-HTP and fenfluramine. *Psychopharmacology* **89**, 216–220.

Fletcher, P. J. and Burton, M. J. (1986b). Microstructural analysis of the anorectic action of peripherally administered 5-HT. *Pharmacol. Biochem. Behav.* **24**, 1133–1136.

Fletcher, P. J. and Yu, P. H. (1989). Enhancement of 5-HT-induced anorexia: a test of the reversibility of monoamine oxidase inhibitors. *Psychopharmacology* **98**, 265–268.

Ford, A. P. D. W. and Clarke, D. E. (1993). The 5-HT$_4$ receptor. *Med. Res. Rev.* **13**, 633–662.

Fozard, J. R. (1989). The development and early clinical evaluation of selective 5-HT$_3$ receptor antagonists. In *The Peripheral Actions of 5-Hydroxytryptamine* (J. R. Fozard, ed.), pp. 354–376. Oxford University Press, Oxford.

Francis, J., Critchley, D. J. P., Dourish, C. T. and Cooper, S. J. (1995). Comparisons between the effects of 5-HT and DL-fenfluramine on food intake and gastric emptying in the rat. *Pharmacol. Biochem. Behav.* **50**, 581–585.

Fregly, M. J. and Rowland, N. E. (1992). Effect of DuP 753, a nonpeptide angiotensin II receptor antagonist, on the drinking responses to acutely administered dipsogenic agents in rats. *Proc. Soc. Exp. Biol. Med.* **199**, 158–164.

Gaddum, J. H. and Picarelli, Z. P. (1957). Two types of tryptamine receptors. *Br. J. Pharmacol.* **12**, 323–328.

Garattini, S., Lamesta, L., Mortari, A., Palma, V. and Valzelli, L. (1961). Pharmacological and biochemical effects of 5-hydroxytryptamine in adrenalectomized rats. *J. Pharm. Pharmacol.* **13**, 385–388.

Garattini, S., Bizzi, A., Caccia, S. and Mennini, T. (1992). Progress report on the anorectic effects of dexfenfluramine, fluoxetine and sertraline. *Int. J. Obes.* **16** (supplement 3), S43–S50.

Geary, N. and Smith, G. P. (1983). Selective hepatic vagotomy blocks pancreatic glucagon's satiety effect. *Physiol. Behav.* **31**, 391–394.

Gershon, M. D., Wade, P. R., Kirchgessner, A. L. and Tamir, H. (1990). 5-HT receptor subtypes outside the central nervous system. *Neuropsychopharmacology* **3**, 385–395.

Gibson, E. L., Kennedy, A. J. and Curzon, G. (1993). D-fenfluramine- and D-norfenfluramine-induced hypophagia: differential mechanisms and involvement of postsynaptic 5-HT receptors. *Eur. J. Pharmacol.* **242**, 83–90.

Grignaschi, G. and Samanin, R. (1992). Role of serotonin and catecholamines in brain in the feeding suppressant effect of fluoxetine. *Neuropharmacology* **31**, 445–449.

Grignaschi, G., Mantelli, B., Fracasso, C., Anelli, M., Caccia, S. and Samanin, R. (1993). Reciprocal interaction of 5-hydroxytryptamine and cholecystokinin in the control of feeding patterns in rats. *Br. J. Pharmacol.* **109**, 491–494.

Gross, P. M., Wall, K. M., Pang, J. J., Shaver, S. W. and Wainman, D. S. (1990). Microvascular specializations promoting rapid interstitial solute dispersion in nucleus tractus solitarius. *Am. J. Physiol.* **259**, R1131–R1138.

Hewson, G., Leighton, G. E., Hill, R. G. and Hughes, J. (1989). Which subtype(s) of 5-HT receptor mediates the anorectic effects of drugs that act via the 5-HT system? *Ann. N. Y. Acad. Sci.* **575**, 525–528.

Higgins, G. A., Tomkins, D. M., Fletcher, P. J. and Sellers, E. M. (1992). Effect of drugs influencing 5-HT function on ethanol drinking and feeding behaviour in rats: studies using a drinkometer system. *Neurosci. Biobehav. Rev.* **16**, 535–552.

Hoyer, D. (1989). 5-Hydroxytryptamine receptors and effector coupling mechanism in peripheral tissues. In *The Peripheral Actions of 5-Hydroxytryptamine* (J. R. Fozard, ed.), pp. 72–99. Oxford University Press, Oxford.

Hoyer, D., Clarke, D. E., Fozard, J. R., Hartig, P. R., Martin, G. R., Mylecharane, E. J., Saxena, P. R. and Humphrey, P. P. A., VII. (1994). International Union of Pharmacology Classification of receptors for 5-hydroxytryptamine (serotonin) *Pharm. Rev.* **46**, 157–203.

Hrupka, B. J., Gietzen, D. W. and Beverly, J. L. (1991). ICS 205–930 and feeding responses to amino acid imbalance: a peripheral effect? *Pharmacol. Biochem. Behav.* **40**, 83–87.

Hubbard, J. I., Lin, N. and Sibbald, J. R. (1989). Subfornical organ lesions in rats abolish hyperdipsic effects of isoproterenol and serotonin. *Brain Res. Bull.* **23**, 41–45.

Jaffe, B. M., Kellum, J. M., Jr., Kopen, D. F. and Stechenberg, L. (1978). Release and physiologic action of serotonin. In *Gut Hormones* (S. R. Bloom, ed.), pp. 515–523. Churchill Livingstone, London.

Johnson, A. K. (1990). Brain mechanisms in the control of body fluid homeostasis. In *Perspectives in Exercise Science and Sports Medicine. Vol. 3: Fluid Homeostasis During Exercise.* (C. V. Gisolfi and D. R. Lamb, eds), pp. 347–419. Benchmark Press, Carmel, IN.

Kalkman, H. O., Engel, G. and Hoyer, D. (1986). Inhibition of 5-carboxamidotryptamine-induced relaxation of guinea-pig ileum correlates with [^{125}I]LSD binding. *Eur. J. Pharmacol.* **129**, 139–145.

Kanarek, R. B. and Dushkin, H. (1988). Peripheral serotonin administration selectively reduces fat intake in rats. *Pharmacol. Biochem. Behav.* **31**, 113–122.

Kellum, J. M. and Jaffe, B. M. (1976). Release of immunoreactive serotonin following acid perfusion of the duodenum. *Ann. Surg.* **184**, 633–638.

Kellum, J., McCabe, M., Schneier, J. and Donowitz, M. (1983). Neural control of acid-induced serotonin release from rabbit duodenum. *Am. J. Physiol.* **245**, G824–G831.

Kennett, G. A. and Curzon, G. (1991). Potencies of antagonists indicate that 5-HT$_{1C}$ receptors mediate 1-3(chlorophenyl)piperazine-induced hypophagia. *Br. J. Pharmacol.* **103**, 2016–2020.

Kennett, G. A. and Grewal, S. S. (1992). Effect of 5-HT$_3$ receptor agonists on rat food intake. *Br. J. Pharmacol.* **105**, 227P.

Kennett, G. A., Wood, M. D., Glen, A., Forbes, I., Gadre, A. and Blackburn, T. P. (1994). *In vivo* properties of SB 200646A, a 5-HT$_{2C/2B}$ receptor antagonist. *Br. J. Pharmacol.* **111**, 797–802.

Key, B. J. and Mehta, V. H. (1977). Changes in electrocortical activity induced by the perfusion of 5-hydroxytryptamine into the nucleus of the solitary tract. *Neuropharmacology* **16**, 99–106.

Kikta, D. C., Threatte, R. M., Barney, C. C., Fregly, M. J., and Greenleaf, J. E. (1981). Peripheral conversion of 1-5-hydroxytryptophan to serotonin induces drinking in rats. *Pharmacol. Biochem. Behav.* **14**, 889–893.

Kikta, D. C., Barney, C. C., Threatte, R. M., Fregly, M. J., Rowland, N. E. and Greenleaf, J. E. (1983). On the mechanism of serotonin-induced dipsogenesis in the rat. *Pharmacol. Biochem. Behav.* **19**, 519–525.

Kilpatrick, G. J. and Rogers, H. (1993). 5-HT$_3$ receptors. In *Serotonin. From Cell Biology to Pharmacology and Therapeutics* (P. M. Vanhoutte, P. R. Saxena, R. Paoletti, Brunello, N. and A. S. Jackson, eds), pp. 99–106. Kluwer Academic, Dordrecht.

Koella, W. P. (1974). Serotonin—a hypnogenic transmitter and an antiwaking agent. *Adv. Biochem. Psychopharmacol.* **11**, 181–186.

Kraly, F. S. and Arias, R. L. (1990). Histamine in brain may have no role for histaminergic control of food-related drinking in the rat. *Physiol. Behav.* **47**, 5–9.

Kraly, F. S., Simansky, K. J., Coogan, L. A. and Trattner, M. S. (1985). Histamine and serotonin independently elicit drinking in the rat. *Physiol. Behav.* **34**, 963–967.

Kursar, J. D., Nelson, D. L., Wainscott, D. B. and Baez, M. (1994). Molecular cloning, functional expression, and mRNA tissue distribution of the human 5-hydroxytryptamine$_{2B}$ receptor. *Mol. Pharm.* **46**, 227–234.

Lanca, A. J. and van der Kooy, D. A. (1985). A serotonin-containing pathway from the area postrema to the parabrachial nucleus in the rat. *Neuroscience* **14**, 1117–1126.

Laporte, A. M., Kidd, E. J., Vergé, D., Gozlan, H. and Hamon, M. (1992). Autoradiographic mapping of central 5-HT$_3$ receptors. In *Central and Peripheral 5-HT$_3$ Receptors* (M. Hamon, ed.), pp. 157–187. Academic Press, London.

Larsson, I., Gronstad, K. O., Dahlstrom, A. and Ahlman, H. (1990). Transport of serotonin from the rat jejunal lumen into mesenteric veins *in vivo*. *Acta Physiol. Scand.* **138**, 403–407.

Lehr, D. and Goldman, W. (1973). Continued pharmacologic analysis of consummatory behavior in the albino rat. *Eur. J. Pharmacol.* **23**, 197–210.

Leibowitz, S. F. (1993). Hypothalamic serotonin in relation to appetite for macronutrients and eating disorders. In *Serotonin: From Cell Biology to Pharmacology and Therapeutics* (P. M. Vanhoutte, P. R. Saxena, R. Paoletti, N. Brunello and A. S. Jackson, eds), pp. 383–391. Kluwer Academic Publishers, Dordrecht.

Leysen, J. E. (1992). 5-HT$_2$-receptors: location, pharmacological, pathological and physiological role. In *Serotonin Receptor Subtypes: Pharmacological Significance and Clinical Implications*. (S. Z. Langer, N. Brunello, G. Racagni and J. Mendlewicz, eds), pp. 31–43. Karger, Basel.

Li, B. and Rowland, N. E. (1994). Cholecystokinin- and dexfenfluramine-induced anorexia compared using devazepide and c-*fos* expression in the rat brain. *Regul. Pept.* **50**, 223–233.

Lind, R. W. (1986). Bi-directional, chemically specified neural connections between the subfornical organ and the midbrain raphe system. *Brain Res.* **384**, 250–261.

Lucki, I., Kreider, M. S. and Simansky, K. J. (1988). Reduction of feeding behavior by the serotonin uptake inhibitor sertraline. *Psychopharmacology* **96**, 289–295.

McCall, R. B. (1990). Role of neurotransmitters in the central regulation of the cardiovascular system. *Prog. Drug Res.* **35**, 25–84.

Massi, M. and Marini, S. (1987). Effect of the 5-HT$_2$ antagonist ritanserin on food intake and on 5-HT-induced anorexia in the rat. *Pharmacol. Biochem. Behav.* **26**, 333–340.

Meyer, D. K., Abele, M. and Hertting, G. (1974). Influence of serotonin on water intake and the renin–angiotensin system in the rat. *Arch. Int. Pharmacodyn.* **212**, 130–140.

Milavec-Krizman, M., Evenou, J. P., Wagner, H., Berthold, R. and Stoll, A. P. (1985). Characterization of beta-adrenoceptor subtypes in rat kidney with new highly selective beta$_1$ blockers and their role in renin release. *Biochem. Pharmacol.* **34**, 3951–3957.

Montgomery, A. M. J. and Burton, M. J. (1986a). Effects of peripheral 5-HT on consumption of flavoured solutions. *Psychopharmacology* **88**, 262–266.

Montgomery, A. M. J. and Burton, M. J. (1986b). Pharmacological investigations of the mechanisms underlying the effects of peripheral 5-HT on flavour consumption and preference. *Psychopharmacology* **89**, 192–197.

Montgomery, A. M. J., Fletcher, P. J. and Burton, M. J. (1986). Behavioural and pharmacological investigations of 5-HT hypophagia and hyperdipsia. *Pharmacol. Biochem. Behav.* **25**, 23–28.

Neill, J. C. and Cooper, S. J. (1989a). Effects of 5-hydroxytryptamine and D-fenfluramine on sham feeding and sham drinking in the gastric-fistulated rat. *Physiol. Behav.* **46**, 949–953.

Neill, J. C. and Cooper, S. J. (1989b). Selective reduction by serotonergic agents of hypertonic saline consumption in rats: evidence for possible 5-HT$_{1C}$ receptor mediation. *Psychopharmacology* **99**, 196–201.

O'Hara, R. S., Fox, R. O. and Cole, J. W. (1959). Serotonin release mediated by intraluminal sucrose solutions. *Surg. Forum* **10**, 215–218.

Oldendorf, W. H. (1971). Brain uptake of radiolabeled aminoacids, amines and hexoses after arterial injection. *Am. J. Physiol.* **221**, 1629–1639.

Ossenkopp, K.-P., Giugno, L. and Sutherland, C. (1985). Conditioned taste aversions induced by 1-5-hydroxytryptophan are mediated by the area postrema. *Prog. Neuropsychopharmacol. Biol. Psychiatry* **9**, 745–748.

Peroutka, S. J. and Snyder, S. H. (1979). Multiple serotonin receptors: differential binding of ^{3}H 5-hydroxytryptamine, ^{3}H lysergic acid diethylamide and ^{3}H spiroperidol. *Mol. Pharmacol.* **16**, 687–699.

Poeschla, B., Gibbs, J., Simansky, K. J. and Smith, G. P. (1992). The 5-HT$_{1A}$ agonist 8-OH-DPAT attenuates the satiating action of cholecystokinin. *Pharmacol. Biochem. Behav.* **42**, 541–543.

Pollock, J. D. and Rowland, N. E. (1981). Peripherally administered serotonin decreases food intake in rats. *Pharmacol. Biochem. Behav.* **15**, 179–183.

Rettig, R., Ganten, D. and Johnson, A. K. (1981). Isoproterenol-induced thirst: renal and extrarenal mechanisms. *Am. J. Physiol.* **241**, R152–R157.

Rezek, M. and Novin, D. (1975). The effects of serotonin on feeding in the rabbit. *Psychopharmacologia (Berl.)* **43**, 255–258.

Richter, G., Stockmann, F., Conlon, J. M. and Creutzfeldt, W. (1986). Serotonin release into blood after food and pentagastrin. *Gastroenterology* **91**, 612–618.

Rittenhouse, P. A., Li Q., Levy A. D. and Van de Kar, L. D. (1992). Neurons in the hypothalamic paraventricular nucleus mediate the serotonergic stimulation of renin secretion. *Brain Res.* **593**, 105–113.

Rowland, N. E. (1980). Impaired drinking to angiotensin II after subdiaphragmatic vagotomy in rats. *Physiol. Behav.* **24**, 1177–1180.

Rowland, N. E. (1988). Water intake of Djungarian and Syrian hamsters treated with various dipsogenic stimuli. *Physiol. Behav.* **43**, 851–854.

Rowland, N., Antelman, S. M. and Kocan, D. (1982). Differences among 'serotonergic' anorectics in a cross-tolerance paradigm: do they all act on serotonin systems? *Eur. J. Pharmacol.* **81**, 57–66.

Rowland, N. E., Caputo, F. A., and Fregly, M. J. (1987). Water intake induced in rats by serotonin and 5-hydroxytryptophan: different mechanisms? *Brain Res. Bull.* **18**, 501–508.

Rubin, W. and Schwartz, B. (1979). An electron microscopic radioautographic identification of the 'enterochromaffin-like' APUD cells in murine oxyntic glands. Demonstration of a metabolic difference between rat and mouse gastric A-like cells. *Gastroenterology* **76**, 437–449.

Samanin, R. and Garattini, S. (1989). Serotonin and the pharmacology of eating disorders. *Ann. N. Y. Acad. Sci.* **575**, 194–208.

Samanin, R., Ghezzi, D., Valzelli, L. and Garattini, S. (1972). The effects of selective lesioning of brain serotonin or catecholamine containing neurons on the anorectic activity of fenfluramine and amphetamine. *Eur. J. Pharmacol.* **19**, 318–322.

Sanger, G. J. (1992). The involvement of 5-HT$_3$ receptors in visceral function. In *Central and Peripheral 5-HT$_3$ Receptors* (M. Hamon, ed.), pp. 207–255. Academic Press, London.

Saxena, P. R. and Lawang, A. (1985). A comparison of cardiovascular and smooth muscle effects of 5-hydroxytryptamine and 5-carboxamidotryptamine, a selective agonist of 5-HT$_1$ receptors. *Arch. Int. Pharmacodyn. Ther.* **277**, 235–252.

Schechter, L. E. and Simansky, K. J. (1988). 1-(2,5-Dimethoxy-4-iodophenyl)-2-aminopropane (DOI) exerts an anorexic action that is blocked by 5-HT$_2$ antagonists in rats. *Psychopharmacology* **94**, 342–346.

Simansky, K. J. (1991). Peripheral 5-carboxamidotryptamine (5-CT) elicits drinking by stimulating 5-HT$_1$-like serotonergic receptors in rats. *Pharmacol. Biochem. Behav.* **38**, 459–462.

Simansky, K. J. (1995). Serotonergic control of the organization of feeding and satiety. *Behav. Brain Res.* **73**.

Simansky, K. J. and Smith, G. P. (1983). Acute abdominal vagotomy reduces drinking to peripheral but not central angiotensin II. *Peptides* **4**, 159–163.

Simansky, K. J., Sisk, F. C., Vaidya, A. H. and Eberle-Wang, K. (1989–1990). Peripherally administered α-methyl-5-hydroxytryptamine and 5-carboxamidotryptamine reduce food intake via different mechanisms in rats. *Behav. Pharmacol.* **1**, 241–246.

Simansky, K. J., Sisk, F. C. and Jakubow, J. (1991). An anorectic action of 2-methylserotonin (2-Me-5-HT) without apparent behavioral toxicity. *Abstr. Soc. Neurosci.* **17**, 144.

Simansky, K. J., Jakubow, J., Sisk, F. C., Vaidya, A. H. and Eberle-Wang, K. (1992). Peripheral serotonin is an incomplete signal for eliciting satiety in sham-feeding rats. *Pharmacol. Biochem. Behav.* **43**, 847–854.

Smith, G. P. (1986). Peripheral mechanisms for the maintenance and termination of drinking in the rat. In *The Physiology of Thirst and Sodium Appetite* (G. de Caro, A. N. Epstein and M. Massi, eds), pp. 265–277. Plenum, New York.

Smith, G. P., Jerome, C., Cushin, B., Eterno, R. and Simansky, K. J. (1981). Abdominal vagotomy blocks the satiety effect of cholecystokinin in the rat. *Science* **213**, 1036–1037.

Smith, G. P., Jerome, C. and Norgren, R. (1985). Afferent axons in abdominal vagus mediate satiety effect of cholecystokinin in rats. *Am. J. Physiol.* **249**, R638–R641.

Soulairac, A. and Soulairac, M. L. (1960). Action de la reserpine, de la serotonine et de l'iproniazide sur le comportement alimentaire du rat. *Comptes Rendus des Séances de la Societé de Biologie et de ses Filliales (Paris)* **154**, 510–513.

Stuckey, J. A., Gibbs, J. and Smith, G. P. (1985). Neural disconnection of gut from brain blocks bombesin-induced satiety. *Peptides* **6**, 1249–1252.

Sykes, R. M., Spyer, K. M. and Izzo, P. N. (1994). Central distribution of substance P, calcitonin gene-related peptide and 5-hydroxytryptamine in vagal sensory afferents in the rat dorsal medulla. *Neuroscience* **59**, 195–210.

Takahashi, T., Hisa, H. and Satoh, S. (1991). Serotonin-induced renin release in the dog kidney. *Eur. J. Pharmacol.* **193**, 315–320.

Thor, K. B., Blitz-Siebert, A. and Helke, C. J. (1992). Autoradiographic localization of 5HT$_1$ binding sites in the medulla oblongata of the rat. *Synapse* **10**, 185–205.

Van de Kar, L. (1991). Neuroendocrine pharmacology of serotonergic (5-HT) neurons. *Annu. Rev. Pharmacol. Toxicol.* **31**, 289–320.

van der Hoek, G. A. and Cooper, S. J. (1994). Ondansetron, a selective 5-HT$_3$ receptor antagonist, reduces palatable food consumption in the nondeprived rat. *Neuropharmacology* **33**, 805–811.

Vane, J. R. (1969). The release and fate of vaso-active hormones in the circulation. *Br. J. Pharmacol.* **35**, 209–242.

Woolley, D. W. and Shaw, E. (1954). A biochemical and pharmacological suggestion about certain mental disorders. *Science* **119**, 587–588.

Zamboni, P. (1965). Azione della enteramina sull'immagazzinamento di acqua nell'organismo. *Arch. Sci. Biol.* **49**, 269–273.

Zamboni, P. (1966). Influenza di amine biogene sul bilancio della acqua nel ratto. *Arch. Sci. Biol.* **50**, 214–220.

5

Insulin and Serotonin Actions and Interactions and the Control of Feeding and Metabolism

MARTINE OROSCO and STELIOS NICOLAÏDIS

Neurobiologie des Régulations, C.N.R.S. URA 1860, Collège de France, 11 place Marcelin-Berthelot, 75231 Paris Cedex 05, France

1 Introduction

There are close relationships between feeding behaviour, insulin secretion and serotonergic activity, relationships that involve both peripheral and central mechanisms. Initially, insulin and serotonin (5-hydroxytryptamine; 5-HT) were studied quite separately, but it is logical to consider the possibility of interactions that may occur between the peptide and the indoleamine. Both insulin and serotonin are known to inhibit feeding behaviour, and potential interactions between their effects form the subject of this chapter.

The 'interaction' could be, in fact, merely the operation of two parallel, but independent, systems with a common end-point, inhibition of food intake. Alternatively, the interaction might be more substantial and involve a cascade-type mechanism, in which a chain of events could begin, for example, with the initial activation of insulin followed by actions of 5-HT leading to an increase in satiety. Parenthetically, such an interaction has already been suggested for 5-HT and another anorexigenic peptide, cholecystokinin (CCK). Thus, the effect of CCK on feeding behaviour was blocked by metergoline, a serotonin antagonist (Stallone *et al.*, 1989). However, in the case of CCK–5-HT inter-action, it was subsequently shown that a CCK antagonist could block the anorexigenic effect of the serotonergic drug fenfluramine (Cooper *et al.*, 1990). This kind of cross-antagonism experiment has yet to be performed to assess whether or not there are also reciprocal interactions between insulin and serotonin. A third type of interaction between insulin and serotonin could be a direct, unidirectional (or reciprocal) action of one on the production and/or release of the other. In this chapter, we shall provide evidence for interactions that may occur both at the level of the pancreas and also centrally.

DRUG RECEPTOR SUBTYPES AND INGESTIVE BEHAVIOUR
ISBN 0-12-187620-9

Other important potential interactions involving insulin and serotonin may occur in relation to metabolism and to the interactions between metabolism and feeding. Feeding enhances metabolic rate and switches the respiratory quotient (RQ) to higher values as early as the first few minutes of ingestion (Nicolaïdis, 1969). Reciprocally, a decrease in metabolism brings about physiological processes underlying hunger and triggers feeding (Nicolaïdis and Even, 1985). The administration of insulin results in an increase (at low doses) or a decrease (at high doses) in metabolism, whilst increasing the value of RQ (Even and Nicolaïdis, 1981).

Above, we introduced the concept of a complex set of interactions, including feeding behaviour, metabolism, insulin and 5-HT; each component is capable of affecting the others. In such a system, we suspect that the close links between feeding behaviour and metabolism depend, at least in part, on the two endogenous substances, insulin and 5-HT. In this chapter, we shall examine the evidence for interactions between insulin and 5-HT with respect to feeding behaviour and (although the evidence is less abundant) metabolism.

2   Respective roles of serotonin and insulin in the control of food intake

2.1   Normal rats

2.1.1   Serotonin

The involvement of brain monoamines in the control of food intake is well established (Grossman, 1960; Hoebel, 1977; Leibowitz and Shor-Posner, 1986). Numerous pharmacological manipulations using precursors, agonists or transmission enhancers have contributed evidence consistent with a role for serotonin in promoting satiety (Samanin et al., 1980; Blundell, 1984). Well-known drugs, such as fenfluramine, exert their anorexigenic effects mainly by means of serotonergic actions (Blundell et al., 1979; Garattini et al., 1979). There is evidence that serotonergic compounds are active in inhibiting feeding in the ventromedial hypothalamus (VMH) and paraventricular nuclei (PVN) of the rat (Hoebel, 1977; Leibowitz, 1980). However, the microinjection approach usually used does not exclude the possible physiological involvement of any amine found in the medial hypothalamus. An alternative approach, involving ex vivo methods for measurement of monoaminergic variations in variously sized brain regions in relation to feeding behaviour, has been more difficult to interpret so far. The reason for this is that ex vivo assays of brain homogenates are of limited functional significance and do not permit corre-lation with behaviour.

The in vivo technique of brain microdialysis solves some of these problems as it allows the concomitant measurement of both the behaviour and the neuro-chemistry. In addition, microdialysis does not confound the intracellular and extracellular monoamine and metabolite content. The pioneering work of

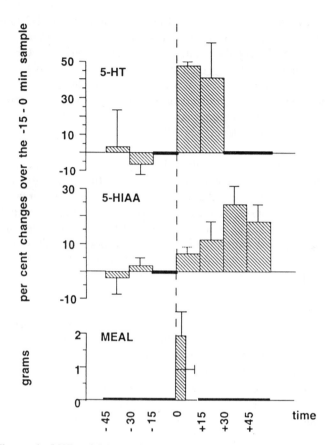

Fig. 1   Changes in 5-HT and 5-HIAA levels in 15-min microdialysates from VMH and PVN around spontaneous feeding in Wistar rats. Results are expressed as mean ± SEM percentage variation of the sample preceding the meal. Mean meal size (g) and duration (min) are represented in the bottom panel.

Hoebel and co-workers has already provided valuable new data concerning the role of serotonin in the medial and lateral hypothalamus in relation to deprivation-induced feeding (D. H. Schwartz *et al.*, 1990). More recently, using microdialysis probes located in both the PVN and VMH, together with simultaneous recording of spontaneous feeding behaviour, we measured the levels of serotonin before, during and after a spontaneously occurring meal (Orosco and Nicolaïdis, 1992). This approach allowed us to identify the changes that occur during the transition from the state of satiety to that of spontaneously occurring hunger. We found increases in 5-HT and 5-hydroxyindolacetic acid (5-HIAA) levels as early as the beginning of the meal, and a further increase in 5-HIAA concentration at the end of the meal (Fig. 1).

What conclusions can be drawn from these changes in 5-HT activity observed in response to both imposed and spontaneous meals? One might predict high levels of the amine or its metabolite as long as the animal is satiated and low levels in the deprived animal, as in Hoebel's experiment. Or one might expect decreasing levels to accompany the transition from satiety to hunger, as in our experiment. Unfortunately, however, this is not exactly what happens. The level of 5-HT drops soon after the end of feeding in both deprivation-induced and spontaneous feeding. As for the metabolite 5-HIAA, there is a long-lasting increase in the level of 5-HT after the end of spontaneous feeding, which suggests a continuation of enhanced 5-HT turnover. However, the return to baseline is not accompanied by a new episode of feeding. Hence, these serotonergic profiles could be associated with the time-course of the process of *satiation* rather than the steady state of *satiety*. Another possibility is that enhancement of serotonergic activity within the medial hypothalamus is more associated with feeding-induced hyperinsulinaemia and the consequent effects on glucose and amino acid metabolic responses. This state of high insulin and high glucose metabolism combined with high satiety can be reproduced experimentally, as discussed below.

2.1.2 Insulin

The role of insulin in the control of food intake and body weight regulation has also attracted considerable interest. The first investigation to show a direct effect of insulin on central structures used slow and prolonged bilateral insulin infusions into the medial hypothalamus of the rat (Nicolaïdis, 1978). These infusions produced hypophagia and, more importantly, a permanent reduction in body weight (Nicolaïdis, 1978). Similar effects of intracerebroventricular and hypothalamic infusions have been reported in both the rat and the baboon (Woods *et al.*, 1979; McGowan *et al.*, 1990).

The results of these experiments, which involved central administration of low doses of insulin, do not necessarily contradict the effects of much higher doses of peripherally active insulin on feeding. In effect, while hypoglycaemic doses of intravenous or subcutaneous insulin bring about glucoprivic feeding in both rats and humans (McKay *et al.*, 1940; Grossman and Stein, 1948), the same doses of insulin inhibit feeding if combined with glucose administration that just prevents hypoglycaemia but has no satiating effect itself (Nicolaïdis and Rowland, 1976; Even and Nicolaïdis, 1986b). The glucoprivic effect of insulin is therefore required for enhanced feeding (for review see Grossman, 1986), while minute doses of insulin applied in the brain or low doses of peripheral insulin, which do not substantially reduce glycaemia, produce a satiety effect (Nicolaïdis and Rowland, 1976; Vanderweele *et al.*, 1980; Even and Nicolaïdis, 1986b). The role of endogenous insulin in the peripheral control of food intake, besides its more well-known effects on glucose metabolism, is better appreciated today (Schwartz *et al.*, 1992).

At the same time, the presence of insulin and of specific insulin receptors in the brain, especially in the hypothalamus, has been well established

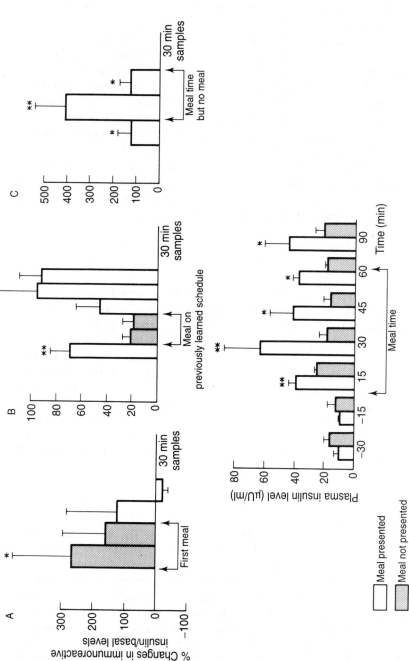

Fig. 2 *Top panel:* Changes in immunoreactive insulin in medial hypothalamic microdialysates: (A) during and after a meal presented for the first time; (B) when the rats have become accustomed to the time course of a scheduled meal; (C) when the rats have been accustomed to this meal, which was skipped on the day of the experiment. Results are expressed as mean ± SEM percentage variation of baseline levels. *$P < 0.05$. **$P < 0.01$ *vs* baseline level. *Bottom panel:* Mean ± SEM plasma insulin levels 30 min before, during and after a scheduled meal when the rats have become accustomed to this meal whether presented or not. *$P < 0.05$, **$P < 0.01$ *vs* baseline level.

(Havrankova *et al.*, 1981; Baskin *et al.*, 1983, Le Roith *et al.*, 1988; Unger *et al.*, 1991). It is generally believed that hypothalamic insulin plays a role in the daily control of food intake and body weight (Schwartz *et al.*, 1992). In a recent study (Orosco *et al.*, 1995a), using microdialysis combined with a very sensitive radioimmunoassay (Gerozissis *et al.*, 1993), we detected immunoreactive insulin (IRI) changes in hypothalamic microdialysates in relation to feeding. There was an increase in the level of IRI during the course of a meal, accompanied by a similar increase in the plasma. This more or less parallel rise in brain and plasma insulin could be due to the transfer of the circulating insulin to the interstitial brain tissue. However, when the animals were accustomed to a scheduled meal, we also observed an increase in the level of IRI in hypothalamic microdialysates, which preceded the meal time whether the meal was finally presented or not. This particular anticipatory increase in IRI concentration was absent in the plasma (Fig. 2).

2.2   Genetically obese rat

2.2.1   Serotonin
In an earlier experiment (Orosco *et al.*, 1986), we found lower levels of hypothalamic 5-HIAA in genetically obese Zucker rats, compared with their lean littermates. More recently, we used microdialysis to measure 5-HT and 5-HIAA in the medial hypothalamus of obese Zucker rats during spontaneous feeding. Despite the lower basal levels found previously, the profile of changes in Zucker rats during feeding was essentially similar to that in Wistar rats, i.e. increases in the levels of 5-HT and 5-HIAA. However, the increase in 5-HT concentration was more pronounced and longer-lasting than that in Wistar rats, while the change in the level of 5-HIAA was proportionally less pronounced. This suggests that greater amounts of the amine are released in the obese rat, possibly because they are required to bring about satiety (Orosco *et al.*, 1995b).

2.2.2   Insulin
Roles for both peripheral and central insulin in the control of food intake and bodyweight have also been confirmed by studies in the genetically obese homozygotic Zucker rat (fa-fa) which shows several abnormalities related to insulin at the peripheral as well as the central level. These disturbances include greater insulin concentrations in both the plasma (Zucker and Antoniades, 1972) and the cerebrospinal fluid (CSF) compared with the lean rats (Fa-fa and Fa-Fa), but a lower ratio of CSF:plasma insulin (Stein *et al.*, 1983), and low hypothalamic insulin content (Baskin *et al.*, 1985). Recently, using microdialysis, we reported enhanced hypothalamic insulin release in response to intravenously infused insulin in the obese rat despite a lower background hypothalamic content when compared with lean rats (Gerozissis *et al.*, 1993) (Fig. 3). This enhancement of the differential values between low (preinfusion)

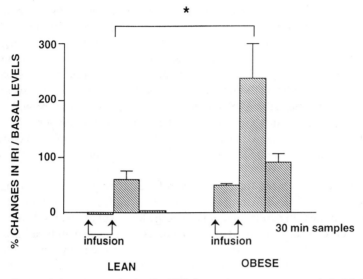

Fig. 3 Changes in immunoreactive insulin (IRI) (mean ± SEM percentage variation) induced by intravenous insulin (0.5 units during 30 min) infusion in lean and obese Zucker rats. *$P < 0.05$ lean vs obese rats.

and high (postinfusion) levels in hypothalamic insulin might reflect an impairment of the central actions of peripheral insulin on feeding. We also showed that insulin infusion did not bring about glucoprivic feeding and that no inhibitory effect was produced by a combined insulin and glucose infusion that reliably suppresses feeding in the normal rat (Orosco et al., 1994). Other altered responses to insulin that are observed in the obese Zucker rat include a peripheral resistance to insulin (Stern et al., 1975; Stein et al., 1987) and a reduced effect of centrally administered insulin in the inhibition of feeding (Ikeda et al., 1986).

3 Respective roles of serotonin and insulin in metabolism

3.1 Serotonin

Significantly, treatments using the prototypical serotonergic anorexigenic drug, fenfluramine, interfere with general metabolism. An early study of the metabolic effects of fenfluramine was performed in the rat using original equipment which separately computed total metabolic rate, the metabolic cost of animals' locomotor effort, and (by factoring out the latter from the former by means of digital filtering of Kalman) the resting (or background) metabolism in free-moving and feeding rats. In addition, the lipogenic vs lipolytic potency and feeding-associated thermogenesis were also computed simultaneously by the same calorimetric system, based on an open circuit-type respiratory gas-exchange measurement system (Even and Nicolaïdis, 1984). This study showed that dexfenfluramine administration produced a progressive release (lipolysis) and enhancement of utilization of endogenous fat reserves. The RQ dropped dramatically and there was a parallel increase in background metabolism (Even and Nicolaïdis, 1986a, 1987). Lipolysis and its consequences for the cellular availability of macronutrients that provide more fuel is the most efficient way of delaying the occurrence of hunger. This is the most physiological of the mechanisms for satiety, and functions as the inverse of the mechanism for hunger which uses the decrease in metabolic rate as its signal.

Earlier, we emphasized the effect of serotonergic activation on feeding, but its effect on metabolic expenditure is also important. An important effect of dexfenfluramine is the enhancement of energy loss. Not only does dexfenfluramine increase meal-associated thermogenesis, but it also induces a higher metabolic cost of muscular contraction and therefore energy spillage during physical exercise (Even and Nicolaïdis, 1987). As a result, the effect of serotonergic activation resulting from drugs like dexfenfluramine is not only anorexigenic, but also leptogenic (*leptos* = lean). It has been shown that dexfenfluramine brings about an expected bodyweight loss, but not indefinitely. Eventually, the rat or human no longer shows the initially observed anorexia and bodyweight loss (Stunkard, 1982; Rowland and Carlton, 1983). Is the loss of the effect simply the result of adaptation? Evidently not, because when the effective doses are administered to a rat that has been previously rendered lean, dexfenfluramine becomes ineffective immediately (Levitsky *et al.*, 1981; Even and Nicolaïdis, 1986a). This provides another reason to believe that serotonergic activation moves bodily reserves towards lower levels, i.e. it has a leptogenic effect.

3.2 Insulin

The effects of intravenous infusions of insulin, or a combination of insulin and glucose, on metabolic parameters have also been assessed (Even and Nicolaïdis, 1981). When insulin is infused alone, it produces an increase in glucose utilization accounted for by a rise in RQ. When insulin is infused in moderate amounts that do not induce dramatic hypoglycaemia, it induces an increase in 'background' metabolism as well. However, the accelerated utilization of the carbohydrate stores leads eventually to their exhaustion and to a drop in the background metabolism. This drop induces the start of a meal, which restores high levels of the background metabolism. The co-infusion of insulin and glucose brings about an increase in background metabolism by providing large amounts of glucose that prevent cellular glucoprivation. However, the combined infusion of insulin allows better utilization of glucose and thus maintains a higher and more steady level of metabolism than is the case when glucose is infused alone. In all instances, there does not seem to be an exclusive role for glucose alone in the control of feeding behaviour: the changes in RQ may never account totally for the changes in glycaemia. For this reason, we have proposed that utilization of all substrates (carbohydrate, fat or amino acids) is necessary for the final result, i.e. the increase or decrease of overall power production by cells that are capable of using all substrates. This hypothesis has been called ischymetric (Greek *ischys* = power) (Nicolaïdis, 1974; Nicolaïdis and Even, 1985).

4 Insulin–serotonin interactions

4.1 Effects of insulin on brain 5-HT metabolism

4.1.1 Peripheral administration of insulin
Peripherally injected insulin is known to affect brain serotonin metabolism. Initial studies used whole or dissected brain homogenates to measure 5-HT, 5-HIAA and sometimes tryptophan content, after intraperitoneal or subcutaneous administration of insulin. The results varied according to the dose, the delay after administration, and the nutritional status of the animals. However, most studies agreed that there was an increase in 5-HT synthesis and metabolism. This effect may be accounted for either by an increase in tryptophan (when assayed), 5-HT and 5-HIAA together (Fernstrom and Wurtman, 1971, 1972a; Juszkiewicz, 1985) or by an increase in tryptophan and 5-HIAA alone (Mackenzie and Trulson, 1978a; Orosco *et al.*, 1991). The parallel increase in tryptophan and 5-HIAA is in better agreement with the idea of enhanced synthesis (for a more detailed explanation, see below) and an accelerated turnover as shown by Juszkiewicz (1985).

These increases in tryptophan and 5-HIAA have also been observed in the case of an enhanced insulin secretion in response to a carbohydrate-rich meal or to glucose force-feeding (Fernstrom and Wurtman, 1971; Tagliamonte *et al.*, 1975), but not when hyperglycaemia reaches too high a level, for example after intravenous glucose infusion. In the latter case, the results may be somewhat different, with a decrease in 5-HIAA (Kolta and Williams, 1984). Similarly, drugs than enhance insulin secretion, such as tolbutamide or phentolamine, do not systematically reproduce the effects of physiological secretion or exogenous administration of insulin (Curzon and Fernando, 1977). In other words, the question of peripheral insulin-induced enhancement of central serotonergic activity is not as simple as was suggested by the initial studies.

Using the *in vivo* technique of microdialysis, it becomes possible to follow the serotonin-enhancing effect of insulin during and after its peripheral administration. Following intraperitoneal injection of insulin, Shimizu and Bray (1990) observed the expected increases in the levels of 5-HT and/or 5-HIAA in the ventromedial and lateral hypothalamus when the animals were not allowed to eat after the treatment. In this experimental model, hypothalamic indoleamines respond to peripheral insulin under more or less severe hypoglycaemic conditions. More recently, we used a model of intra-venous infusions of either insulin, which induces feeding, or insulin combined with glucose, which induces satiety, to compare the induced changes in the serotonergic system in medial hypothalamic structures, including VMH and PVN. With both treatments, we observed a regular, long-lasting increase in 5-HIAA concentration during and after the infusion period, together with a mirror-image decrease in 5-HT levels (Orosco and Nicolaïdis, 1994) (Fig. 4). The increase in 5-HIAA is in agreement with the result usually observed in both tissue homogenates (Orosco *et al.*, 1991) and the CSF (Danguir *et al.*, 1984), and reflects an enhanced synthesis of the amine. The decrease in 5-HT concentration, although not expected, is not inconsistent with an enhanced synthesis because, according to microdialysis principles, released rather than intracellular amines are measured with this method (Kalen *et al.*, 1988). This finding is interesting because a decrease in the concentration of 5-HT, com-bined with an increase in that of its metabolite 5-HIAA, may account for an accelerated reuptake and thus an accelerated turnover of serotonin.

4.1.2   Local cerebral administration of insulin
Although few studies have dealt with this aspect of insulin action, insulin seems to have no direct serotonergic effect when administered into the brain. Mackenzie and Trulson (1978b) were the first to infuse insulin intracisternally and to measure brain serotonergic metabolism. They found no change in the activity of tryptophan, 5-HT or 5-HIAA, contrary to their findings in parallel experiments using intraperitoneal injection. However, it is questionable whether extracerebral material infused intracisternally is capable of reaching structures that line the third ventricle located further up in the CSF stream.

Using *in vivo* techniques (push–pull perfusions), Myers and co-workers have studied the effect of locally (in the push–pull vehicle) applied insulin on hypothalamic monoamine release in relation to the nutritional state (Myers *et al.*, 1988; Minano *et al.*, 1989). These authors found changes in 5-HT and 5-HIAA concentration in the medial and lateral hypothalamus, but these were decreases. It is difficult to interpret these changes: they are opposite to those observed after peripheral administration of insulin and glucose, which have an anorexigenic effect like local hypothalamic insulin infusion. In addition, the conditions used in the experiment (20–22 h food deprivation) make their interpretation difficult.

4.1.3   Proposed mechanisms
The mechanism of action of insulin on brain serotonin, or of manipulations that enhance insulin secretion, is based on the work of Fernstrom and Wurtman (1971, 1972a). These authors described an increase in serotonin synthesis due to insulin following enhanced uptake of the precursor amino acid, tryptophan, into the brain (Fig. 5). This enhanced uptake is due mainly to the increase in the

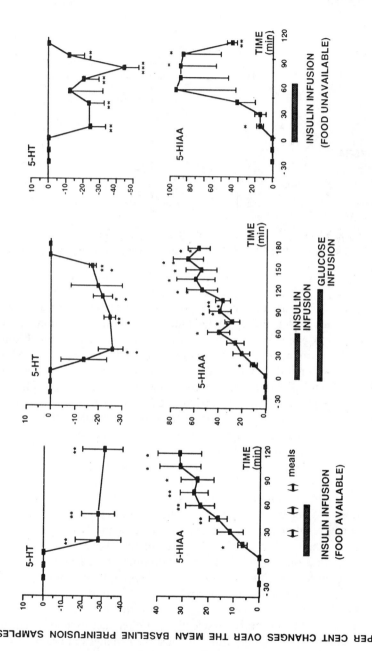

Fig. 4 Changes in 5-HT and 5-HIAA in 15-min microdialysates, during and after intravenous insulin (1 unit during 1 h) infusion or concomitant intravenous insulin and glucose infusion (glucose: 5.1 g over 2 h) or intravenous insulin infusion when food is not available. Insulin-induced feeding is indicated. Results are expressed as mean ± SEM percentage variations of the baseline samples preceding the infusion. *$P < 0.05$, **$P < 0.01$, ***$P < 0.001$ vs baseline level.

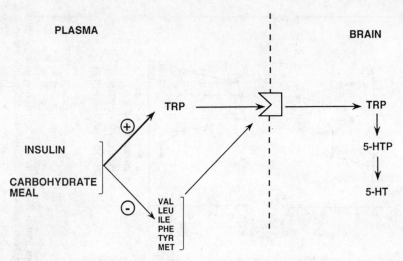

Fig. 5 Schematic representation of the mechanism of action of insulin on brain 5-HT as proposed by Fernstrom and Wurtman (1971, 1972a). TRP, tryptophan; 5-HT, 5-hydroxytryptamine; 5-HTP, 5-hydroxytryptophan.

plasma concentration of tryptophan as opposed to other large neutral amino acids (valine, leucine, isoleucine, phenylalanine, tyrosine and methionine) that compete with tryptophan for a common transport system into the brain (Fernstrom and Wurtman, 1972b). These competitor amino acids are taken up by peripheral organs, mainly striated muscle, by a mechanism that is enhanced by insulin (Manchester, 1970). In the meantime, insulin exerts other peripheral effects, such as inhibition of tryptophan pyrrolase (Sadler et al., 1983) or of the production of free fatty acids. Both of these effects of insulin allow the binding of plasma tryptophan to albumin and thus preserve it temporarily from the fate of the other competitor amino acids (Fernstrom, 1983).

This enhanced serotonin synthesis is due primarily to peripheral insulin mechanisms. This may explain the lack of effect of central administration, or, if effects are found, they are different from those that follow peripheral administration of insulin. Whether dominant or exclusive, the effect of peripheral insulin on central serotonergic activity reminds us that the latter should be related directly to the feeding behaviour of the animal. However, not all the data favour the idea of a simple, linear relationship: β cell activation $\rightarrow$ peripheral metabolic effects of insulin $\rightarrow$ selective brain uptake of monoamine precursors $\rightarrow$ related activation of selected amines $\rightarrow$ central indicators of peripheral (metabolic) events $\rightarrow$ switching on and off the relevant behavioural response (feeding and macronutrient selection). Other factors may perturb these linear relationships, and therefore the observed changes in brain tissue may reflect peripheral metabolic events that contribute towards, but do not entirely determine, feeding behaviour.

4.1.4   Diabetes and 5-HT

The fact that islet-derived insulin is able to affect central serotonergic activity raises the question of the role of a 5-HT–insulin interaction in diabetes. To measure the effect of diabetes on brain serotonin content and metabolism, several authors have produced diabetic animals by treating them with strepto-zotocin (Mackenzie and Trulson, 1978a; Chu et al., 1986; Bitar et al., 1987). The results may differ, depending on the time after streptozotocin adminis-tration and dosage, but they all indicate reduced synthesis and/or metabolism of 5-HT. These changes can be reversed by insulin injection or by insulin pretreatment, in which case the streptozotocin-induced deficiency does not appear (Oliver et al., 1989).

4.2   Effects of 5-HT on insulin secretion

The reciprocal interaction, i.e. effects of 5-HT on insulin, has also been demonstrated. Dexfenfluramine has been extensively studied in this regard. Among its various effects, dexfenfluramine has been shown to ameliorate fat diet-induced insulin resistance in rats (Storlien et al., 1989), to decrease both serum glucose and insulin levels in JCR-LA corpulent rats (Brindley et al., 1992) and to increase insulin efficiency in obese patients with non-insulin-dependent diabetes mellitus (Scheen et al., 1991). These two effects, leading to a decrease in both insulin secretion and resistance, are not contradictory since obese and diabetic patients, or animal models, are often both hyperinsulinae-mic and resistant to insulin. Thus, the reduction of exaggerated insulin secretion may ameliorate the sensitivity of the residual fraction (review by Brindley, 1992). However, the most plausible mechanism underlying these observations seems to be a direct effect of dexfenfluramine on the insulin receptor, as shown by Harrison et al. (1975) and Jorgensen (1977). The beneficial effects of dexfenfluramine are not due solely to its anorexigenic effect, because pair-feeding in non-treated rats does not decrease glucose and insulin levels as much as dexfenfluramine does. In addition, the serotonergic drug benfluorex (mainly prescribed in diabetes therapy) is more effective in diabetes, but less effective in inhibiting feeding, than dexfenfluramine (Brin-dley et al., 1988, 1991). A similar insulinagogue action in obese diabetic humans has been observed with fluoxetine (Potter van Loon et al., 1992).

The primary site of action for the effects of serotonergic drugs on insulin is far from established. Both central and peripheral mechanisms may exist.

4.2.1   Central mechanism

The above-mentioned serotonergic drugs, dexfenfluramine, fluoxetine and benfluorex, which increase both the release and action of insulin, share the property of releasing 5-HT while inhibiting its reuptake. What is the effect on insulin of drugs acting at the level of 5-HT receptors?

Whenever agonist activity occurs at different subtypes of 5-HT receptor, the results may be different. For instance, injection of the 5-HT_{1A} agonist, 8-hydroxy-2-(di-*n*-propylamino) tetralin (8-OH-DPAT), which inhibits 5-HT release by activating presynaptic autoreceptors and has orexigenic rather than anorexigenic effects, increases glycaemia and decreases insulin secretion (Chaouloff and Jeanrenaud, 1987). Administration of the 5-HT_2 agonist, 1-(2,5-dimethoxy-4-iodophenyl)-2-aminopropane (DOI), increases glycaemia without changing insulin levels. In contrast, 1-(3-chlorophenyl)-piperazine (mCPP) and 1-(3-(trifluoromethyl)phenyl)piperazine (TFMPP) do not affect glucose levels but reverse DOI-induced hyperglycaemia. In addition, hyperglycaemia without increase in insulin level may suggest a direct inhibition of insulin secretion by DOI (Chaouloff *et al.*, 1990).

4.2.2 Peripheral mechanisms

Alternatively, it is possible that serotonergic manipulations that affect insulin produce effects at the level of the gastrointestinal tract. It must be borne in mind that serotonin was first discovered in the intestinal mucosa (Erspamer and Asero, 1952) and may play a role in the control of food intake at this level. Thus, endogenous 5-HT is released by pressure applied on the intestinal mucosa (Bulbring and Crema, 1959) and by infusion of glucose into the duodenum (Drapanas *et al.*, 1962); 5-HT from stomach and intestine is increased by food deprivation (Bubenik *et al.*, 1992); and peripheral 5-HT administration brings about satiation although, in principle, 5-HT cannot cross the blood–brain barrier (Pollock and Rowland, 1981; Fletcher, 1987). In the same way, it has been proposed that the anorexigenic effect of fenfluramine could partly involve a peripheral mechanism through the inhibition of gastric emptying (Davies *et al.*, 1983; Rowland and Carlton, 1984). A possible mode of action of fenfluramine may be via the release of 5-HT in the gut since the ileal contraction that fenfluramine produces can be blocked by 5-HT antagonists (Mottram and Patel, 1979). In addition, 5-HT has been found in the pancreas at the level of nerve fibres adjacent to the exocrine or endocrine cells, depending on the species (Ding *et al.*, 1991). This suggests a regulatory role for 5-HT in pancreatic function.

Given these peripheral actions of 5-HT on digestive and metabolic processes, it is possible that part of the 5-HT–insulin interaction takes place extracerebrally. A few findings favour this possibility. Insulin release in response to glucose stimulation is decreased by 5-HT *in vivo* (Telib *et al.*, 1968) and *in vitro* using a perfused rat pancreas when fenfluramine is added to the perfusate (Barseghian *et al.*, 1983). Fenfluramine has been shown to bind directly to insulin receptors and to stimulate glucose oxidation both in adipocytes (Harrison *et al.*, 1975) and in an isolated hemidiaphragm (Jorgensen, 1977). However, there are opposing arguments: destruction of the intrapancreatic 5-HT nerves by 5,7-dihydroxytryptamine alters neither the basal release of insulin nor its response to a glucose challenge (Jansson *et al.*, 1985). More recently, pharmacological manipulations used by Chaouloff *et al.*

(1990) have allowed discrimination between central and peripheral primary sites of action of 5-HT agonists on plasma insulin levels and activity. As described above, the centrally acting 5-HT$_2$ agonist, DOI, increases glycaemia without changing insulin levels. Also, the peripherally acting 5-HT$_2$ agonist, α-methyl-5-HT, elicits hyperglycaemia with a parallel increase in insulin levels. Hence, the authors conclude that inhibition of hyperglycaemia-induced insulin release by DOI is of central origin.

Taken together, these studies indicate that interactions between 5-HT and insulin do not reflect a single phenomenon. The main challenge is to discover the physiological significance of these interactions.

5 Meaning of the 5-HT–insulin interaction

5.1 Involvement of the 5-HT–insulin interaction in the control of feeding

5.1.1 The Wurtman and Wurtman hypothesis

The most prominent argument in favour of an interaction between 5-HT and insulin in the control of feeding lies in a hypothesis proposed by Wurtman and Wurtman (1977), based on previous findings by Fernstrom and Wurtman (1971, 1972a,b). This proposes that consumption of a carbohydrate-rich meal and the secretion of insulin that it induces shifts preference towards a protein-rich meal via activation of the serotonergic system. This change in preference for a macronutrient has been reported in several studies in which pharmacological manipulations produced an enhancement of 5-HT activity (Wurtman and Wurtman, 1977, 1979; Garattini et al., 1979; Samanin et al., 1980; Blundell, 1984; Fernstrom, 1985). Conversely, a protein-rich meal should provide the brain with a small amount of tryptophan and a larger amount of competitor amino acids, the proportion of which is much more abundant in proteins. The decrease in 5-HT synthesis induced by a protein-rich meal should lead to a switch in preference for carbohydrates by the next meal (Fig. 6). This hypothesis has been substantiated by other authors (Li and Anderson, 1982, 1983). However, although attractive, it must be recognized that this regulation loop works only under certain experimental conditions and contradictory evidence has also been found (Ashley et al., 1982; Ashley and Leathwood, 1984).

5.1.2 The case of the obese Zucker rat

The model of the genetically obese Zucker rat may also provide an argument in favour of 5-HT–insulin interaction in the control of feeding. As mentioned above, the obese Zucker rat is relatively insensitive to a number of actions of insulin. In previous work, we administered insulin subcutaneously to the three genotypes of the Zucker strain, the lean homozygous Fa-Fa, the lean heterozygous Fa-fa and the obese homozygous fa-fa. We found, as did other authors

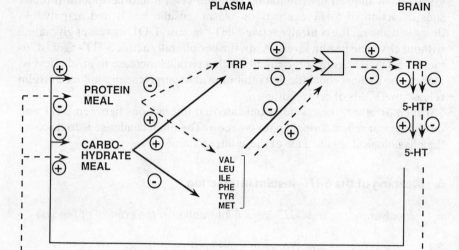

Fig. 6 Illustration of the theory proposed by Wurtman and Wurtman (1977) concerning the involvement of the 5-HT–insulin interaction in the choice of macronutrients. TRP, tryptophan; 5-HT, 5-hydroxytryptamine; 5-HPT, 5-hydroxytryptophan.

with normal rats, an increase in hypothalamic tryptophan and 5-HIAA levels in Fa-Fa and Fa-fa rats, but not in the obese fa-fa (Fig. 7). Given the resistance to insulin of the obese rats, we concluded that insulin was not able to activate the hypothalamic satiety mechanism which involves 5-HT. We proposed that this deficit in serotonergic activity could contribute to the hyperphagia of the obese Zucker rat (Orosco *et al.*, 1991).

5.2 Arguments against involvement of the 5-HT–insulin interaction in the control of ingestion

5.2.1 Parallel assessment of feeding behaviour and 5-HT activity during insulin or combined insulin and glucose infusions
As mentioned above, we used microdialysis to assess dynamic changes in hypothalamic 5-HT and 5-HIAA activity induced by intravenous infusion of either insulin, known to promote feeding, or insulin and glucose, known to promote satiety (Nicolaïdis and Rowland, 1976; Even and Nicolaïdis, 1986b). All three protocols in this work (i.e. insulin in the presence or absence of food, and insulin combined with glucose) were designed mainly to induce a state of either hunger or satiety, and thus to assess whether monoaminergic changes at the level of VMH and PVN are related to these motivational states, rather than to the metabolic events that accompany feeding (rise in glucose, insulin or other hormones, or gastrointestinal motility and secretion, etc.). In this work,

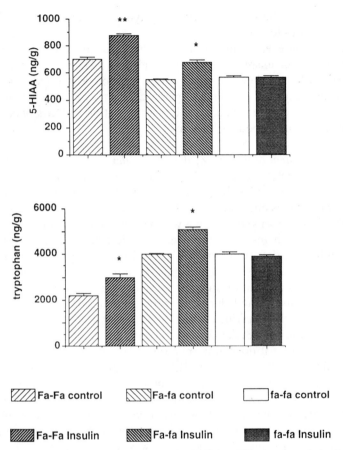

Fig. 7 Effect of insulin (10 units/kg subcutaneously, 2 h before killing) on hypothalamic 5-HIAA (top) and tryptophan (bottom) levels (ng/g tissue, mean ± SEM) in Fa-Fa, Fa-fa and fa-fa Zucker rats. $*P < 0.05$, $**P < 0.001$ vs respective control.

the infusions triggered rapid and, unexpectedly, rather uniform monoaminergic changes. In all cases (when insulin was infused alone, or with glucose, and in the presence or in the absence of food) 5-HT levels decreased while 5-HIAA levels increased (see Fig. 4). When insulin was infused in the presence of food, the superimposed episodes of feeding have practically no influence on infusion-induced changes, in contrast to the increases in 5-HT and 5-HIAA levels that occur during spontaneous feeding (Orosco and Nicolaïdis, 1992).

The fact that the insulin-induced hunger and satiety induced by insulin and glucose co-infusion were not accompanied by the monoaminergic changes in the PVN–VMH characteristic of spontaneous hunger–satiety was confirmed by the changes in dopamine (DA) and dihydroxyphenylacetic acid (DOPAC) measured in the same microdialysis samples in parallel to indoles. None of these compounds showed the profile they typically show before, during and after spontaneous feeding.

Hence, in these experiments, insulin did not act on feeding through a serotonergic mechanism because hypothalamic 5-HT and 5-HIAA levels varied similarly whether the intravenous infusion was orexigenic (insulin alone) or anorexigenic (insulin and glucose). Moreover, these changes were different from those observed when hunger, satiation and satiety occurred in the context of spontaneous behaviour.

5.2.2   Reassessment of the case of the obese Zucker rat

The same protocol of either insulin or a combination of insulin and glucose infusions was conducted in the obese Zucker rat to see whether peculiarities in central monoamines might account for the behavioural anomalies that characterize this model. In this context, it is worth recalling the resistance of the obese Zucker rat to both insulin-induced glucoprivic feeding and to insulin plus glucose-induced satiety (Orosco et al., 1994). In this group, the meals observed in the course of the infusions were similar in both size and frequency to those observed in vehicle-infused animals. Because they were not influenced by either insulin or insulin and glucose infusions, we considered that all the meals were spontaneously occurring events.

Insulin infusion induces the same global profile of monoamine changes in the obese Zucker rat as it does in normal rats (Orosco and Nicolaïdis, 1994). A decrease in 5-HT and increase in 5-HIAA levels appears in both groups as soon as the infusion begins. However, in the obese rat, the magnitude of variations is larger and the time-course shorter. Examination of each individual profile revealed that the changes that usually accompany spontaneous meals (increases in 5-HT and 5-HIAA levels) were superimposed over insulin-induced changes. The same kind of phenomenon was observed with the insulin and glucose co-infusion, which does not inhibit feeding in the Zucker rat. This was particularly evident when the two effects (of infusion and feeding) were in opposing directions, as was the case for 5-HT, and less clearly for 5-HIAA which just exaggerated an already established moderate increase (Fig. 8). From these data, it appears that the obese Zucker rat is not completely resistant to the serotonergic effect of insulin at the hypothalamic level, despite the results of our previous studies using hypothalamic homogenates (Orosco et al., 1991). The insulin-induced effects in the Zucker rat are not very 'strong', however, since they can be transiently reversed by physiological or behavioural events such as feeding. In other words, intravenous insulin infusion produces changes in hypothalamic 5-HT and 5-HIAA activity which are similar in both normal and obese Zucker rats. However, only in the latter do meals produce changes that are added algebraically to the infusion-induced changes. The response of the obese Zucker rat provides further evidence that the effects of insulin on the serotonergic system and on feeding can be dissociated. The differences that we observed in the hypothalamic profile of both insulin and

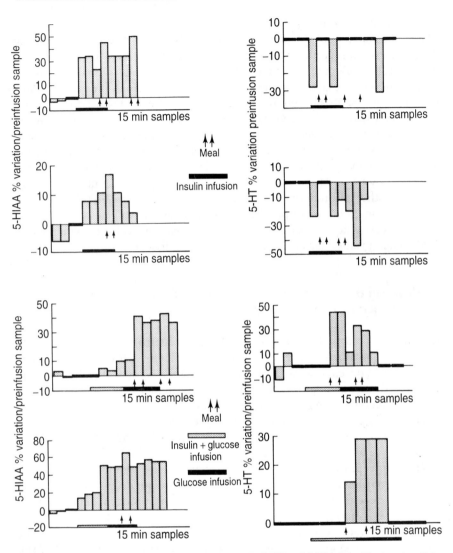

Fig. 8 Characteristic individual profiles of changes in 5-HT and 5-HIAA in 15-min microdialysates, during and after intravenous insulin (1 unit during 1 h) infusion or concomitant intravenous insulin and glucose infusion (insulin: 1 unit over 1 h; glucose: 5.1 g over 2 h) in obese Zucker rats. Spontaneously occurring feeding episodes are indicated. Results are expressed as mean percentage variations over the baseline sample preceding the infusion.

monoamines in the obese Zucker rat may be relevant to its impaired regulation of food intake, by means either of independent mechanisms or of some final common factor. A candidate for such a 'common factor' could be endogenous brain insulin or a brain insulin-like peptide such as one of the brain-located growth factors.

5.2.3   Effects of anorexigenic drugs

The studies cited above dealing with the effects of serotonergic anorexigenic drugs on insulin secretion and activity could lead to a hasty conclusion of a direct 5-HT–insulin interaction in feeding. In fact, as discussed above, careful examination of the data do not argue in favour of such an interaction. Pair-feeding experiments showed that the insulinergic effects of these drugs are not secondary to their reduction of feeding. Rather, they are parallel effects, beneficial for pathologies related to obesity (diabetes, insulin resistance, glucose intolerance), and have an additional advantage to the therapeutic indications of these drugs. It seems that 5-HT, the synaptic activity of which is enhanced by these drugs, induces positive effects on glucose metabolism. In addition, other serotonergic substances acting at postsynaptic receptors also reduce feeding, but do not produce the same beneficial effects on insulin and glucose levels as do releasers or reuptake blockers. This is further evidence that feeding and insulinergic effects of 5-HT must be dissociated.

6   How can the arguments for and against the involvement of insulin–5-HT interaction in feeding be reconciled?

It seems clear that 5-HT and insulin may directly control short-term feeding by themselves, but not necessarily in an interactive manner. However, undeniable links exist between insulin, 5-HT and metabolic events (glucose and lipid utilization) surrounding feeding or pathologies (impairment of insulin action) related to feeding. Even the most cogent argument in favour of a 5-HT–insulin interaction in the control of short-term feeding, i.e. the hypothesis of Wurtman and Wurtman, suffers numerous gaps and cannot be applied in all circumstances and experimental conditions.

The results in the Zucker rat from our earlier experiments (Orosco *et al.*, 1991) and more recent studies mentioned above are not necessarily contradictory. Our recent study, using a dynamic *in vivo* approach, allowed us to visualize short-term 5-HT variations concomitantly with the recording of feeding behaviour, while the previous work, *ex vivo*, gave access only to more global effects assessed at a single time-point after the injection of insulin. It is possible that the lack of global change in 5-HT may be the cause of hyperphagia in the obese. Alternatively, it is possible that the abnormal profile of 5-HT in the obese is due to other metabolic abnormalities in these animals. The independence of the feeding effects of insulin and brain 5-HT, respectively, was suggested in our aforementioned experiments in which (a) the insulin-resistant Zucker rat showed no feeding but a 5-HT response to insulin and to combined insulin and glucose infusions, and (b) the normal rat showed the expected feeding response, but brain 5-HT responses were similar in the case of insulin and insulin plus glucose infusions, but different in the case of spontaneous feeding.

7 Conclusions

The possibility of an interaction between 5-HT and insulin in the control of feeding was first raised when it was thought that peripheral insulin depended on a brain transmitter to mediate its anorexigenic effect. Nowadays, the question is somewhat different in the light of recent evidence, however controversial, about the direct effect of insulin in the brain. Since our original work on brain insulin and its relation to peripheral insulin, the question remains the subject of controversy. Some authors believe that peripheral insulin first reaches the CSF and from there the hypothalamic structures (Woods and Porte, 1977; Vanderweele *et al.*, 1980). Dynamic assays of CSF insulin suggested that peripheral insulin could reach the brain tissue following a 'dumped and delayed' profile via its passage through the cerebroventricular space (Woods and Porte, 1977). The most recent hypothesis from this group is that delivery of insulin to the neuropil may be due to a specialized brain transport system of transcytosis (Schwartz *et al.*, 1991). Others propose that the blood–brain barrier prevents entry of insulin into the brain (Havrankova *et al.*, 1981). The production of endogenous brain insulin is compatible with the finding that messenger RNA coding for insulin is present in the hypothalamic cells of rats and humans (Giddins *et al.*, 1985; Young, 1986; Schechter *et al.*, 1990).

Our own data are compatible with the idea that another brain insulin-like peptide, such as brain growth factor, generated beyond the blood–brain barrier, could replace insulin or act with it for similar functions. In our recent study on immunoreactive insulin (IRI) changes in hypothalamic microdialysates in relation to feeding (Orosco *et al.*, 1995a), we tried to understand the origin of brain insulin. The prandial increase in IRI we observed, more or less in parallel with hyperinsulinaemia, is consistent with the idea that hypothalamic insulin originates from the plasma insulin, in agreement with the suggested saturable transcytosis transport through the blood–brain barrier (Woods and Porte, 1977; Partridge, 1986; Schwartz *et al.*, 1991). In contrast, the active transport mechanism is less capable of accounting for the anticipatory increase in IRI, which is enhanced as a function of animal's expectation of food, while plasma insulin does not rise under these conditions (Orosco *et al.*, 1995a). In our other report about hypothalamic IRI in obese Zucker rats in response to intravenous insulin infusion (Gerozissis *et al.*, 1993), the dramatic increase observed was far from being a simple reflection in brain tissue of the increase in plasma insulin concentration. One explanation of our data assumes the production of insulin by brain cells themselves, as some authors have suggested (Young, 1986). The IRI changes could be also accounted for by a selective process of capacitance-like transport (Hachiya *et al.*, 1988; M. W. Schwartz *et al.*, 1990; Yang *et al.*, 1989) capable of accumulating and releasing insulin depending on local management of the peptide.

Finally, we should consider three cases. First, brain insulin results from the passage of peripheral insulin into the brain where it may be either directly active or stored until requirement. Second, brain insulin may be synthesized locally in response to a peripheral signal in parallel or not with peripheral insulin itself. These two hypotheses do not exclude each other. In both cases, brain insulin, whatever its origin, is a mediator between peripheral events and brain messengers. Third, brain and peripheral insulin are independently regulated in response to similar but not identical events.

In our present state of knowledge, it seems reasonable to consider two separate but complementary mechanisms of interaction: one that links peripheral insulin with brain insulin, whatever its actual identity and site of production, and another that links peripheral insulin and serotonin. Such interactions could be involved in the inhibition of feeding in a co-active way: the peptide would need the indoleamine (and perhaps other amines) to become an efficient modulator at the level of the hypothalamic structures involved in satiety.

References

Ashley, D. V. M. and Leathwood, P. D. (1984). A high carbohydrate protein-free meal, either at breakfast or in the evening does not alter plasma tryptophan to large neutral amino acids ratios in healthy men. In *Progress in Tryptophan and Serotonin Research* (H. G. Schlossberger, W. Kochen, B. Linzen and H. Steinhart, eds), pp. 591–594. De Gruyter, Berlin.

Ashley, D. V. M., Barclay, D. V., Chauffard, F. A., Moennoz, D. and Leathwood, P. D. (1982). Plasma amino acid responses in humans to evening meals of different nutritional composition. *Am. J. Clin. Nutr.* 36, 143–153.

Barseghian, G., Lev-Ran, A., Hwang, D., Josefsberg, Z. and Tomkinson, C. (1983). Fenfluramine inhibits insulin secretion and potentiates glucagon release by the perfused rat pancreas. *Eur. J. Pharmacol.* 96, 53–59.

Baskin, D. G., Porte, D. J., Guest, K. and Dorsa, D. M. (1983). Regional concentrations of insulin in the rat brain. *Endocrinology* 112, 898–903.

Baskin, D. G., Stein, L. J., Ikeda, H., Woods, S. C., Figlewicz, D. P., Porte, D., Jr., Greenwood, M. R. C. and Dorsa, D. M. (1985). Genetically obese Zucker rats have abnormally low brain insulin content. *Life Sci.* 36, 627–633.

Baskin, D. G., Wilcox, B. J., Figlewicz, D. P. and Dorsa, D. M. (1988). Insulin and insulin-like growth factors in the CNS. *Trends Neurosci.* 11, 107–111.

Bitar, M. S., Koulu, M. and Linnoila, M. (1987). Diabetes-induced changes in monoamine concentrations of rat hypothalamic nuclei. *Brain Res.* 409, 236–242.

Blundell, J. E. (1984). Serotonin and appetite. *Neuropharmacology* 23, 1537–1552.

Blundell, J. E., Latham, C. J., McArthur, R. A., Moniz, E. and Rogers, P. J. (1979). Structural analysis of the actions of amphetamine and fenfluramine on food intake and feeding behaviour in animals and man. *Curr. Med. Res. Opin.* 6, 34–54.

Brindley, D. N. (1992). Neuroendocrine regulation and obesity. *Int. J. Obes.* 16 (supplement 3), S73–S79.

Brindley, D. N., Akester, H., Derrick, G. P., Irvine, D. D., Patmore, R. D., Spencer, H., Yule-Smith, A., Finnerty, C., Saxton, J., Macdonald, I. A. and Rolland, Y. (1988). Effects of chronic administration of benfluorex to rats, on the metabolism of corticosterone, glucose, triacylglycerols, glycerol and fatty acids. *Biochem. Pharmacol.* 37, 695–705.

Brindley, D. N., Hales, P., Al-Sieni, A. I. I. and Russell, J. C. (1991). Decreased serum lipids, serum insulin and triacylglycerol synthesis in adipose tissue of JCR:LA-corpulent rats treated with benfluorex. *Biochim. Biophys. Acta* **1085**, 119–125.

Brindley, D. N., Hales, P., Al-Sieni, A. I. I. and Russell, J. C. (1992). Sustained decreases in weight and serum insulin, glucose, triacylglycerol and cholesterol in JCR:LA-corpulent rats treated with D-fenfluramine. *Br. J. Pharmacol.* **105**, 679–685.

Bubenik, G. A., Ball, R. O. and Pang, S. F. (1992). The effect of food deprivation on brain and gastrointestinal tissue levels of tryptophan, serotonin, 5-hydroxyindolacetic acid and melatonin. *J. Pineal Res.* **12**, 7–16.

Bulbring, E. and Crema, A. (1959). The release of 5-hydroxytryptamine in relation to pressure exerted on the intestinal mucosa. *J. Physiol. (Lond.)* **192**, 823–846.

Chaouloff, F. and Jeanrenaud, B. (1987). 5-HT1A and alpha-2 adrenergic receptors mediate the hyperglycemic and hypoinsulinemic effects of 8-hydroxy-2-(di-*n*-propylamino)tetralin in the conscious rat. *J. Pharmacol. Exp. Ther.* **243**, 1159–1166.

Chaouloff, F., Laude, D. and Baudrie, V. (1990). Effects of the 5-HT1c/5-HT2 receptor agonists DOI and alpha-methyl-5-HT on plasma glucose and insulin levels in the rat. *Eur. J. Pharmacol.* **187**, 435–443.

Chu, P. C., Lin, M. T., Shian, L. R. and Leu, S. Y. (1986). Alterations in physiologic functions and in brain monoamine content in streptozotocin-diabetic rats. *Diabetes* **35**, 481–485.

Cooper, S. J., Dourish, C. T. and Barber, D. J. (1990). Reversal of the anorectic effect of (+)-fenfluramine in the rat by the selective cholecystokinin antagonist MK-329. *Br. J. Pharmacol.* **99**, 65–70.

Curzon, G. and Fernando, J. C. R. (1977). Drugs altering insulin secretion: effects on plasma and brain concentrations of aromatic amino acids and on brain 5-hydroxytryptamine turnover. *Br. J. Pharmacol.* **60**, 401–408.

Danguir, J., Elghozi, J. L. and Laude, D. (1984). Increased dopamine and serotonin metabolites in the CSF during severe insulin-induced hypoglycemia in freely-moving rats. *Neurochem. Int.* **6**, 71–75.

Davies, R. F., Rossi, J., Panksepp, J., Bean, N. J. and Zolovick A. J. (1983). Fenfluramine anorexia: a peripheral locus of action. *Physiol. Behav.* **30**, 723–730.

Ding, W. G., Fujimura, M., Tooyama, Y. and Kimura, H. (1991). Phylogenetic study of serotonin-immunoreactive structures in the pancreas of various vertebrates. *Cell Tissue Res.* **263**, 237–243.

Drapanas, T., McDonald, J. C. and Stewart, J. D. (1962). Serotonin release following instillation of hypertonic glucose into the proximal intestine. *Ann. Surg.* **156**, 528–536.

Erspamer, V. and Asero, B. (1952). Identification of enteramine, the specific hormone of the enterochromaffin cells, as 5-hydroxytryptamine. *Nature* **169**, 800–801.

Even, P. and Nicolaïdis, S. (1981). Effet orexigénique ou anorexigénique de l'insuline: mécanisme ischymétrique? *J. Physiol. (Paris)* **77**, 17A.

Even, P. and Nicolaïdis, S. (1984). Le métabolisme de fond: définition et dispositif de sa mesure. *Compte Rendu de l'Académie des Sciences (Paris)* **298**, 261–266.

Even, P. and Nicolaïdis, S. (1986a). Metabolic mechanism of the anorectic and leptogenic effects of the serotonin agonist fenfluramine. In *Serotoninergic System, Feeding and Body Weight Regulation* (S. Nicolaïdis, ed.), pp. 141–163. Academic Press, London.

Even, P. and Nicolaïdis, S. (1986b). Short-term control of feeding: limitation of the glucostatic theory. *Brain Res. Bull.* **17**, 621–626.

Even, P. and Nicolaïdis, S. (1987). Metabolic mechanism of the anorectic and leptogenic effects of the serotonin agonist fenfluramine. *Appetite* **7** (**supplement**), 141–163.

Fernstrom, J. D. (1983). Role of precursor availability in control of monoamine biosynthesis in brain. *Physiol. Rev.* **63**, 484–546.

Fernstrom, J. D. (1985). Dietary effects on brain serotonin synthesis: relationship to appetite regulation. *Am. J. Clin. Nutr.* **42**, 1072–1082.

Fernstrom, J. D. and Wurtman, R. J. (1971). Brain serotonin content: increase following ingestion of carbohydrate diet. *Science* **174**, 197–204.

Fernstrom, J. D. and Wurtman, R. J. (1972a). Elevation of plasma tryptophan by insulin in the rat. *Metabolism* **21**, 337–342.

Fernstrom, J. D. and Wurtman, R. J. (1972b). Brain serotonin content: physiological regulation by plasma neutral amino-acids. *Science* **178**, 414–416.

Fletcher, P. J. (1987). The anorectic action of peripheral 5-HT examined in the runway: evidence for an action on satiation. *Psychopharmacology* **93**, 498–501.

Garattini, S., Caccia, S., Mennini, T., Samanin, R., Consolo, S. and Ladinsky, H. (1979). Biochemical pharmacology of the anorectic drug fenfluramine. A review. *Curr. Med. Res. Opin.* **6 (supplement 1)**, 15–27.

Gerozissis, K., Orosco, M., Rouch, C. and Nicolaïdis, S. (1993). Basal and hyperinsulinemia-induced immunoreactive hypothalamic insulin changes in lean and genetically obese Zucker rats revealed by microdialysis. *Brain Res.* **611**, 258–263.

Giddins, S., Chirgwin, J. and Permutt, M. (1985). Evaluation of rat insulin messenger RNA in pancreatic and extrapancreatic tissues. *Diabetologia* **28**, 343–347.

Grossman, S. P. (1960). Eating or drinking elicited by direct adrenergic or cholinergic stimulation of hypothalamus. *Science* **132**, 301–302.

Grossman, S. P. (1986). The role of glucose, insulin and glucagon in the regulation of food intake and body weight. *Neurosci. Biobehav. Rev.* **10**, 295–315.

Grossman, S. P. and Stein, J. F. (1948). Vagotomy and the hunger producing action of insulin in man. *J. Appl. Physiol.* **1**, 263–267.

Hachiya, H. L., Halban, P. A. and King, G. L. (1988). Intracellular pathways of insulin transport across vascular endothelial cells. *Am. J. Physiol.* **255**, C459–C464.

Harrison, L. C., Martin, F. I. R., King-Roach, A. and Melick, R. A. (1975). The effect of fenfluramine on insulin binding and on basal and insulin-stimulated oxidation of 1-^{14}C glucose by human adipose tissue. *Postgrad. Med. J.* **51 (supplement 1)**, 110–114.

Havrankova, J. M., Brownstein, M. and Roth, J. (1981). Insulin and insulin receptors in rodents brains. *Diabetologia* **supplement 20**, 268–273.

Hoebel, B. G. (1977). The pharmacology of feeding. In *Handbook of Psychopharmacology* (L. L. Iversen, S. D. Iversen and S. H. Snyder, eds), pp. 55–129. Plenum Press, New York.

Ikeda, H., West, D. B., Pustek, J. J., Figlewicz, D. P., Greenwood, M. R. C., Porte, D., Jr. and Woods, S. C. (1986). Intraventricular insulin reduces food intake and body weight of lean but not obese Zucker rats. *Appetite* **7**, 381–386.

Jansson, L., Leung, P. E. and McEvoy, R. C. (1985). Ablation of serotonergic nerves in the rat pancreas. Lack of effects on hormone secretion and intrinsic blood flow. *Acta Endocrinol.* **110**, 515–521.

Jorgensen, K. D. (1977). Actions of fenfluramine on glucose uptake *in vitro* and *in vivo*. *Acta Pharmacol. Toxicol.* **40**, 401–417.

Juszkiewicz, M. (1985). The effect of insulin on the central serotonergic system of the rat. *Pol. J. Pharmacol. Pharm.* **37**, 591–600.

Kalen, P., Strecker, R. E., Rosengren, E. and Björklund, A. (1988). Endogenous release of neuronal serotonin and 5-hydroxyindolacetic acid in the caudate-putamen of the rat revealed by intracerebral dialysis coupled to high-performance chromatography with fluorimetric detection. *J. Neurochem.* **51**, 1422–1435.

Kolta, M. G. and Williams, B. B. (1984). Effect of hyperglycemia on biogenic amines, β-endorphin and insulin of the rat brain. *Horm. Metab. Res.* **16**, 16–20.

Leibowitz, S. F. (1980). Neurochemical systems of the hypothalamus. Control of feeding and drinking behavior and water-electrolyte excretion. In *Handbook of the Hypothalamus* (P. J. Morgane and J. Panksepp, eds), pp. 299–437. Marcel Dekker, New York.

Leibowitz, S. F. and Shor-Posner, G. (1986). Brain serotonin and eating behaviour. *Appetite* **7**, 1–14.

Le Roith, D., Rojeski, M. and Roth, J. (1988). Insulin receptors in brain and other tissues: similarities and differences. *Neurochem. Int.* **12**, 419–423.

Levitsky, D., Strupp, B. and Lupoli, J. (1981). Tolerance to anorectic drugs: pharmacological or artifactual. *Pharmacol. Biochem. Behav.* **14**, 661–667.

Li, E. T. S. and Anderson, G. H. (1982). Meal composition influences subsequent food selection in the young rat. *Physiol. Behav.* **29**, 779–783.

Li, E. T. S. and Anderson, G. H. (1983). 5-Hydroxytryptamine control of meal to meal composition chosen by rats. *Fed. Proc.* **42**, 548–554.

McGowan, M. K., Andrews, K. M., Kelly, J. and Grossman, S. P. (1990). Effect of chronic intrahypothalamic infusion of insulin on food intake and diurnal meal patterning in the rat. *Behav. Neurosci.* **104**, 371–383.

McKay, E. M., Callaway, J. W. and Barnes, R. H. (1940). Hyperalimentation in normal animals produced by protamine zinc insulin. *Nutrition* **20**, 59–66.

Mackenzie, R. G. and Trulson, M. E. (1978a). Effects of insulin and streptozotocin-induced diabetes on brain tryptophan and serotonin metabolism in rats. *J. Neurochem.* **30**, 205–211.

Mackenzie, R. G. and Trulson, M. E. (1978b). Does insulin act directly on the brain to increase tryptophan levels? *J. Neurochem.* **30**, 1205–1208.

Manchester, K. L. (1970). The control by insulin of amino acid accumulation in muscle. *Biochem. J.* **117**, 457–465.

Minano, F. J., Peinado, J. M. and Myers, R. D. (1989). Profile of NE, DA and 5-HT activity shifts in medial hypothalamus perfused by 2-DG and insulin in the sated or fasted rat. *Brain Res. Bull.* **22**, 695–704.

Mottram, D. R. and Patel, R. J. (1979). Peripheral effects of fenfluramine mediated via the release of 5-hydroxytryptamine. *Gen. Pharmacol.* **10**, 441–444.

Myers, R. D., Peinado, J. M. and Minano, F. J. (1988). Monoamine transmitter activity in lateral hypothalamus during its perfusion with insulin or 2-DG in sated and fasted rats. *Physiol. Behav.* **44**, 633–643.

Nicolaïdis, S. (1969). Early systemic response to oro-gastric stimulation in the regulation of food and water balance. Functional and electrophysiological data. *Ann. N. Y. Acad. Sci.* **157**, 1176–1203.

Nicolaïdis, S. (1974). Short term and long term regulation of energy balance. *Proceedings of the XXVI International Union of Physiological Sciences, New Delhi*, pp. 122–123.

Nicolaïdis, S. (1978). Mécanisme nerveux de l'équilibre énergétique. *Journées Annuelles de Diabetologie de l'Hotel Dieu de Paris* **1**, 152–156.

Nicolaïdis, S. and Even, P. (1985). Physiological determinant of hunger, satiation and satiety. *Am. J. Clin. Nutr.* **42**, 1083–1092.

Nicolaïdis, S. and Rowland, N. (1976). Metering of intravenous *versus* oral nutrients. *Am. J. Physiol.* **231**, 661–668.

Oliver, E. H., Sartin, J. L., Dieberg, G., Rahe, C. H., Marple, D. N. and Kemppainen, R. H. (1989). Effects of acute insulin deficiency on catecholamine and indoleamine content and catecholamine turnover in microdissected hypothalamic nuclei in streptozotocin-diabetic rats. *Acta Endocrinol.* **120**, 343–350.

Orosco, M. and Nicolaïdis, S. (1992). Spontaneous feeding-related monoaminergic changes in the rostromedial hypothalamus revealed by microdialysis. *Physiol. Behav.* **52**, 1015–1019.

Orosco, M. and Nicolaïdis, S. (1994). Insulin and glucose-induced changes in feeding and medial hypothalamic monoamines revealed by microdialysis in rats. *Brain Res. Bull.* **33**, 289–297.

Orosco, M., Trouvin, J. H., Cohen, Y. and Jacquot, C. (1986). Ontogeny of brain monoamines in lean and obese Zucker rats. *Physiol. Behav.* **36**, 853–856.

Orosco, M., Rouch, C., Gripois, D., Blouquit, M. F., Roffi, J., Jacquot, C. and Cohen, Y. (1991). Effects of insulin on brain monoamine metabolism in the Zucker rat: influence of genotype and age. *Psychoneuroendocrinology* **16**, 537–546.

Orosco, M., Rouch, C. and Nicolaïdis, S. (1994). Resistance of the obese Zucker rat to insulin-induced feeding and to satiety induced by coinfusion of insulin and glucose. *Appetite* **23**, 209–218.

Orosco, M., Gerozissis, K., Rouch, C. and Nicolaïdis, S. (1995a). Feeding-related immunoreactive insulin changes in the PVN–VMH revealed by microdialysis. *Brain Res.* **671**, 149–158.

Orosco, M., Rouch, C., Meile, M. J. and Nicolaïdis, S. (1995b). Spontaneous feeding-related monoamine changes in rostromedial hypothalamus of the obese Zucker rat: a microdialysis study. *Physiol. Behav.* **57**, 1103–1106.

Partridge, W. M. (1986). Receptor-mediated peptide transport through the blood–brain barrier. *Endocrinol. Rev.* **7**, 314–330.

Pollock, J. D. and Rowland, N. (1981). Peripherally administered serotonin decreases food intake in rats. *Pharmacol. Biochem. Behav.* **15**, 179–183.

Potter van Loon, B. J., Radder, J. K., Frölich, M., Krans, H. M. J., Zwinderman, A. H. and Meinders, A. E. (1992). Fluoxetine increases insulin action in obese non-insulin dependent diabetic individuals. *Int. J. Obesity* **16**, 79–85.

Rowland, N. and Carlton, J. (1983). Different behavioral mechanisms underlie tolerance to the anorectic effects of fenfluramine and quipazine. *Psychopharmacology* **81**, 155–157.

Rowland, N. and Carlton, J. (1984). Inhibition of gastric emptying by peripheral and central fenfluramine in rats: correlation with anorexia. *Life Sci.* **34**, 2495–2499.

Sadler, E., Weiner, M. and Buterbaugh, G. G. (1983). Effect of streptozotocin-induced diabetes on tryptophan oxygenase activity and brain tryptophan levels in rats. *Res. Commun. Chem. Pathol. Pharmacol.* **42**, 37–58.

Samanin, R., Mennini, T. and Garattini, S. (1980). Evidence that it is possible to cause anorexia by increasing release and/or directly stimulating postsynaptic serotonin receptors in the brain. *Prog. Neuropsychopharmacol.* **4**, 363–369.

Schechter, R., Sadiq, H. F. and Devaskar, S. U. (1990). Insulin and insulin mRNA are detected in neuronal cell cultures maintained in an insulin-free/serum-free medium. *J. Histochem. Cytochem.* **38**, 829–836.

Scheen, A. J., Paolisso, G., Salvatore, T. and Lefebvre, P. J. (1991). Improvement of insulin-induced glucose disposal in obese patients with NIDDM after 1-week treatment with D-fenfluramine. *Diabetes Care* **14**, 325–332.

Schwartz, D. H., Hernandez, L. and Hoebel, B. G. (1990). Serotonin release in lateral and medial hypothalamus during feeding and its anticipation. *Brain Res. Bull.* **25**, 797–802.

Schwartz, M. W., Sipols, A. J., Kahn, S. E., Lattemann, D. P., Taborsky, G. J., Bergman, R. N., Woods, S. C. and Porte, D. J. (1990). Kinetics and specificity of insulin uptake from plasma into cerebrospinal fluid. *Am. J. Physiol.* **259**, E378–E383.

Schwartz, M. W., Bergman, R. N., Kahn, S. E., Taborsky, G. J., Fisher, L. D., Sipols, A. J., Woods, S. C., Steil, G. M. and Porte, D. J. (1991). Evidence for entry of plasma insulin into cerebrospinal fluid through an intermediate compartment in dogs. Quantitative aspects and implications for transport. *J. Clin. Invest.* **88**, 1272–1281.

Schwartz, M. W., Figlewicz, D. P., Baskin, D. G., Woods, S. C. and Porte, D., Jr. (1992). Insulin in the brain: a hormonal regulator of energy balance. *Endocr. Rev.* **13**, 387–414.

Shimizu, H. and Bray, G. A. (1990). Effects of insulin on hypothalamic monoamine metabolism. *Brain Res.* **510**, 251–258.

Stallone, D., Nicolaïdis, S. and Gibbs, J. (1989). Cholecystokinin anorexia depends upon serotoninergic function. *Am. J. Physiol.* **256**, R1138–R1141.

Stein, L. J., Dorsa, D. M., Baskin, D. G., Figlewicz, D. P., Ikeda, H., Frankman, S. P., Greenwood, M. R. C., Porte, D., Jr. and Woods, S. C. (1983). Immunoreactive insulin levels are elevated in the cerebrospinal fluid of genetically obese Zucker rats. *Endocrinology* **113**, 2299–2301.

Stein, L. J., Dorsa, D. M., Baskin, D. G., Figlewicz, D. P., Porte, D., Jr. and Woods, S. C. (1987). Reduced effect of experimental peripheral hyperinsulinemia to elevate cerebrospinal fluid insulin concentrations of obese Zucker rats. *Endocrinology* **121**, 1611–1615.

Stern, J. S., Johnson, P. R., Batchelor, B., Zucker, L. and Hirsch, J. (1975). Pancreatic insulin release and peripheral tissue resistance in Zucker obese rats fed high and low carbohydrate diets. *Am. J. Physiol.* **228**, 543–548.

Storlien, L. H., Thorburn, A. W., Smythe, G. A., Jenkins, A. B., Chishilm, D. J. and Kraeger, E. W. (1989). Effect of D-fenfluramine on basal glucose turnover and fat-feeding-induced insulin resistance in rats. *Diabetes* **38**, 499–503.

Stunkard, A. (1982). Anorectic agents lower a body weight set point. *Life Sci.* **30**, 2043–2055.

Tagliamonte, A., Demontis, M. G., Olianas, M., Onali, P. L. and Gessa, G. L. (1975). Possible role of insulin in the transport of tyrosine and tryptophan from blood to brain. *Pharmacol. Res. Commun.* **7**, 493–499.

Telib, M., Raptis, S., Schroder, K. E. and Pfeiffer, E. F. (1968). Serotonin and insulin release *in vivo. Diabetologia* **4**, 253–256.

Unger, J. W., Livingston, J. N. and Moss, A. M. (1991). Insulin receptors in the central nervous system: localization, signalling mechanisms and functional aspects. *Prog. Neurobiol.* **36**, 343–362.

Vanderweele, D. A., Pi-Sunyer, F. X., Novin, D. and Bush, M. J. (1980). Chronic insulin infusion suppresses food ingestion and body weight gain in rats. *Brain Res. Bull.* **5**, 7–11.

Woods, S. C. and Porte, D., Jr. (1977). Relationship between plasma and cerebrospinal insulin levels of dogs. *Am. J. Physiol.* **233**, E331–E334.

Woods, S. C., Lotter, E. C., McKay, D. and Porte, D. (1979). Chronic intracerebroventricular infusion of insulin reduces food intake and body weight in baboons. *Nature* **282**, 503–505.

Wurtman, J. J. and Wurtman, R. J. (1977). Fenfluramine and fluoxetine spare protein consumption while suppressing caloric intake by rats. *Science* **198**, 1178–1180.

Wurtman, J. J. and Wurtman, R. J. (1979). Drugs that enhance central serotoninergic transmission diminish elective carbohydrate consumption by rats. *Life Sci.* **24**, 895–904.

Yang, Y. J., Hope, I. D., Ader, M. and Bergman, R. N. (1989). Insulin transport across capillaries is rate limiting for insulin action in dogs. *J. Clin. Invest.* **84**, 1620–1628.

Young, W. S. (1986). Periventricular hypothalamic cells in the rat brain contain insulin mRNA. *Neuropeptides* **8**, 93–97.

Zucker, L. M. and Antoniades, H. N. (1972). Insulin and obesity in the Zucker genetically obese rat 'fatty'. *Endocrinology* **90**, 1320–1330.

6

Opioid Receptor Subtype Antagonists and Ingestion

RICHARD J. BODNAR

Department of Psychology and Neuropsychology Doctoral Sub-Program, Queens College, City University of New York, 65-30 Kissena Boulevard, Flushing, New York 11367-0904, USA

A role for the endogenous opioid systems in ingestive behaviour has been confirmed by the observations that opioid agonists typically stimulate intake and opioid antagonists typically inhibit intake (for reviews see Morley *et al.*, 1983; Levine *et al.*, 1985; Leibowitz, 1987; Cooper and Kirkham, 1992). This chapter focuses on the selective effects of specific opioid receptor subtype antagonists within different feeding and drinking situations. Following a brief description of opioid gene-related families, receptor subtypes, and prototypical agonists and antagonists, there is a summary of the effects of opioid receptor subtype antagonists across a series of ingestive situations, including spontaneous intake and body weight control, deprivation-induced feeding, glucoprivic feeding, palatable and stress-induced intake, and water intake under challenge conditions.

1 Opioid ligands, receptor subtypes and selective antagonists

Identification of multiple endogenous opioid ligands and gene-related families (pre-pro-enkephalin, pre-pro-dynorphin and pro-opiomelanocortin; for review see Akil *et al.*, 1984) and multiple opioid receptor subtypes (μ, δ and κ; Martin *et al.*, 1976; Lord *et al.*, 1977) led to the development of highly selective opioid receptor subtype agonists and antagonists.

1.1 Mu receptors

The μ receptor is subdivided into μ_1 and μ_2 subtypes (for review see Pasternak and Wood, 1986). The μ_1 receptor binds opiates and most enkephalins with similar high affinities and has been characterized using the irreversible

DRUG RECEPTOR SUBTYPES AND INGESTIVE BEHAVIOUR
ISBN 0-12-187620-9

μ_1-selective antagonist, naloxonazine (e.g. Hahn *et al.*, 1982). The μ_2 site is the prototypical site for morphine binding (Pasternak and Wood, 1986). μ-Selective drugs with activity at both μ_1 and μ_2 binding sites include the irreversible antagonist, β-funaltrexamine (β-FNA; Portoghese *et al.*, 1980) and the reversible antagonist, Cys^2-Tyr^3-Orn^5-Pen^7-amide (CTOP; Gulya *et al.*, 1986). While equally sensitive ingestive responses to β-FNA ($\mu_1 + \mu_2$) and naloxonazine (μ_1) suggest μ_1 mediation of that response, selective sensitivity to β-FNA ($\mu_1 + \mu_2$), but not to naloxonazine (μ_1) suggests μ_2 mediation.

1.2 Delta receptors

The δ receptor was initially characterized by its greater binding potency for enkephalins relative to morphine (Lord *et al.*, 1977), although some δ-selective enkephalin analogues (e.g. D-Ala^2, D-Leu^5-enkephalin (DADL); D-Ser^2, Leu^5-enkephalin-Thr^6 (DSLET)) also display high affinity for the μ_1 receptor (Hazum *et al.*, 1981; Itzhak and Pasternak, 1987). The δ receptor has been subdivided into δ_1 and δ_2 subtypes (Negri *et al.*, 1991) based on the δ_1 antagonist actions of D-Ala^2, Leu^5, Cys^6-enkephalin (DALCE; Bowen *et al.*, 1987) and the δ_2 antagonist actions of naltrindole isothiocyanate (NTII; Portoghese *et al.*, 1990). Indeed, the δ_1 and δ_2 subtypes have been dissociated from each other in analgesic assays (e.g. Jiang *et al.*, 1991; Mattia *et al.*, 1991, 1992).

1.3 Kappa receptors

The κ receptor was initially described using the narcotics, ketocyclazocine and ethylketocyclazocine (Martin *et al.*, 1976), but subsequent binding studies indicated the existence of at least four κ receptor subtypes (Nock *et al.*, 1988; Zukin *et al.*, 1988; Clark *et al.*, 1989; Rothman *et al.*, 1990). While the κ_1 receptor subtype has been characterized by the selective antagonist, norbinaltorphimine (Nor-BNI; Portoghese *et al.*, 1987), the phenylpiperidines (e.g. LY255582) have been postulated as selective antagonists for the κ_2 receptor subtype (Rothman *et al.*, 1993). While the κ_3 receptor subtype is characterized by the agonist, naloxone benzoylhydrazone (NalBzOH; Clark *et al.*, 1989), a selective antagonist is not available.

2 Spontaneous feeding and body weight control

The general short-acting opioid antagonists, naloxone and naltrexone, decrease spontaneous *ad libitum* food intake and the hyperphagic response following food deprivation (e.g. Holtzman, 1974; Brown and Holtzman, 1979; Frenk and Rogers, 1979; Cooper, 1980). Similarly, acute administration of the general irreversible opioid antagonist, β-chlornaltrexamine reduces spontaneous food intake and body weight over 2–4 days (Gosnell *et al.*, 1987).

Table 1 Reduction in spontaneous food intake and body weight following acute or chronic administration of selective opioid receptor subtype antagonists

Receptor subtype	Antagonist	Acute intake change (%)	Acute weight change (%)	Chronic weight change (%)
μ	β-FNA	41*	7*	9*
μ_1	Naloxonazine	32*	7*	11*
δ_1	DALCE	n.s.	5*	7*
δ_2	NTII	—	—	6*
κ_1	Nor-BNI	54†	3*	n.s.
κ_2	LY255582	50*	3*	n.s.

*$P < 0.05$; n.s., not significant.
†2-h intake measurement; all others after 24 h.
References: Simone et al., (1985), Mann et al., (1988), Arjune and Bodnar (1990), Arjune et al. (1990, 1991), Levine et al. (1991a), Cole et al. (1995).

2.1 Mu receptors and spontaneous intake

It appears that μ, κ and δ receptors are each involved in spontaneous food intake and control of body weight (Table 1). Acute central administration of the μ antagonist β-FNA produces a short-term (2–6 h) increase and longer-term (24–48 h) decrease in spontaneous food intake, which corresponds with its short-acting κ agonist and longer-term irreversible μ antagonist properties (Ukai and Holtzman, 1988a; Arjune et al., 1990). Indeed, β-FNA's short-acting hyperphagia is blocked by κ receptor antagonism (Arjune et al., 1990). Whereas acute administration of β-FNA concomitantly reduces body weight between 24 and 72 h (Arjune et al., 1990), chronic administration reduces body weight and food intake over 11 days (Cole et al., 1995). Similarly, both systemic and central administration of the μ_1 antagonist naloxonazine reduces spontaneous intake after 24 h following acute administration, reduces intake and weight following chronic administration in adult rats, and significantly reduces the rate of body weight gain of adolescent rats in a stage of dynamic growth (Simone et al., 1985; Mann et al., 1988; Cole et al., 1995).

2.2 Delta receptors and spontaneous intake

In contrast, centrally administered DALCE produces a short-term (2–10 h) increase in food intake without altering longer-term (24–72 h) intake, corresponding with the respective δ_1 agonist and antagonist properties of the analogue (Arjune et al., 1991). However, DALCE significantly reduces body weight following either acute (Arjune et al., 1991) or chronic (Cole et al., 1995) administration. Central administration of the δ_2-selective antagonist NTII significantly reduces spontaneous intake and body weight following acute and chronic administration (Cole et al., 1995).

2.3   Kappa receptors and spontaneous intake

Central administration of the κ_1 antagonist Nor-BNI significantly reduces nocturnal intake and body weight following acute administration, but fails to alter body weight significantly following chronic administration (Arjune and Bodnar, 1990; Cole et al., 1995). Central administration of the κ_2 antagonist LY255582 displays an identical pattern of effects on spontaneous intake and body weight as Nor-BNI (Shaw et al., 1990, 1991; Levine et al., 1991b). Thus, while all opioid receptor subtype antagonists reduce body weight following acute administration, selective μ and δ antagonists appear to have more persistent effects following chronic treatment.

3   Intake following food deprivation

3.1   Opioid antagonists and food deprivation

It appears that μ antagonists are typically the most potent in reducing the compensatory intake response following food deprivation (Table 2). The μ antagonist β-FNA significantly reduced deprivation-induced intake by 42–50%, exerting effects for up to 4 h following food reintroduction across studies (Arjune et al., 1990; Levine et al., 1991a; Koch and Bodnar, 1994). Similarly, the μ_1 antagonist naloxonazine significantly reduced deprivation-induced intake following systemic (34%; Simone et al., 1985) or central (47–75%; Koch and Bodnar, 1994) administration. In contrast, central administration of the κ_1 antagonist Nor-BNI produced a marginally significant (28%) reduction in deprivation-induced intake (Levine et al., 1990). Neither the δ antagonist naltrindole nor the δ_1 antagonist DALCE altered food intake in deprived animals following central administration (Arjune et al., 1991; Koch and Bodnar, 1994). In assessing intracerebral sites of action for these deprivation effects, it appears that both β-FNA and Nor-BNI significantly reduce

Table 2   Reduction in food intake and macronutrient choice following selective opioid receptor subtype antagonists in deprived rats

Receptor subtype	Antagonist	Total change (%)	Carbohydrate change (%)	Fat change (%)
μ	β-FNA	42–50*	53*	38*
μ_1	Naloxonazine	34–75*	46–92*	52–62*
κ_1	Nor-BNI	28*	n.s.	n.s.
δ	Naltrindole	n.s.	n.s.	n.s.
δ_1	DALCE	n.s.	n.s.	n.s.

$*P < 0.05$; n.s., not significant.
References: Simone et al. (1985), Arjune et al. (1990, 1991), Levine et al. (1990, 1991b), Koch and Bodnar (1994).

deprivation-induced intake following microinjection into either the hypothalamic paraventricular nucleus (PVN) or nucleus accumbens (Bless and
Kelley, 1994; Koch et al., 1995).

3.2 Macronutrient or preference effects?

Two hypotheses have been advanced to explain the nutritive mechanism by
which the endogenous opioid system modulates food consumption: (a) selective modulation of fat intake (e.g. Marks-Kaufman and Kanarek, 1980, 1981,
1990; Marks-Kaufman et al., 1985); and (b) altered intake of the macronutrient
that the animal prefers (Gosnell et al., 1990; Gosnell and Krahn, 1992, 1993).
To assess the two hypotheses, one must determine not only whether specific
macronutrients are reduced by specific antagonists in a given ingestive situation, but also whether such reductions co-vary with the animal's baseline
preference in that ingestive situation. Following the work of Gosnell's laboratory in evaluating these questions for morphine hyperphagia (Gosnell et al.,
1990; Gosnell and Krahn, 1992, 1993), our laboratory (Koch and Bodnar,
1994) first established the intake preferences for carbohydrate, fat and protein
under spontaneous intake conditions and compared changes in preferences
following either food deprivation or 2-deoxy-D-glucose hyperphagia (see
Section 4). Whereas only protein preference was significantly reduced in
deprived rats relative to spontaneous intake, glucoprivic rats displayed a
significant increase in carbohydrate preference and a significant decrease in fat
preference relative to spontaneous intake. In evaluating these hypotheses in
terms of selective opioid antagonist effects upon deprivation-induced intake
(Table 2), β-FNA and naloxonazine each significantly reduced overall carbohydrate and fat intake, but not protein intake in deprived rats (Koch and
Bodnar, 1994). To determine antagonist-induced shifts in preferences in
deprived rats, carbohydrate preference and fat preference were used as
covariates relative to the overall antagonist alterations. Both carbohydrate and
fat preference significantly increased the amount of explained variance for both
μ and μ_1 antagonist effects upon deprivation-induced intake. In contrast,
neither κ_1, δ nor δ_1 antagonists significantly altered intake of specific macronutrients in deprived rats and were not affected by preference covariance. This
strongly suggests that the potent effects of selective μ and μ_1 antagonists on
macronutrient intake in deprived rats are better explained by the hypothesis
that opioids alter the macronutrient that the animals prefer rather than having
a selective action on fat intake.

4 Glucoprivic feeding

Glucoprivic feeding has been studied using administration of either insulin
(e.g. Booth and Brookover, 1968; Booth, 1972), which produces both intracellular and extracellular hypoglycaemia, or the antimetabolic glucose

analogue, 2-deoxy-D-glucose (2DG; e.g. Smith and Epstein, 1969), which produces intracellular, but not extracellular, hypoglycaemia. These two gluco-privic responses have been dissociated from each other on the basis of lesion and vagotomy effects (e.g. Booth, 1972; Sclafani et al., 1975; Walsh and Grossman, 1975; Rowland and Engle, 1978). General opioid antagonists are far more effective and potent in reducing 2DG-induced compared with insulin-induced hyperphagia (Lowy et al., 1980; Levine and Morley, 1981; Ostrowski et al., 1981; Rowland and Bartness, 1982). A similar pattern of potency differences in reducing the two glucoprivic responses is observed following administration of selective opioid antagonists, as well as differences in the relative participation of specific subtypes in each glucoprivic response.

4.1 Mu receptors and glucoprivation

The μ antagonist β-FNA significantly reduces both 2DG- and insulin-induced hyperphagia (Table 3; Arjune et al., 1990; Beczkowska and Bodnar, 1991; Koch and Bodnar, 1994). The more pronounced reductions in 2DG-induced hyperphagia by β-FNA were due to a decline in both carbohydrate and fat intake, but not in protein intake (Koch and Bodnar, 1994). Again, carbo-hydrate and fat preference used as covariates significantly increased the amount of explained variance for β-FNA's effects on 2DG-induced intake, indicating a μ action in altering the macronutrient that the animal prefers in glucoprivic rats. In contrast, the μ_1-selective antagonist naloxonazine failed to alter either 2DG-induced (Simone et al., 1985) or insulin-induced (Becz-kowska and Bodnar, 1991) hyperphagia, and failed significantly to alter either carbohydrate or fat intake in 2DG-pretreated rats (Koch and Bodnar, 1994). Thus, unlike spontaneous or deprivation intake conditions under which μ and μ_1 antagonists were equieffective, the respective ability of β-FNA ($\mu_1 + \mu_2$) and inability of naloxonazine (μ_1) to affect both forms of glucoprivic hyperphagia strongly suggests that the μ_2 opioid receptor subtype modulates both gluco-

Table 3 Reduction in food intake and macronutrient choice following selective opioid receptor subtype antagonists in glucoprivic rats

Receptor subtype	Antagonist	Insulin total change (%)	2DG total change (%)	2DG carbohydrate change (%)	2DG fat change (%)
μ	β-FNA	40–54*	58–90*	51*	63–89*
μ_1	Naloxonazine	n.s.	n.s.	n.s.	n.s.
κ_1	Nor-BNI	n.s.	40–68*	n.s.	51–88*
δ_1	DALCE	n.s.	n.s.	n.s.	n.s.

*$P < 0.05$; n.s., not significant.
References: Simone et al. (1985), Arjune and Bodnar (1990), Arjune et al. (1990, 1991), Beczkowska and Bodnar (1991), Koch and Bodnar (1994).

privic ingestive responses. Evaluation of intracerebral loci of action indicates that β-FNA microinjected into either the PVN or nucleus accumbens reduces 2DG-induced hyperphagia (Koch et al., 1995).

4.2 Kappa and delta receptors and glucoprivation

The κ_1 antagonist Nor-BNI potently and significantly reduces 2DG-induced hyperphagia (Arjune and Bodnar, 1990; Koch and Bodnar, 1994), yet fails to alter insulin hyperphagia (Beczkowska and Bodnar, 1991) (Table 3). The reductions in 2DG-induced hyperphagia by Nor-BNI are due to selective reductions in fat intake (Koch and Bodnar, 1994). Thus, it appears that κ_1-mediated effects on macronutrient intake in glucoprivic rats are better explained by the hypothesis that opioids selectively alter fat intake. Again, evaluation of intracerebral loci of action indicates that Nor-BNI microinjected into either the PVN or nucleus accumbens reduces 2DG-induced hyperphagia (Koch et al., 1995). Finally, δ_1 antagonism with DALCE fails to alter either 2DG- or insulin-induced hyperphagia, or either carbohydrate or fat intake, in 2DG-pretreated rats (Arjune et al., 1991; Beczkowska and Bodnar, 1991; Koch and Bodnar, 1994).

5   Palatable and stress-induced intake

5.1 Opioid antagonists and high fat intake

The first part of this section will review selective opioid antagonist effects on the increased intake of a high-fat diet in spontaneously feeding rats (e.g. Sclafani, 1978). General opioid antagonists reduce intake of a high-fat diet (Cooper et al., 1985; Islam and Bodnar, 1990), and opioids have been implicated in modulating food intake by selectively affecting fat intake (Marks-Kaufman and Kanarek, 1980, 1981, 1990; Marks-Kaufman et al., 1985). The μ antagonist β-FNA significantly reduces intake of a high-fat diet, while the μ_1 antagonist naloxonazine is ineffective, suggesting a role for the μ_2 opioid-binding site in this ingestive response (Table 4; Islam and Bodnar, 1990). The κ_1 receptor antagonist Nor-BNI also significantly reduces intake of a high-fat diet (Arjune and Bodnar, 1990), while neither δ (ICI174864; Arjune and Bodnar, 1990) nor δ_1 (DALCE; Arjune et al., 1991) receptor antagonists are effective.

5.2 Mu receptors and palatability

Increased spontaneous intake has been observed for liquids containing either simple sugars (e.g. sucrose; Ackroff and Sclafani, 1988; Ramirez, 1990), complex carbohydrates (e.g. maltose dextrin, Polycose: Sclafani, 1987; Ramirez, 1990) or artificial sweeteners (e.g. saccharin). The opioid system

Table 4 Reduction in palatable intake and stress-induced intake following selective
opioid receptor subtype antagonists

Receptor subtype	Antagonist	High fat intake change (%)	Sucrose intake change (%)	Saccharin intake change (%)	MD intake change (%)	TP intake change (%)
μ	β-FNA	37*	34*	n.s.	39–44*	28*
μ_1	Naloxonazine	n.s.	n.s.	n.s.	n.s.	32*
κ_1	Nor-BNI	33–79*	55*	n.s.	n.s.	n.s.
δ_1	DALCE	n.s.	n.s.	61†	n.s.	n.s.
δ	ICI174864	n.s.	—	—	—	—
	Naltrindole	—	n.s.	75–94*	n.s.	n.s.

*$P < 0.05$; n.s., not significant.
†Effect was transitory (5 min).
MD, maltose dextrin; TP, tail pinch.
References: Simone *et al.* (1985), Arjune and Bodnar (1990), Arjune *et al.* (1990, 1991),
Beczkowska and Bodnar (1991), Koch and Bodnar (1993), Koch and Bodnar (1994).

appears to mediate each of these ingestive responses since general opioid
antagonists produce reduced intake (e.g. LeMagnen *et al.*, 1980; Cooper, 1983;
Siviy and Reid, 1983; Lynch, 1986; Beczkowska *et al.*, 1992). Indeed, centrally
administered general antagonists are quite potent, as measured by the dose
necessary to produce a 40% inhibition of intake (ID_{40}): sucrose (ID_{40} 6 nmol),
maltose dextrin (ID_{40} 25 nmol) and saccharin (ID_{40} 29 nmol). Further, general
opioid antagonists appear to act by interfering with the maintenance rather
than the initiation of intake (e.g. Kirkham and Blundell, 1984). The μ
antagonist β-FNA significantly reduces sucrose and maltose dextrin intake, but
not that of saccharin (Table 4; Beczkowska *et al.*, 1992, 1993). Like general
antagonists, β-FNA displays delayed effects, suggesting interference with meal
maintenance. However, β-FNA is far less potent than naltrexone in inhibiting
sucrose ($ID_{40} = 508$ nmol) and maltose dextrin ($ID_{40} = 763$ nmol). These data
suggest that μ receptor antagonism of simple and complex carbohydrate intake
may be altering intake *per se*, and not the hedonic qualities associated with the
ingesta. It appears that the μ_2 opioid binding site was responsible for these
actions since the μ_1 antagonist naloxonazine failed to alter either sucrose,
maltose dextrin or saccharin intake (Beczkowska *et al.*, 1992, 1993).

5.3 Kappa receptors and palatability

The κ_1 receptor antagonist Nor-BNI selectively and significantly reduces
sucrose intake, but not that of saccharin or maltose dextrin (Table 4; Beczkowska *et al.*, 1992, 1993). Again, Nor-BNI's effects are delayed, suggesting
interference with meal maintenance. Interestingly, the potency of κ_1 antagon-

ist effects on sucrose intake (ID_{40} 4 nmol) is comparable to that observed for general opioid antagonism, an effect in keeping with a κ-mediated role in palatability (Morley *et al.*, 1982, 1985; Cooper *et al.*, 1985; Levine *et al.*, 1985). However, the potent ability of Nor-BNI to reduce high-fat or sucrose intake is tempered by its inability to alter either saccharin or maltose dextrin intake, suggesting that κ_1-mediated effects may be limited to certain classes of palatable ingesta.

5.4 Delta receptors and palatability

δ and, to a lesser degree, δ_1 antagonists also exerted selective effects on palatable intake in that they significantly reduced saccharin, but not sucrose or maltose dextrin, intake (Table 4; Beczkowska *et al.*, 1992, 1993). However, the potency of naltrindole's effects on saccharin intake (ID_{40} = 60 nmol) was threefold less than the observed for naltrexone. Further, naltrindole's inhibition of saccharin intake was immediate, a temporal profile different from that of other general and specific antagonists. Given the non-nutritive characteristics of saccharin, it suggests that δ antagonist effects may be acting through an indirect modulatory role on ingestion, possibly altering the orosensory characteristics of the tastant.

5.5 Opioid antagonists and sham intake

To analyse whether selective opioid antagonist effects upon palatable (e.g. sucrose) intake are due to alterations in orosensory characteristics or in postingestive effects, the sham-feeding preparation can be employed to minimize the influence of gastric and intestinal factors normally leading to satiation (Young *et al.*, 1974; Weingarten and Watson, 1982). General opioid antagonists significantly and stereospecifically reduce sucrose intake in sham-feeding rats (Rockwood and Reid, 1982; Kirkham and Cooper, 1988a,b). Sucrose intake in sham-feeding rats is significantly reduced by β-FNA (44%) and Nor-BNI (62%), but not by naloxonazine, naltrindole or DALCE (Leventhal *et al.*, 1995). The reductions in sham sucrose intake of a 20% solution by μ and κ antagonism were similar in pattern and magnitude to diluting sucrose concentration from 20% to 10% in untreated sham-feeding rats. Since both intact and sham-feeding rats shared identical patterns of specificity, magnitudes and potencies of opioid effects, this suggests that central μ and κ antagonism acts on orosensory mechanisms supporting sucrose intake.

5.6 Opioid antagonists and sodium chloride

Rats will also ingest dilute sodium chloride solutions as a function of the solute concentration (e.g. Fregly *et al.*, 1965; Khavari, 1970), and increased intake will occur following water deprivation. Whereas systemic naloxone reduces saline intake at both hypotonic (0.6%) and hypertonic (1.7%) concentrations in deprived rats (Cooper and Gilbert, 1984), central naloxone reduced hypotonic saline intake only in deprived rats (Gosnell and Majchrzak, 1990). In assessing selective opioid receptor subtype antagonist effects on saline and water intake in a two-bottle choice situation in water-deprived rats (Bodnar *et al.*, 1995), neigher hypotonic nor hypertonic saline intake was affected by either μ, μ_1, κ_1, δ or δ_1 antagonists. The integrity of saline drinking was preserved despite the fact that μ (β-FNA, 53%) and κ (Nor-BNI, 31%) antagonists significantly reduced water intake. Thus, it appears that no specific opioid receptor subtype is primarily responsible for the general antagonist reduction in saline intake, suggesting that combinations of these receptor subtypes may be responsible for this modulation.

5.7   Opioid antagonists and stress intake

The hyperphagic response following tail-pinch stress (e.g. Antelman and Szechtman, 1975) is reduced by administration of general opioid antagonists (Lowy *et al.*, 1980; Morley and Levine, 1980; Bertiere *et al.*, 1984; but see Antelman and Rowland, 1981). Tail-pinch stress is significantly reduced by either reversible (CTOP; Hawkins *et al.*, 1992) μ antagonists in the substantia nigra or irreversible (β-FNA; Koch and Bodnar, 1993) μ antagonists administered into the ventricles (Table 4). Further, the μ_1 antagonist naloxonazine also significantly reduces tail-pinch feeding. In contrast, neither κ_1, δ nor δ_1 antagonism significantly affects tail-pinch feeding. It should be noted that this form of tail-pinch feeding is only marginally affected by general, μ and μ_1 antagonists, suggesting that the endogenous opioid system plays a less significant role in this ingestive response than for the other responses described above.

6   Water intake under challenge situations

Water intake is increased under a variety of situations, including water deprivation and administration of hypertonic saline (e.g. Fitzsimons, 1961), angiotensin II (ANG II; e.g. Epstein *et al.*, 1970) or the β-adrenergic receptor agonist isoproterenol (e.g. Gutman *et al.*, 1971; Houpt and Epstein, 1971). General opioid antagonists are capable of significantly reducing water intake following water deprivation (e.g. Maickel *et al.*, 1977; Brown and Holtzman, 1979) or administration of hypertonic saline (Brown and Holtzman, 1980; Brown *et al.*, 1980; Czech and Stein, 1980), ANG II (Ostrowski *et al.*, 1981; Rowland, 1982) and isoproterenol (Brown and Holtzman, 1981; Wilson *et al.*, 1984). Analysis of selective opioid receptor subtype antagonist effects on these different water intake challenge situations reveals differential modulation of the antagonists as a function of the challenge (Table 5). Thus, the μ antagonist β-FNA significantly reduces water intake following either water deprivation,

Table 5 Reduction in water intake under challenge situations following selective opioid receptor subtype antagonists

Receptor subtype	Antagonist	Water deprivation change (%)	Hypertonic saline change (%)	Angiotensin change (%)	Isoproterenol change (%)
μ	β-FNA	50*	n.s.	62*	77*
μ_1	Naloxonazine	n.s.	n.s.	n.s.	n.s.
κ_1	Nor-BNI	n.s.	66*	70*	100*
δ_1	DALCE	n.s.	n.s.	50*	100*
δ	Naltrindole	n.s.	n.s.	n.s.	—

*$P < 0.05$; n.s., not significant.
References: Beczkowska et al. (1992), Glass et al. (1994), Ruegg et al. (1994).

ANG II administration or isoproterenol administration, but only transiently altered hyperdipsia induced by hypertonic saline administration (Beczkowska et al., 1992; Glass et al., 1994; Ruegg et al., 1994). In contrast, the μ_1 antagonist naloxonazine fails to alter any of these hyperdipsic responses, indicating that μ mediation of hyperdipsic challenges acts through the μ_2 opioid binding site. The κ_1 receptor antagonist Nor-BNI significantly reduces water intake following administration of hypertonic saline, ANG II or isoproterenol, but fails significantly to alter deprivation-induced water intake (Beczkowska et al., 1992; Glass et al., 1994; Ruegg et al., 1994). Finally, the δ_1 antagonist DALCE, but not the δ antagonist naltrindole, significantly reduces hyperdipsia induced by ANG II or isoproterenol, suggesting δ_1, but not δ_2, mediation of these water-intake responses. In contrast, neither δ antagonist altered water intake following either water deprivation or hypertonic saline administration (Beczkowska et al., 1992; Glass et al., 1994; Ruegg et al., 1994).

Thus, different fluid challenges activate different subsets of opioid receptor subtypes. Water deprivation is significantly reduced by μ but not μ_1, κ_1, δ or δ_1 antagonists (Beczkowska et al., 1992), suggesting that the μ_2 site is implicated in this hyperdipsic challenge, and parallels effects observed for food deprivation. Hyperdipsia following hypertonic saline administration is significantly reduced by κ_1 but not by μ, μ_1, δ or δ_1 antagonists (Ruegg et al., 1994), suggesting that the κ_1 site is implicated in this hyperdipsic challenge, and parallels the role of κ agonists in stimulating spontaneous water intake (Sanger and McCarthy, 1981; Ukai and Holtzman, 1988b). The hyperdipsic responses following either ANG II or isoproterenol administration were each significantly reduced by either μ, κ_1 or δ_1 antagonists, but not μ_1 or δ_2 antagonists (Glass et al., 1994; Ruegg et al., 1994), indicating that multiple, yet specific, opioid receptor subtypes participate in these responses. Interestingly, isoproterenol drinking is thought to be mediated through the ANG II system, based on the effects of nephrectomy (e.g. Houpt and Epstein, 1971, Rettig et al.,

1981), ANG II-converting enzyme inhibition (e.g. Katovich *et al.*, 1979) and lesions placed in either the subfornical organ (Simpson and Routtenberg, 1975; Hubbard *et al.*, 1989), anteroventral third ventricle (e.g. Buggy and Johnson, 1978; Lind and Johnson, 1981), lateral parabrachial nucleus (Ohman and Johnson, 1986) or dorsal hindbrain (Edwards and Ritter, 1982). Thus, the parallels of the efficaciousness of different opioid receptor subtype antagonists upon ANG II and isoproterenol drinking further reinforces the common pathways that these two dipsogens utilize. In contrast, hyperdipsia following hypertonic saline is not affected by ANG II antagonists (Fregly and Rowland, 1992), and lesion studies indicate dissociations between drinking induced by either hypertonic saline or ANG II (for review see Ramsay and Thrasher, 1990). Dissociations in the pattern of opioid receptor subtype mediation between these two dipsogenic responses further reinforce the different pathways that they utilize to produce drinking.

7 Summary

This chapter has highlighted a series of interesting differences in the involvement of different opioid receptor subtypes across different ingestive situations. Such data are summarized as a function of the effects of each receptor antagonist across ingestive responses (Table 6).

μ_1 receptor antagonism with either β-FNA or CTOP significantly reduces spontaneous intake and body weight, deprivation-induced feeding, glucoprivic feeding induced by either 2DG or insulin, high-fat intake, sucrose and maltose dextrin intake, tail-pinch feeding, and drinking following water deprivation or administration of ANG II or isoproterenol. These μ antagonists fail to alter either saccharin or water intake following hypertonic saline administration. The μ-mediated effects follow a pattern, suggesting modulation of weight maintenance and regulatory challenges rather than the palatable or hedonic qualities of ingesta.

μ_1 receptor antagonism with naloxonazine significantly reduces spontaneous intake and body weight, and deprivation-induced and tail-pinch feeding. Naloxonazine fails to alter either type of glucoprivic feeding, high-fat intake, sucrose, maltose dextrin or saccharin intake, or drinking following water deprivation or administration of hypertonic saline, ANG II or isoproterenol. These data highlight the important distinctions between μ_1 and μ_2 binding sites in opioid modulation of intake.

κ_1 receptor antagonism with Nor-BNI significantly reduces spontaneous intake, 2DG hyperphagia, high-fat intake, sucrose intake and drinking following administration of hypertonic saline, ANG II or isoproterenol. Nor-BNI marginally affects deprivation-induced feeding and body weight, and fails to alter insulin hyperphagia, maltose dextrin or saccharin intake, or drinking following water deprivation. The less pronounced effects of κ_1 antagonists on deprivation and weight control is in keeping with a proposed role for the κ

Table 6 Summary of opioid receptor subtype antagonist reductions as a function of ingestive situations

Ingestive situation	Opioid receptor subtype antagonist					
	β-FNA (μ)(%)	Naloxonazine (μ_1)(%)	Nor-BNI (κ_1)(%)	Naltrindole (δ)(%)	DALCE (δ_1)(%)	NTII (δ_2)(%)
Spontaneous feeding						
Intake	41*	32*	54*	n.s.	n.s.	—
Weight	9*	11*	n.s.	—	7*	6*
Deprivation feeding						
Overall	50*	75*	28*	n.s.	n.s.	n.s.
Carbohydrate	53*	92*	n.s.	n.s.	n.s.	—
Fat	38*	62*	n.s.	n.s.	n.s.	—
Glucoprivic feeding						
Insulin overall	54*	n.s.	n.s.	—	n.s.	—
2DG overall	90*	n.s.	68*	n.s.	n.s.	—
2DG carbohydrate	51*	n.s.	n.s.	n.s.	n.s.	—
2DG fat	89*	n.s.	88*	n.s.	n.s.	—
Palatable or stress feeding						
High fat	37*	n.s.	79*	n.s.	n.s.	—
Sucrose	34*	n.s.	55*	n.s.	n.s.	—
Saccharin	n.s.	n.s.	n.s.	94*	n.s.	—
Maltose dextrin	44*	n.s.	n.s.	n.s.	n.s.	—
Tail pinch	28*	32*	n.s.	n.s.	n.s.	—
Drinking challenges						
Water deprivation	50*	n.s.	n.s.	n.s.	n.s.	—
Hypertonic saline	n.s.	n.s.	66*	n.s.	n.s.	—
Angiotensin II	62*	n.s.	70*	n.s.	50*	—
Isoproterenol	77*	n.s.	100*	—	100*	—

*$P < 0.05$; n.s., not significant.

receptor in palatability, but its selective effects suggest that it may mediate only certain subclasses of palatable ingesta.

Receptor antagonism with LY255582 significantly reduces spontaneous intake but not body weight over longer periods. The recent association of this antagonist with the κ_2 site has precluded further study of the extent of its ingestive effects.

Antagonism with naltrindole or ICI174864 significantly reduces saccharin intake, but fails to affect many of the other ingestive responses. The short actions of these antagonists necessitate analysis of the irreversible and more selective δ_1 and δ_2 antagonists.

Antagonism with DALCE significantly reduces chronic spontaneous intake and body weight, as well as drinking following administration of ANG II or isoproterenol. Its ineffectiveness in all of the other ingestive situations suggests a limited role for this receptor subtype in ingestive processes.

Antagonism with NTII significantly reduces chronic spontaneous intake and body weight, but its recent association with the δ_2 site has precluded further study.

Acknowledgements

This research was supported by a NIH-NIDA grant (DA04194). I thank the following former and present graduate students and postdoctoral fellows for their valuable contributions to this work: Dr Dulmanie Arjune, Dr Iwona Beczkowska, Jessica Cole, Michael Glass, Dr Anita Islam, Dr Jim Koch, Liza Leventhal, Dr Phyllis Mann, Hildegard Ruegg and Dr Don Simone.

References

Ackroff, K. and Sclafani, A. (1988). Sucrose-induced hyperphagia and obesity in rats fed a macronutrient self-selection diet. *Physiol. Behav.* **44**, 181–187.

Akil, H., Watson, S. J., Young, E., Lewis, M. E., Khachaturian, H. and Walker, J. M. (1984). Endogenous opioids: biology and function. *Annu. Rev. Neurosci.* **7**, 223–255.

Antelman, S. M. and Rowland, N. (1981). Endogenous opiates and stress-induced feeding. *Science* **214**, 1149.

Antelman, S. M. and Szechtman, H. (1975). Tail pinch induces eating in sated rats which appears to depend on nigrostriatal dopamine. *Science* **189**, 731–733.

Arjune, D. and Bodnar, R. J. (1990). Suppression of nocturnal, palatable and glucoprivic intake in rats by the κ opioid antagonist, nor-binaltorphamine. *Brain Res.* **534**, 313–316.

Arjune, D., Standifer, K. M., Pasternak, G. W. and Bodnar, R. J. (1990). Reduction by central β-funaltrexamine of food intake in rats under freely-feeding, deprivation and glucoprivic conditions. *Brain Res.* **535**, 101–109.

Arjune, D., Bowen, W. D. and Bodnar, R. J. (1991). Ingestive behavior following central [D-Ala2, Leu5, Cys6]-enkephalin (DALCE), a short-acting agonist and long-acting antagonist at the δ opioid receptor. *Pharmacol. Biochem. Behav.* **39**, 429–436.

Beczkowska, I. W. and Bodnar, R. J. (1991). Mediation of insulin hyperphagia by specific central opiate receptor antagonists. *Brain Res.* **547**, 315–318.

Beczkowska, I. W., Bowen, W. D. and Bodnar, R. J. (1992). Central opioid receptor subtype antagonists differentially alter sucrose and deprivation-induced water intake in rats. *Brain Res.* **589**, 291–301.

Beczkowska, I. W., Koch, J. E., Bostock, M. E., Leibowitz, S. F. and Bodnar, R. J. (1993). Central opioid receptor subtype antagonists differentially reduce intake of saccharin and maltose dextrin solutions in rats. *Brain Res.* **618**, 261–270.

Bertiere, M. C., Mame Sy, T., Baigts, F., Mandenoff, A. and Apfelbaum, M. (1984). Stress and sucrose hyperphagia: role of endogenous opiates. *Pharmacol. Biochem. Behav.* **20**, 675–679.

Bless, E. P. and Kelley, A. E. (1994). Differential effects of μ, δ and κ opiate receptor blockade in the nucleus accumbens on feeding behavior. *Soc. Neurosci. Abstr.* **20**, 382.

Bodnar, R. J., Glass, M. J. and Koch, J. E. (1995). Analysis of central opioid receptor subtype antagonism of hypotonic and hypertonic saline intake in water-deprived rats. *Brain Res. Bull.* **36**, 293–300.

Booth, D. A. (1972). Modulation of the feeding response to peripheral insulin, 2-deoxy-D-glucose or 3-O-methoxy-glucose injections. *Physiol. Behav.* **8**, 1066–1076.

Booth, D. A. and Brookover, T. (1968). Hunger elicited in the rat by a single injection of bovine crystalline insulin. *Physiol. Behav.* **3**, 439–446.

Bowen, W. D., Hellewell, S. B., Kelemen, M., Huey, R. and Steward, D. (1987). Affinity labelling of δ-opiate receptors using [D-Ala-2, Leu-5, Cys-6]-enkephalin: covalent attachment via thiosulfide exchange. *J. Biol. Chem.* **262**, 13 434–13 439.

Brown, D. R. and Holtzman, S. J. (1979). Suppression of deprivation induced food and water intake in rats and mice by naloxone. *Pharmacol. Biochem. Behav.* **11**, 567–583.

Brown, D. R. and Holtzman, S. G. (1980). Evidence that opiate receptors mediate suppression of hypertonic saline-induced drinking in the mouse by narcotic antagonists. *Life Sci.* **26**, 1543–1550.

Brown, D. R. and Holtzman, S. G. (1981). Opiate antagonists: central sites of action in suppressing water intake of the rat. *Brain Res.* **221**, 432–436.

Brown, D. R., Blank, M. S. and Holtzman, S. G. (1980). Suppression by naloxone of water intake induced by deprivation and hypertonic saline in intact and hypophysectomized rats. *Life Sci.* **26**, 1535–1542.

Buggy, J. and Johnson, A. K. (1978). Angiotensin-induced thirst: effects of third ventricle obstruction and periventricular ablation. *Brain Res.* **149**, 117–128.

Clark, J. A., Liu, L., Price, M., Hersh, B., Edelson, M. and Pasternak, G. W. (1989). Kappa opiate receptor multiplicity: evidence for two U50,488H-sensitive K-1 subtypes and a novel K-3 subtype. *J. Pharmacol. Exp. Ther.* **251**, 461–468.

Cole, J. L., Leventhal, L., Pasternak, G. W., Bowen, W. D. and Bodnar, R. J. (1995). Reductions in body weight following chronic central opioid receptor subtype antagonists during development of dietary obesity in rats. *Brain Res.* **678**, 168–176.

Cooper, S. J. (1980). Naloxone: effects on food and water consumption in the non-deprived and deprived rat. *Psychopharmacology* **71**, 1–6.

Cooper, S. J. (1983). Effects of opiate agonists and antagonists on fluid intake and saccharin choice in the rat. *Neuropharmacology* **22**, 323–328.

Cooper, S. J. and Gilbert, D. B. (1984). Naloxone suppresses fluid consumption in tests of choice between sodium chloride solutions and water in male and female water-deprived rats. *Psychopharmacology* **84**, 362–367.

Cooper, S. J. and Kirkham, T. C. (1992). Opioid mechanisms in the control of food consumption and taste preferences. In *Handbook of Experimental Pharmacology* (A. Herz, H. Akil and E. Simon, eds), pp. 239–262. Springer, Berlin.

Cooper, S. J., Jackson, A., Morgan, R. and Carter, R. (1985). Evidence for opiate receptor involvement in the consumption of a high palatability diet in non-deprived rats. *Neuropeptides* **5**, 345–348.

Czech, D. A. and Stein, E. A. (1980). Naloxone suppresses osmoregulatory drinking in rats. *Pharmacol. Biochem. Behav.* **12**, 987–989.

Edwards, G. L. and Ritter, R. C. (1982). Area postrema lesions increase drinking to angiotensin and extracellular dehydration. *Physiol. Behav.* **29**, 943–947.

Epstein, A. N., Fitzsimons, J. P. and Rolls, B. J. (1970). Drinking induced by injection of angiotensin into the brain of the rat. *J. Physiol. (Lond.)* **210**, 457–474.

Fitzsimons, J. T. (1961). Drinking by nephrectomized rats injected with various substances. *J. Physiol. (Lond.)* **155**, 563–579.

Fregly, M. J. and Rowland, N. E. (1992). Effect of DuP 753, a nonpeptide angiotensin II receptor antagonist, on the drinking responses to acutely administered dipsogenic agents in rats. *Proc. Soc. Exp. Biol. Med.* **199**, 158–164.

Fregly, M. J., Harper, J. M. and Radford, E. P. (1965). Regulation of sodium chloride intake by rats. *Am. J. Physiol.* **209**, 287–292.

Frenk, H. and Rogers, G. H. (1979). The suppressant effects of naloxone on food and water intake in the rat. *Behav. Neural. Biol.* **26**, 23–40.

Glass, M. J., Hahn, B., Joseph, A. and Bodnar, R. J. (1994). Central opioid receptor subtype mediation of isoproterenol-induced drinking in rats. *Brain Res.* **657**, 310–314.

Gosnell, B. A. and Krahn, D. D. (1992). The effects of continuous naltrexone infusions on diet preferences are modulated by adaptation to the diets. *Physiol. Behav.* **51**, 239–244.

Gosnell, B. A. and Krahn, D. D. (1993). The effects of chronic morphine infusion on diet selection and body weight. *Physiol. Behav.* **54**, 853–859.

Gosnell, B. A. and Majchrzak, M. J. (1990). Effects of a selective μ opioid receptor agonist and naloxone on the intake of sodium chloride solutions. *Psychopharmacology* **100**, 66–71.

Gosnell, B. A., Grace, M. and Levine, A. S. (1987). Effects of β-chlornaltrexamine on food intake, body weight and opioid-induced feeding. *Life Sci.* **40**, 1459–1467.

Gosnell, B. A., Krahn, D. D. and Majchrzak, M. J. (1990). The effects of morphine on diet selection are dependent upon baseline diet preferences. *Pharmacol. Biochem. Behav.* **37**, 207–212.

Gulya, K., Pelton, J. T., Hruby, V. J. and Yamamura, H. I. (1986). Cyclic somatostatin octapeptide analogues with high affinity and selectivity towards μ opioid receptors. *Life Sci.* **38**, 2221–2229.

Gutman, Y., Benzakein, F. and Livneh, P. (1971). Polydipsia induced by isoprenaline and by lithium: relation to kidneys and renin. *Eur. J. Pharmacol.* **16**, 380–384.

Hahn, E. F., Carroll-Buatti, M. and Pasternak, G. W. (1982). Irreversible opiate agonists and antagonists: the 14-hydroxydihydromorphinone azines. *J. Neurosci.* **2**, 572–576.

Hawkins, M. F., Cubic, B., Baumeister, A. A. and Bartin, C. (1992). Microinjection of opioid antagonists into the substantia nigra reduces stress-induced eating in rats. *Brain Res.* **584**, 261–265.

Hazum, E., Chang, K. J., Cuatrescasas, P. and Pasternak, G. W. (1981). Naloxazone irreversibility inhibits the high-affinity binding of $[I^{125}]$-$[D\text{-Ala}^2\text{-}D\text{-Leu}^5]$-enkephalin. *Life Sci.* **28**, 2973–2979.

Holtzman, S. J. (1974). Behavioral effects of separate and combined administration of naloxone and D-amphetamine. *J. Pharmacol. Exp. Ther.* **189**, 51–60.

Houpt, K. A. and Epstein, A. N. (1971). The complete dependence of β-adrenergic drinking on the renal dipsogen. *Physiol. Behav.* **7**, 897–902.

Hubbard, J. I., Lin, N. and Sibbald, J. R. (1989). Subfornical organ lesions in rats abolish hyperdipsic effects of isoproterenol and serotonin. *Brain Res. Bull.* **23**, 41–45.

Islam, A. K. and Bodnar, R. J. (1990). Selective opioid receptor antagonist effects upon intake of a high-fat diet in rats. *Brain Res.* **508**, 293–296.

Itzhak, Y. and Pasternak, G. W. (1987). Interaction of [D-Ser^2, Leu^5]-enkephalin-Thr^6 (DSLET), a relatively selective δ ligand, with μ_1 opioid binding sites. *Life Sci.* **40**, 307–311.

Jiang, Q., Takemori, A. E., Sultana, M., Portoghese, P. S., Bowen, W. D., Mosberg, H. I. and Porreca, F. (1991). Differential antagonism of opioid δ antinociception by [D-Ala^2, Leu^5, Cys^6]-enkephalin (DALCE) and naltrindole 5'-isothiocyanate (5'-NTII): evidence for δ receptor subtypes. *J. Pharmacol. Exp. Ther.* **257**, 1069–1075.

Katovich, M. J., Barney, C. C., Fregly, M. J. and McCaa, R. E. (1979). Effect of an angiotensin converting enzyme inhibitor (SQ 14 225) on β-adrenergic and angiotensin-induced thirsts. *Eur. J. Pharmacol.* **56**, 123–130.

Khavari, K. (1970). Some parameters of sucrose and saline ingestion. *Physiol. Behav.* **5**, 663–666.

Kirkham, T. C. and Blundell, J. E. (1984). Dual action of naloxone on feeding revealed by behavioral analysis: separate effects on initiation and termination of eating. *Appetite* **5**, 45–52.

Kirkham, T. C. and Cooper, S. J. (1988a). Attenuation of sham feeding by naltrexone is stereospecific: evidence for opioid mediation of orosensory reward. *Physiol. Behav.* **43**, 845–847.

Kirkham, T. C. and Cooper, S. J. (1988b). Naloxone attenuation of sham feeding is modified by manipulation of sucrose concentration. *Physiol. Behav.* **44**, 491–494.

Koch, J. E. and Bodnar, R. J. (1993). Involvement of mu-1 and mu-2 opioid receptor subtypes in tail-pinch feeding in rats. *Physiol. Behav.* **53**, 603–605.

Koch, J. E. and Bodnar, R. J. (1994). Selective alterations in macronutrient intake of food-deprived or glucoprivic rats by centrally-administered opioid receptor subtype antagonists in rats. *Brain Res.* **657**, 191–201.

Koch, J. E., Glass, M. J., Cooper, M. L. and Bodnar, R. J. (1995). Alterations in deprivation, glucoprivic and sucrose intake following general, μ and κ opioid antagonists in the hypothalamic paraventricular nucleus of rats. *Neurosci.* **66**, 951–957.

Leibowitz, S. F. (1987). Opioid, α-2-noradrenergic and adrenocorticotropin systems of hypothalamic paraventricular nucleus. In *Perspectives on Behavioral Medicine* (A. Baum, ed.), pp. 113–136. Lawrence Erlbaum, New Jersey.

LeMagnen, J., Marfaing-Jallat, P., Micelli, D. and Devos, M. (1980). Pain modulating and reward systems: a single brain mechanism. *Pharmacol. Biochem. Behav.* **12**, 729–733.

Leventhal, L., Kirkham, T. C., Cole, J. L. and Bodnar, R. J. (1995). Selective actions of central μ and κ opioid antagonists upon sucrose intake in sham-feeding rats. *Brain Res.* **685**, 205–210.

Levine, A. S. and Morley, J. E. (1981). Peptidergic control of insulin-induced feeding. *Peptides* **2**, 261–264.

Levine, A. S., Morley, J. E., Gosnell, B. A., Billington, C. J. and Bartness, T. J. (1985). Opioids and consummatory behavior. *Brain Res. Bull.* **14**, 663–672.

Levine, A. S., Grace, M., Billington, C. J. and Portoghese, P. S. (1990). Norbinaltorphamine decreases deprivation and opioid-induced feeding. *Brain Res.* **534**, 60–64.

Levine, A. S., Grace, M. and Billington, C. J. (1991a). B-funaltrexamine (B-FNA) decreases deprivation and opioid-induced feeding. *Brain Res.* **562**, 281–284.

Levine, A. S., Grace, M., Billington, C. J. and Zimmerman, D. M. (1991b). Central administration of the opioid antagonist LY255582 decreases short- and long-term food intake in rats. *Brain Res.* **566**, 193–197.

Lind, R. W. and Johnson, A. K. (1981). Periventricular preoptic–hypothalamic lesions: effects on isoproterenol-induced thirst. *Pharmacol. Biochem. Behav.* **15**, 563–565.

Lord, J. A. H., Waterfield, A. A., Hughes, J. and Kosterlitz, H. (1977). Endogenous opioid peptides: multiple agonists and receptors. *Nature* **267**, 495–499.

Lowy, M. T., Maickel, R. P. and Yim, G. K. W. (1980). Naloxone reduction of stress-related feeding. *Life Sci.* **26**, 2113–2118.

Lynch, W. C. (1986). Opiate blockade inhibits saccharin intake and blocks normal preference acquisition. *Pharmacol. Biochem. Behav.* **24**, 833–836.

Maickel, R. P., Braude, M. C. and Zabik, J. E. (1977). The effects of various narcotic agonists and antagonists on deprivation-induced fluid consumption. *Neuropharmacology,* **16**, 863–866.

Mann, P. E., Pasternak, G. W., Hahn, E. F., Curreri, G., Lubin, E. and Bodnar, R. J. (1988). Comparison of chronic naloxone and naloxonazine effects upon food intake and body weight maintenance in rats. *Neuropharmacology* **27**, 349–355.

Marks-Kaufman, R. and Kanarek, R. (1980). Morphine selectively influences macronutrient intake in the rat. *Pharmacol. Biochem. Behav.* **12**, 427–430.

Marks-Kaufman, R. and Kanarek, R. (1981). Modifications of nutrient selection by naloxone in rats. *Psychopharmacology* **74**, 321–324.

Marks-Kaufman, R. and Kanarek, R. (1990). Diet selection following a chronic morphine and naloxone regimen. *Pharmacol. Biochem. Behav.* **35**, 665–669.

Marks-Kaufman, R., Plager, A. and Kanarek, R. (1985). Central and peripheral contributions of endogenous opioid systems to nutrient selection in rats. *Psychopharmacology* **85**, 414–418.

Martin, W. R., Eades, C. G., Thompson, J. A., Huppler, R. E. and Gilbert, P. E. (1976). The effects of morphine- and nalorphine-like drugs in the nondependent and morphine-dependent chronic spinal dog. *J. Pharmacol. Exp. Ther.* **197**, 517–532.

Mattia, A., Vanderah, T., Mosberg, H. I. and Porreca, F. (1991). Lack of antinociceptive cross-tolerance between [D-Pen^2, D-Pen^5]-enkephalin and [D-Ala^2]-deltorphan II in mice: evidence for δ receptor subtypes. *J. Pharmacol. Exp. Ther.* **258**, 583–587.

Mattia, A., Farmer, S. C., Takemori, A. E., Sultana, M., Portoghese, P. S., Mosberg, H. I., Bowen, W. D. and Porreca, F. (1992). Spinal opioid δ antinociception in the mouse: mediation by a 5′-NTII-sensitive δ receptor subtype. *J. Pharmacol. Exp. Ther.* **260**, 518–525.

Morley, J. E. and Levine, A. S. (1980). Stress-induced eating is mediated through endogenous opiates. *Science* **209**, 1259–1261.

Morley, J. E., Levine, A. S., Grace, M. and Kneip, J. (1982). An investigation of the role of κ opiate receptors in the initiation of feeding. *Life Sci.* **31**, 2617–2626.

Morley, J. E., Levine, A. S., Yim, G. K. W. and Lowy, M. T. (1983). Opioid modulation of appetite. *Neurosci. Biobehav. Rev.* **7**, 281–305.

Morley, J. E., Levine, A. S., Kneip, J., Grace, M., Zeugner, H. and Shearman, G. T. (1985). The κ opioid receptor and food intake. *Eur. J. Pharmacol.* **112**, 17–25.

Negri, L., Potenza, R. L., Corsi, R. and Melchiorri, P. (1991). Evidence for two subtypes of δ receptors in rat brain. *Eur. J. Pharmacol.* **196**, 335–336.

Nock, B., Rajpara, A., O'Connor, L. H. and Cicero, T. J. (1988). [3-H]-U69593 labels a subtype of opiate receptor with characteristics different from that labelled by [3-H]-ethylketocyclazocine. *Life Sci.* **42**, 2403–2412.

Ohman, L. E. and Johnson, A. K. (1986). Lesions in the lateral parabrachial nucleus enhance drinking to angiotensin II and isoproterenol. *Am. J. Physiol.* **251**, R504–R509.

Ostrowski, N. L., Rowland, N., Foley, T. L., Nelson, J. L. and Reid, L. D. (1981). Morphine antagonists and consummatory behaviors. *Pharmacol. Biochem. Behav.* **14**, 549–559.

Pasternak, G. W. and Wood, P. L. (1986). Multiple μ opiate receptors. *Life Sci.* **38**, 1889–1896.

Portoghese, P. S., Larson, D. L., Sayre, L. M., Fries, D. S. and Takemori, A. E. (1980). A novel opioid receptor site directed alkylating agent with irreversible narcotic antagonistic and reversible agonistic activities. *J. Med. Chem.* **23**, 233–234.

Portoghese, P. S., Lipkowski, A. W. and Takemori, A. E. (1987). Binaltorphamine and nor-binaltorphamine, potent and selective κ-opioid receptor antagonists. *Life Sci.* **40**, 1287–1292.

Portoghese, P. S., Sultana, M. and Takemori, A. E. (1990). Naltrindole 5′-isothiocyanate: a non-equilibrium, highly selective δ opioid receptor antagonist. *J. Med. Chem.* **33**, 1547–1548.

Ramirez, I. (1990). Why do sugars taste good? *Neurosci. Biobehav. Rev.* **14**, 125–134.

Ramsay, D. J. and Thrasher, T. N. (1990). Thirst and water balance. In *Handbook of Behavioral Neurobiology* (E. M. Stricker, ed.), pp. 353–386 Plenum, New York.

Rettig, R., Ganten, D. and Johnson, A. K. (1981). Isoproterenol-induced thirst: renal and extrarenal mechanisms. *Am. J. Physiol.* **241**, R152–R157.

Rockwood, G. A. and Reid, L. D. (1982). Naloxone modifies sugar–water intake in rats drinking with open gastric fistulas. *Physiol. Behav.* **29**, 1175–1178.

Rothman, R. B., Bykov, V., deCosta, B. R., Jacobson, A. E., Rice, K. C. and Brady, L. S. (1990). Interaction of endogenous opioid peptides and other drugs with four κ opioid binding sites in guinea pig brain. *Peptides* **11**, 311–331.

Rothman, R. B., Xu, H., Char, G. U., Kim, A., DeCosta, B. R., Rice, K. C. and Zimmerman, D. M. (1993). Phenylpiperidine opioid antagonists that promote weight loss in rats have high affinity for the K-2B (enkephalin-sensitive) binding site. *Peptides* **14**, 17–20.

Rowland, N. (1982). Comparison of the suppression by naloxone of water intake induced in rats by hyperosmolarity, hypovolemia and angiotensin. *Pharmacol. Biochem. Behav.* **16**, 87–91.

Rowland, N. and Bartness, T. J. (1982). Naloxone suppresses insulin-induced food intake in novel and familiar environments, but does not affect hypoglycemia. *Pharmacol. Biochem. Behav.* **16**, 1001–1003.

Rowland, N. and Engle, D. J. (1978). Hypothalamic hyperphagia prevented by prior subdiagphragmatic vagotomy: insulin hyperphagia is unaffected. *Physiol. Behav.* **21**, 685–689.

Ruegg, H., Hahn, B., Koch, J. E. and Bodnar, R. J. (1994). Differential modulation of angiotensin II and hypertonic saline-induced drinking by opioid receptor subtype antagonists in rats. *Brain Res.* **635**, 203–210.

Sanger, D. J. and McCarthy, P. S. (1981). Increased food and water intake produced by rats by opiate receptor agonists. *Psychopharmacology* **74**, 217–220.

Sclafani, A. (1978). Dietary obesity. In *Recent Advances in Obesity Research: II* (G. A. Bray, ed.), pp. 123–132. Newman, London.

Sclafani, A. (1987). Carbohydrate taste, appetite and obesity: an overview. *Neurosci. Biobehav. Rev.* **11**, 131–153.

Sclafani, A., Gale, S. K. and Springer, D. (1975). Effects of hypothalamic knife cuts on the ingestive responses to glucose and insulin. *Physiol. Behav.* **15**, 63–70.

Shaw, W. N., Mitch, C. H., Leander, J. D. and Zimmerman, D. M. (1990). Effect of phenylpiperidine opioid antagonists on food consumption and weight gain of the obese Zucker rat. *J. Pharmacol. Exp. Ther.* **253**, 85–89.

Shaw, W. N., Mitch, C. H., Leander, J. D., Mendelsohn, L. G. and Zimmerman, D. M. (1991). The effect of the opioid antagonist LY255582 on body weight of the obese Zucker rat. *Int. J. Obes.* **15**, 387–395.

Simone, D. A., Bodnar, R. J., Goldman, E. J. and Pasternak, G. W. (1985). Involvement of opioid receptor subtypes in rat feeding behavior. *Life Sci.* **36**, 829–833.

Simpson, J. B. and Routtenberg, A. (1975). Subfornical organ lesions reduce intravenous angiotensin-induced drinking. *Brain Res.* **88**, 154–161.

Siviy, S. M. and Reid, L. D. (1983). Endorphinergic modulation of acceptability of putative reinforcers. *Appetite* **4**, 249–257.

Smith, G. P. and Epstein, A. N. (1969). Increased feeding response to decreased glucose utilization in the rat and monkey. *Am. J. Physiol.* **217**, 1083–1087.

Ukai, M. and Holtzman, S. G. (1988a). Effects of β-funaltrexamine on ingestive behaviors in the rat. *Eur. J. Pharmacol.* **153**, 161–165.

Ukai, M. and Holtzman, S. G. (1988b). Effects of intrahypothalamic administration of opioid peptides selective for μ, κ and δ receptors on different schedules of water intake in rats. *Brain Res.* **459**, 275–281.

Walsh, L. L. and Grossman, S. P. (1975). Loss of feeding in response to 2-deoxy-D-glucose but not insulin after zona incerta lesions in the rat. *Physiol. Behav.* **15**, 481–485.

Weingarten, H. P. and Watson, S. D. (1982). Sham feeding as a procedure for assessing the influence of diet palatability on food intake. *Physiol. Behav.* **28**, 401–407.

Wilson, K. M., Rowland, N. and Fregly, M. J. (1984). Drinking: a final common pathway. *Appetite* **5**, 31–38.

Young, R. C., Gibbs, J., Antin, J., Holt, J. and Smith, G. P. (1974). Absence of satiety during sham-feeding in the rat. *J. Comp. Physiol. Psychol.* **87**, 795–800.

Zukin, R. S., Eghbalai, M., Olive, D., Unterwald, E. M. and Tempel, A. (1988). Characterization and visualization of rat and guinea pig brain K opioid receptors: evidence for K-1 and K-2 opioid receptors. *Proc. Natl. Acad. Sci. U S A* **85**, 4061–4065.

7

Stimulation of Ingestive Behaviour by Preferential and Selective Opioid Agonists

BLAKE A. GOSNELL[1] and ALLEN S. LEVINE[2]

[1]Department of Psychiatry, University of Wisconsin–Madison, 6001 Research Park Blvd, Madison, WI 53719, USA
[2]Departments of Psychiatry and Food Science and Nutrition, University of Minnesota, St Paul, MN 55417, and Veterans Administration Medical Center, Minneapolis, MN, USA

1 Introduction

Observations on the ability of morphine to influence ingestive behaviour preceded the identification of opioid receptors and opioid peptides in the brain (Martin et al., 1963; Pert and Snyder, 1973; Simon et al., 1973; Hughes et al., 1975). Further studies with opioid agonists and antagonists suggest that endogenous opioids participate in the regulation of ingestion. Various aspects of this role of opioids have been investigated. These include issues such as species differences, environmental variables, hormonal modulation and sites of action (for reviews see Morley et al., 1983b; Levine et al., 1985; Reid, 1985; Gosnell, 1987; Cooper et al., 1988). It is now known that there are at least three types of opioid receptors (μ, δ and κ) and a number of endogenous ligands with varying degrees of selectivity for these receptors (see Akil et al., 1984; Mansour et al., 1987). This multiplicity of opioid peptides and receptors, together with their diverse distribution within the central nervous system, suggests that they may contribute differentially to a number of physiological and behavioural processes. The primary aim of this chapter is to review reports involving the use of opioid agonists that, either directly or when compared and contrasted with other studies, address the issue of differential receptor involvement in the regulation of ingestive behaviour. A discussion of the literature with an emphasis on the effects of opioid antagonists can be found elsewhere in this volume (see Chapter 6).

Several limitations may apply to an attempt to identify the relevant receptors mediating a particular behaviour based on studies comparing the effects of

---

selectively acting drugs. In addition to differences in profiles of receptor selectivity, drugs may differ in receptor binding affinity, solubility, degradation or elimination, time course of action and the production of other effects. Differences in the relative effectiveness of opioid agonists in eliciting food intake may be due to differences in any or all of these properties. Nevertheless, an examination of the literature for consistent patterns both within and across studies may permit tentative conclusions about the receptors involved and identify areas for further study. The design of this chapter is to review, in separate sections, studies dealing primarily with systemic, intracerebroventricular and localized injections of opioid agonists.

2 Studies with systemically administered opioids

Martin *et al.* (1963) first demonstrated that food intake increased in rats after they were given daily peripheral morphine injections. Others found that chronically administered heroin, codeine and levorphanol initially decrease, then increase, feeding, resulting in an increase in daytime feeding and a shift in the usual circadian feeding pattern (Kumar *et al.*, 1971; Thornhill *et al.*, 1976, 1978). Morphine also increases feeding in non-dependent, non-food deprived rats (Sanger and McCarthy, 1980; Morley *et al.*, 1982; Lowy and Yim, 1983). In some cases, feeding induced by repeated injection of morphine and other opiates is greater than that observed after the first injection (Jalowiec *et al.*, 1981; Morley *et al.*, 1982; Thornhill and Saunders, 1983; Rudski *et al.*, 1992). This may be due to the development of tolerance to the sedative effects of opiates, thereby allowing greater manifestation of the feeding effects.

Attempts have been made to determine which opioid receptors are involved in feeding behaviour by using peripherally administered opiate agonists with selective receptor profiles. The cyclazocine compounds, thought to be partial κ ligands, increase food or milk intake during the light phase of the light–dark cycle in satiated rats (Sanger and McCarthy, 1981; Locke *et al.*, 1982; Morley *et al.*, 1982; Lowy and Yim, 1983). Tifluadom, a novel opiate with a benzo-diazepine-like structure and preferential activity at the κ opiate receptor, has been shown to increase food intake (Morley *et al.*, 1983a, 1985; Cooper *et al.*, 1985). Based on studies of the ability of various opioid antagonists to block tifluadom-induced feeding, Jackson and Sewell (1984) suggested that the effects of this agonist on feeding involved κ and/or μ receptors but not δ receptors. The mixed agonist–antagonist butorphanol tartrate and tifluadom are more potent stimulators of feeding than the cyclazocine compounds or morphine (Levine and Morley, 1983; Morley *et al.*, 1983a, 1985; Cooper *et al.*, 1985; Levine *et al.*, 1994). The more selective κ ligands such as bremazocine and U-50 488H also increase feeding after peripheral injection; the effects of bremazocine are not as strong as those of other κ agonists (Morley and Levine, 1983; Cooper *et al.*, 1985; Jackson and Cooper, 1985; Morley *et al.*, 1985). Subtypes of κ opioid receptors have been reported (Clark *et al.*, 1989), and agonists of both κ_1 (U-50 488H) and κ_3 (naloxone benzoylhydrazone) receptors have been reported to stimulate food intake (Koch et al., 1992).

Cross-tolerance studies have also been used in an attempt to dissect the effects of opioid ligands on food intake. Ligands of both the μ and κ receptors have more reliable and potent effects on feeding behaviour in rats after repeated injection. Morphine (μ) and bremazocine (κ) were used in one cross-tolerance study to evaluate receptor specificity related to food intake (Morley et al., 1985). When bremazocine was administered for 8 consecutive days, food intake subsequent to the injection on the eighth day was greater than that observed on the first day. When these rats were injected with morphine on the ninth day, intake was not increased relative to that of controls or the first bremazocine injection day. Complementary results were obtained when morphine was injected for 8 days and bremazocine on the ninth day: prior morphine injection facilitated morphine- but not bremazocine-induced hyperphagia. These studies suggest that separate subpopulations of opioid receptors may be involved in the regulation of food intake. N-allylnormetazocine (NANM), a σ receptor agonist, also increases feeding in rats after peripheral administration (Gosnell et al., 1983). Cross tolerance was measured in rats given repeated injections of NANM and then tested for feeding responses to ketocyclazocine (κ) or morphine (μ). Ketocyclazocine injections increased feeding more in NANM-experienced rats than in NANM-naive rats. However, experience with NANM failed to alter the effect of morphine on feeding.

The above studies indicate that compounds somewhat selective for the μ, σ and κ receptors increase feeding after peripheral administration. A peripherally active selective δ agonist has been synthesized (Chang et al., 1993); to our knowledge, however, the effects of this compound on food intake have not been reported. In some cases, the less selective compounds are more effective at stimulating food intake than more receptor-selective compounds. For example, butorphanol tartrate, a morphinan congener, increases short-term food intake more effectively than most other opiate–opioid agonists (Levine and Morley, 1983; Morley et al., 1983a, 1985). We originally thought that these effects of butorphanol were related to the κ opioid receptor, since butorphanol was thought to be a κ agonist. However, the current literature presents a more confusing picture of butorphanol's receptor profile. Butorphanol appears to act as an agonist or antagonist at both the κ and μ opioid receptors, depending on the assay. It partially or completely substitutes for μ agonists in drug discrimination procedures (Shannon and Holtzman, 1977; Schaefer and Holtzman, 1981; White and Holtzman, 1983; Picker and Dykstra, 1989). However, butorphanol antagonizes the analgesic effects of methadone (Dykstra, 1990) and precipitates withdrawal in morphine-dependent rats (Woods and Gmerek, 1985; Gmerek et al., 1987). It increases urination (Leander, 1982, 1983), a κ effect, and acts like other κ agents in drug-dependence studies (Woods and Gmerek, 1985). Butorphanol acts as a κ antagonist in morphine-tolerant rats by antagonizing bremazocine's (κ) rate-decreasing effects in an operant environment (Picker *et al.*, 1990). One study suggested that δ opioid receptors may be involved in mediating butorphanol dependence (Jaw *et al.*, 1993). Thus, the drug has a complex receptor profile, dependent on the type of assay used. We recently used selective opioid antagonists in an attempt to evaluate the receptor profile of butorphanol on feeding (Levine *et al.*, 1994). Intracerebroventricular injection of nor-binaltorphamine (nor-BNI) reduced the feeding effects of butorphanol (8 mg/kg subcutaneously) at doses of 1, 10 and 100 nmol at the 1–2-h time points and decreased feeding at all time points for the 10-nmol dose. The 100-nmol dose of nor-BNI decreased butorphanol-induced feeding by about 72% during the first hour of the study. In contrast, only the highest dose (50 nmol) of β-funaltrexamine (β-FNA), a selective μ antagonist, decreased butorphanol-induced feeding. The δ opioid antagonist, naltrindole, had no effect on butorphanol-induced feeding. It is also interesting to note that central administration of butorphanol did not increase feeding nearly as well as peripheral injection; this suggests that a metabolite of the drug may be involved in increasing food intake. Recently, Rudski *et al.* (1995) found that buprenorphine, which has a similar behaviour profile to butorphanol, also increased food intake. Both butorphanol and buprenorphine also increase operant-contingent food intake in satiated rats (Rudski *et al.*, 1994, 1995).

3   Studies with intracerebroventricular administration of opioids

Studies involving injections of opioids into the lateral ventricles have provided strong evidence that opioids influence feeding at a central rather than peripheral site. Such studies have not, however, identified any one receptor type as being the primary mediator of the effect. Intracerebroventricular injections of selective agonists of μ, δ and κ receptors have all been shown to cause increased food intake (Morley and Levine, 1983; Jackson and Sewell, 1985; Gosnell *et al.*, 1986a; Imura *et al.*, 1986; Robert *et al.*, 1989; Levine *et al.*, 1991). Nevertheless, there are some differences in the time course of the feeding effects of agonists of different receptor types. The effects of κ and δ agonists tend to occur sooner than those of μ agonists, possibly due to the sedative effects of μ agonists (e.g. Levine *et al.*, 1991). This difference has also been observed after systemic and localized microinjection of opioids (e.g. Morley *et al.*, 1982; Tepperman and Hirst, 1983; Bakshi and Kelley, 1993b). It is also interesting to note that, in some cases, injection of the preferential κ agonist dynorphin caused postural asymmetries and 'barrel-rolling' (Herman *et al.*, 1980; Walker *et al.*, 1980; Gosnell *et al.*, 1986a). Furthermore, there is some evidence that dynorphin is rapidly broken down into a fragment that produces non-opioid effects (Walker *et al.*, 1982; Young *et al.*, 1987). As mentioned in the introduction, such differences may limit the use of direct comparisons of the feeding effects of agonists to make inferences regarding the receptor types involved. A role for κ receptors in the regulation of food intake is still indicated by the effectiveness of non-peptide selective κ agonists when injected peripherally or intracerebroventricularly.

Levine and co-workers (1990) evaluated the effect of the κ antagonist, norbinaltorphamine (nor-BNI) on deprivation and opioid-induced feeding. Central (intracerebroventricular) injection of nor-BNI (100 nmol) decreased deprivation-induced feeding in a relatively weak fashion (maximum decrease 28%). However, nor-BNI (1, 10 and 100 nmol) decreased feeding induced by the κ ligand U-50 488H by about 85% during the first hour of the study. Nor-BNI also decreased feeding induced by the preferential δ agonist [D-Ser^2]-leucine enkephalin-Thr (DSLET) and the selective μ agonist [D-Ala^2,N-Me-Phe^4,Gly^5-ol]-enkephalin (DAMGO). If one assumes that nor-BNI is a highly selective κ antagonist, it appears that not only κ but also δ- and μ-induced feeding are dependent on an active κ opioid receptor. Recent evidence, however, has called into question the receptor selectivity of nor-BNI. Spanagel *et al.* (1994) have reported that repeated injection of nor-BNI (twice daily for 10 days) blocked the antinociceptive effects of μ, δ and κ ligands. However, only the κ effects were long lasting, affecting the analgesia produced by the κ ligand U69593 for 20 days. In a study similar to that involving nor-BNI, Levine *et al.* (1991) found that the selective μ antagonist β-FNA decreased deprivation induced feeding by 24–50% at doses ranging from 0.1 to 20 nmol. Central (intracerebroventricular) injection of β-FNA (0.1, 1 and 10 nmol) decreased feeding induced by the μ opioid agonist DAMGO by 57%, 60% and 71% during the 2–4-h period of a 4-h study. Feeding induced by the δ agonist, DSLET, was also decreased by pretreatment with β-FNA. However, this occurred only at the 1–2-h time point, a period when only a small amount of food was ingested. β-FNA did not attenuate feeding stimulated by U-50 488H, a κ opioid agonist. Based on such receptor antagonist studies it appears that feeding stimulated by a selective opioid agonist may involve more than one opioid receptor.

In addition to studies in which food intake was measured, several studies have examined the effects of selective opioid agonists on the intake of palatable fluids. Studies with systemic injection of morphine and naloxone indicated that opioids can increase and decrease, respectively, the intake of or preference for palatable fluids (Cooper, 1983; Siviy and Reid, 1983; Cooper and Gilbert, 1984; Czirr and Reid, 1986; Bertino *et al.*, 1988). These studies suggested that opioids may alter ingestive behaviour by enhancing the palatability or reward value of foods and fluids (see Reid, 1985; Cooper *et al.*, 1988). Gosnell and Majchrzak (1989) tested the effects of intracerebroventricular injection of selective opioid agonists on the intake of saccharin solutions. They found that the μ agonist DAMGO and the δ agonist [D-Thr^2]-leucine enkephalin-Thr (DTLET) caused an increase in intake, but that the κ agonist U-50 488H had no effect. Similar effects were observed when rats were required to press a lever (fixed ratio-1 schedule) to obtain the solution (Gosnell and Patel, 1993). μ and δ agonists were also more effective than κ agonists in increasing the intake of sodium chloride solutions (Gosnell and Majchrzak, 1990; Gosnell *et al.*, 1990). These studies contrast with the effects of κ agonists on food intake (see above) and the observation that subcutaneous administration of U-50 488H increased the intake of a sucrose solution (Lynch and Burns, 1990). The pattern of results, however, is similar to that observed when selective agonists are injected into specific regions of the brain (see below).

4 Studies with localized injections of opioids

The effects of intracerebroventricular injections of opioid agonists and antagonists provide strong support for a central site of action for their effects on feeding. However, they can provide little indication of the specific neural structures involved. Microinjection studies have provided a clearer picture of the sites at which opioids may act to modulate feeding. A number of sites have been investigated; naturally, those sites that had previously been identified as playing a role in the mediation of taste, feeding and/or reward have received the most attention. In the following section, we discuss the sites that have received the most attention and/or those for which some indication of a differential involvement of μ, δ and κ receptors is suggested. A summary of the results of studies dealing with five major injection sites is presented in Table 1.

4.1 Hypothalamus

Given the accepted role of the hypothalamus in the regulation of a number of behaviours linked to homoeostasis, it is not surprising that this structure has received considerable attention in studies on the role of opioids in feeding. Grandison and Guidotti (1977) reported in a preliminary note that injections of β-endorphin (a μ–δ agonist) into the ventromedial hypothalamus (VMH) stimulated feeding in satiated rats. Since this report, several studies have reported increased feeding after injection of a number of opioid agonists. Tepperman and Hirst (1982) reported that morphine and levorphanol stimulated intake after injection into the VMH. Equivalent doses (in nmol) of dextrorphan, the κ agonist ketocyclazocine, and the σ agonist phencyclidine were ineffective. These results indicated a role for μ receptors in the VMH in the regulation of feeding. In a subsequent paper (Tepperman and Hirst, 1983) the feeding effects of morphine were compared with those of the preferential δ agonist [D-Ala^2,D-Leu^5] enkephalin (DADLE). The authors concluded that DADLE was more potent than morphine and that δ receptors in the VMH may also contribute to the control of food intake. On the other hand, Gosnell *et al.* (1986b) found that VMH injection of dynorphin stimulated food intake, whereas similar doses of DADLE or β-endorphin were ineffective. Thus, a role for κ receptors was suggested. It should be noted that negative results have also been reported for VMH injections of morphine, [D-Ala^2]Met-enkephalin-amide (DALA) and MR2034 (Woods and Leibowitz, 1985; Stanley *et al.*,

1989). Conflicting results regarding the effects of morphine may possibly be explained by differences in dose and/or the type of diet used: doses of 2.7–10.6 nmol stimulated the intake of standard lab chow (Tepperman *et al.*, 1981; Tepperman and Hirst 1982, 1983), whereas injection of 25 nmol did not increase the intake of a sweetened mash diet (Woods and Leibowitz, 1985; Stanley *et al.*, 1989).

These studies suggest that the feeding effects of peripherally administered opioids may be due in part to their action at opioid receptors in the VMH. Further, the effects of opioid antagonists injected into the VMH suggests that endogenous opioid activity in this area may be involved in the regulation of food intake (Thornhill and Saunders, 1984; Woods and Leibowitz, 1985; Gosnell *et al.*, 1986b). However, conflicting data and the lack of information on the effects of more selective agonists do not permit any statements to be made about the relative roles of the various receptors in the VMH in relation to feeding.

The paraventricular nucleus (PVN) of the hypothalamus is also thought to be involved in the regulation of food intake (Gold *et al.*, 1977; Leibowitz and Hor, 1982). Agonists of all three opioid receptor types have been reported to stimulate food intake when injected into the PVN. These include the μ agonist morphine, the preferential δ agonists DALA and DADLE, the κ agonist dynorphin and the μ–δ agonist β-endorphin (see Table 1). Injections of dynorphin or DAMGO into a region just posterior to the PVN was also effective in stimulating food intake (Gosnell, 1988). McLean and Hoebel (1983) reported that injections of DALA and morphine into the PVN stimulated food intake. Although the effects of DALA appeared sooner after injection than those of morphine, the minimum effective dose of morphine (0.1 μg, 0.15 nmol) was less than that of DALA (2 μg, 3.4 nmol). In a study of water intake (food not available during the test). Ukai and Holtzman (1988) reported that PVN injection of DAMGO tended to increase water intake in non-deprived rats, whereas selective κ and δ agonists had no effect. Gosnell and colleagues (1986b) reported that PVN injection of dynorphin stimulated food intake, whereas equivalent doses (1.5–1.7 nmol) of β-endorphin or DADLE were ineffective. However, Leibowitz and Hor (1982) did observe a significant increase in food intake after a 1-nmol injection of β-endorphin into the PVN. As with the VMH, then, it is difficult at this point to rule out any of the opioid receptors from being involved in the regulation of feeding in the PVN.

Other hypothalamic sites that have been examined in relation to opioid-induced feeding include the perifornical area, the lateral hypothalamus and the dorsomedial nucleus. Stanley *et al.* (1989) reported that morphine and DALA stimulated food intake when injected into the latter two areas but not into the perifornical area. Woods and Leibowitz (1985), however, found that morphine did stimulate intake when injected into the perifornical area. Naloxone injection into this area caused a reduction in intake, whereas no effect was observed after injection into the dorsomedial nucleus (Woods and Leibowitz,

Table 1   Effects of site-specific injection of opioid agonists on ingestive behaviour

Effective	Ineffective	Bilateral or unilateral	Reference
Ventromedial hypothalamic nucleus			
β-Endorphin (1.46 nmol)		Unilateral	Grandison and Guidotti (1977)
Morphine (2.7 nmol)		Unilateral	Tepperman et al. (1981)
Morphine (5.3 nmol)	Ketocyclazocine (5.3 nmol) Phencyclidine (5.3 nmol)	Unilateral	Tepperman and Hirst (1982)
DADLE (0.7 nmol) Morphine (5.3 nmol)		Unilateral	Tepperman and Hirst (1983)
	Morphine (25 nmol)	Unilateral	Woods and Leibowitz (1985)
Dynorphin A (1.63 nmol)	β-Endorphin (1.43 nmol) DADLE (1.75–4.39 nmol)	Unilateral	Gosnell et al. (1986b)
	Morphine (25 nmol) DALA (6.8 nmol) MR2034 (8.6 nmol)	Unilateral	Stanley et al. (1989)
Paraventricular hypothalamic nucleus			
β-Endorphin (1 nmol)		Unilateral	Leibowitz and Hor (1982)
Morphine (0.15 nmol) DALA (3.4 nmol)		Unilateral	McLean and Hoebel (1983)
Morphine (1.56 nmol)		Unilateral	Woods and Leibowitz (1985)
Dynorphin A (0.47 nmol) DADLE (4.39 nmol)	β-Endorphin (1.43 nmol)	Unilateral	Gosnell et al. (1986b)
Dynorphin A (2 nmol) DAMGO (2 nmol)		Unilateral	Gosnell (1988)
Morphine (25 nmol) DALA (6.8 nmol)	MR2034 (8.6 nmol)	Unilateral	Stanley et al. (1989)
Amygdala			
DAMGO (1 nmol)	Dynorphin A (0.3–3 nmol) DSLET (0.3–3 nmol)	Unilateral	Gosnell (1988)
Morphine (25 nmol) DALA (6.8 nmol)	MR2034 (8.6 nmol)	Unilateral	Stanley et al. (1989)

Continued

Table 1 *Continued*

Effective	Ineffective	Bilateral or unilateral	Reference
Ventral tegmental area			
Morphine (0.1 nmol)		Bilateral	Mucha and Iverson (1986)
Morphine (8 nmol)[a]		Unilateral	Jenck *et al.* (1987b)
DPDPE (8 nmol)[a]			
U-50 488H (8 nmol)[a]			
Dynorphin 1–13 (0.3 pmol)[b]		Unilateral	Hamilton and Bozarth (1988)
Morphine (3 nmol)[b]			
	Morphine (25 nmol)	Unilateral	Stanley *et al.* (1989)
	DALA (6.8 nmol)		
	MR2034 (8.6 nmol)		
Morphine (1 nmol)	U-50 488H (10 pmol to 10 nmol)	Bilateral	Nencini and Stewart (1990)
Morphine (10 nmol)[c]	U-50 488H (0.1–10 nmol)	Unilateral	Noel and Wise (1993)
DAMGO (0.1 nmol)[c]		Unilateral	Noel and Wise (1995)
DPDPE (10 nmol)[c]			
DAMGO (0.01–0.1 nmol)[d]	DPDPE (0.1–10 nmol)	Unilateral	Badiani *et al.* (1995)
	U-50 488H (0.1–10 nmol)		
Nucleus accumbens			
Morphine (0.1 nmol)		Bilateral	Mucha and Iverson (1986)
Morphine (2 nmol)	U-50 488H (2–100 nmol)	Bilateral	Majeed *et al.* (1986)
DADLE (2 nmol)	Bremazocine (2–100 nmol)		
DPDPE (2 nmol)			
β-Endorphin (2 nmol)			
α-Neo-endorphin (5 nmol)			
Dynorphin (10 nmol)			
Morphine (1.5 nmol)		Bilateral	Evans and Vaccarino (1990)
Morphine (0.75 nmol)		Bilateral	Bakshi and Kelley (1993a)
DAMGO (4 nmol)	U-50 488H (0.4–8 nmol)	Bilateral	Bakshi and Kelley (1993b)
DPDPE (4 nmol)			

Doses in parentheses refer to the lowest dose reported to cause a significant increase in food intake, unless noted otherwise. See text for full names of abbreviated compounds.
[a]Significant effect was a facilitation of lateral hypothalamic electrical stimulation-induced feeding.
[b]Significant effect was an increased time spent eating in a 15-min trial.
[c]Significant effect was an increase in eating speed in a series of short test sessions.
[d]Significant effects were an increase in time spent eating and number of feeding bouts, and a decreased latency to start feeding.

1985). Thornhill and Saunders (1984) reported reduced lever pressing for food after naloxone injection into the lateral hypothalamus of food-deprived rats; Gosnell *et al.* (1986b) did not observe this effect in a free-feeding test after food deprivation.

To summarize, studies of the role of the hypothalamus have dealt primarily with the PVN and the VMH. Preferential or selective agonists of μ, δ and κ receptors have been found to cause an increase in feeding when injected into these nuclei, and injections of antagonists cause a decrease in feeding.

4.2 Amygdala

The amygdala is another structure that is thought to play a role in the control of food intake. Nuclei within the amygdala project to regions of the hypothalamus considered important in the control of feeding, and lesions and electrical stimulation of the amygdala are known to affect food and water intake (Grossman and Grossman, 1963; Krettek and Price, 1978; Berk and Finkelstein). In electrophysiological studies, Nakano *et al.* (1986) identified feeding-related neurons in the amygdala of the monkey that were morphine sensitive. Stanley *et al.* (1989) found that amygdalar injections of morphine or DALA caused an increase in food intake, whereas the agonist MR2034 was ineffective. Gosnell (1988) reported that injection of the selective μ agonist DAMGO into the central nucleus of the amygdala caused a naloxone-reversible increase in food intake. Injections of dynorphin and DSLET (preferential κ and δ agonists, respectively) were without effect. The apparent ineffectiveness of δ and κ agonists contrasts with effects observed after injection into the hypothalamus, where a role for all three receptor types has been proposed (see above).

4.3 Parabrachial nucleus

The parabrachial nucleus (PBN), at least in the rat, receives gustatory input from the nucleus of the solitary tract (Norgren, 1977). In light of the possibility that opioids may influence ingestive behaviour through an influence on palatability, this nucleus is a potential site of action for the effects of opioids on ingestive behaviour. Evoked responses of taste-sensitive neurons in the PBN were found to be morphine sensitive (Hermann and Novin, 1980). Few studies, however, have examined this area in relation to opioid-induced feeding. The threshold for eliciting feeding through electrical stimulation of the lateral hypothalamus has been shown to be opioid sensitive, and Carr *et al.* (1991) reported that injection of naloxone into the PBN increased this threshold. The κ antagonist nor-BNI, however, did not. They suggest that μ receptors in the PBN may contribute to the regulation of feeding. In contrast to the typical observation of an increase in saccharin intake or preference after opioid treatments, Moufid-Bellancourt and Velley (1994) reported that injection of morphine into the PBN caused a decrease in saccharin preference. Further, they found that ibotenic acid lesions of the lateral hypothalamus eliminated the baseline preference for saccharin and caused an increased saccharin preference in response to PBN morphine injections. Additional studies will be required to investigate this possible lateral hypothalamus–PBN interaction in more detail and to reconcile the finding of a morphine-induced decrease in saccharin preference with the more numerous reports of opioid-induced increases in saccharin preference (see above).

4.4 Nucleus accumbens and ventral tegmental area

The ventral tegmental area (VTA) has received considerable attention in studies on the neural mechanisms of drug reinforcement. This area contains cell bodies of dopaminergic neurons that project to a number of brain regions, including the nucleus accumbens, the amygdala and the medial prefrontal cortex (see Oades and Halliday, 1987). Activation of these neurons, and the subsequent increase in extracellular dopamine in the nucleus accumbens, is associated with the reinforcing effects of a number of drugs of abuse (see Wise, 1987, 1989; Di Chiara et al., 1992). Furthermore, this neural pathway may be involved in mediating the reinforcing effects of food, water and saccharin (Wise, 1987, 1989; Hernandez and Hoebel, 1988; Mark et al., 1991; Yoshida et al., 1992). As mentioned above, it is thought that opioids enhance palatability or the rewarding value of food. The VTA, therefore, and structures associated with it are potentially the neural structures mediating the effects of opioids on feeding.

Morphine injection into the VTA produced an increase in food intake, and naloxone injection decreased the intake of a sweetened solution (Mucha and Iverson, 1986; Segall and Margules, 1989). Noel and Wise (1993, 1995) found that VTA injections of morphine, DAMGO and the selective δ agonist [D-Pen^{2,5}]enkephalin (DPDPE) increased eating speed in food-deprived rats; the κ agonist U-50 488H had no significant effect. Similarly, Nencini and Stewart (1990) observed that VTA injections of morphine but not of U-50 488H increased food intake in non-deprived rats. On the other hand, Stanley et al. (1989) found no significant effects of VTA injections of DALA, morphine or MR2034 on food intake. Badiani et al. (1995) tested the effects of VTA opioid injections under a number of conditions. In 15-min test sessions in novel test cages, VTA injection of DAMGO increased the amount of time rats spent eating, increased the number of feeding bouts, and decreased the latency to begin feeding. Injections of U-50 488H and DPDPE had no significant effect. When objects in addition to food (balsa wood and a drinking spout) were present in the test cages, DAMGO caused an increase in the amount of time spent gnawing. The authors suggest that the effects of DAMGO may reflect a 'general activation of mouthing behavior directed towards incentive stimuli' (p. 273). When rats were tested in an apparatus in which they were required to enter a tunnel to gain access to food, VTA injection of DAMGO had no effect on feeding behaviour.

In contrast to the lack of effect of VTA injections of the κ agonist U-50 488H on feeding behaviour, Hamilton and Bozarth (1988) reported that VTA injections of dynorphin (1–13) (a preferential κ ligand) were much more potent than morphine in eliciting feeding in satiated rats. The discrepancy between this finding and the lack of effect of U-50 488H may be due to the hunger status of the animals at the time of testing, to the testing procedures or to the non-opioid effects of dynorphin or fragments of dynorphin (Walker et al., 1982; Young et al., 1987). Whereas Hamilton and Bozarth (1988) measured the time spent eating in a 15-min test session, Nencini and Stewart (1990) measured the amount of food consumed in 5-h tests, and Noel and Wise (1993) measured the speed of eating a given amount of food (five 45-mg pellets) in a series of 36-s test sessions. With procedures similar to those of Hamilton and Bozarth (1988) (measurement of free-feeding behaviour of non-deprived rats in a 15-min period), Badiani et al. (1995) found no significant effects of U-50 488H on feeding behaviour. Clearly, additional studies will be necessary to determine the precise role of the VTA in opioid-mediated feeding and the types of receptors involved.

Jenck et al. (1987b) used another approach in their investigation of the role of opioids in the VTA in relation to feeding. Electrical stimulation of the hypothalamus was used to induce feeding. VTA injection of μ, δ and κ agonists was found to facilitate this stimulation-induced feeding, as reflected by a reduction in the minimum stimulation frequency required to stimulate the intake of a small amount of food within a certain amount of time. In a separate report, Jenck et al. (1987a) measured the effects of VTA opioid injections on electrical self-stimulation of the lateral hypothalamus. Morphine and the selective δ agonist DPDPE reduced self-stimulation thresholds, whereas the κ agonist U-50 488H had no effect. Based on these results, the authors suggested that μ and δ receptors in the VTA are involved in feeding and brain stimulation reward, whereas κ receptors in this area are involved in feeding but not reward.

The nucleus accumbens is one of the primary terminal fields of dopaminergic neurons projecting from the VTA. As mentioned above, increased extracellular dopamine in the nucleus accumbens has been linked to the reinforcing effects of a number of drugs as well as that of food, water and saccharin. It is therefore a potentially important structure in mediating the postulated effect of opioids on palatability. Mucha and Iversen (1986) found that injections of morphine into the nucleus accumbens caused an increase in food intake. Additional experiments indicated that the effect was opioid receptor mediated and could be distinguished from effects on water intake. Evans and Vaccarino (1990) also injected morphine into the nucleus accumbens and observed an increase in intake. In diet-selection experiments, they found that morphine injection increased the intake of the preferred diet rather than that of a specific macronutrient. In a mapping study of the striatum in relation to morphine-induced feeding, Bakshi and Kelley (1993a) identified the nucleus accumbens and the ventromedial striatum as the sites at which injections were most effective. In a further study, Bakshi and Kelley (1993b) found that injections of the selective μ agonist DAMGO stimulated intake when injected into the nucleus accumbens, ventromedial striatum or ventrolateral striatum. The selective δ agonist DPDPE also stimulated food intake when injected into the nucleus accumbens and ventrolateral striatum; injection of the κ agonist U-50 488H had no effect. The effects of DPDPE were smaller, but occurred earlier, than those of DAMGO. These results closely resemble those of Majeed et al. (1986), who found that injections of μ and δ agonists into the nucleus accumbens was more effective in stimulating intake than κ agonists.

Self and Stein (1992) reviewed the literature on self-administration, conditioned place preference and brain stimulation reinforcement in relation to opioids. They concluded that μ and δ receptors play a role in mediating the reinforcing effects of opioids and that κ receptors do not. The pattern of effects on feeding of opioids injected into the nucleus accumbens is similar: μ and δ agonists are more effective than κ agonists. After opioid injection into the lateral ventricles or the VTA, this pattern has also been observed for dopamine release in the nucleus accumbens (Spanagel et al., 1990; Devine et al., 1993). As discussed above, μ and δ agonists, but not κ agonists, were found to increase the intake of saccharin and sodium chloride solutions. These findings are consistent with the findings of Jenck et al. (1987a, 1987b) that μ and δ but not κ agonists facilitate lateral hypothalamic brain stimulation reward, and the suggestion by Noel and Wise (1993) that κ-mediated feeding may be independent of dopaminergic mechanisms. Thus, it is possible that the ingestive behaviour induced by μ and δ agonists may be due in part to activation of the mesolimbic dopaminergic system. The use of selective blockade and/or depletion of dopamine might permit a more detailed examination of the relative involvement of dopaminergic systems in mediating the effects of μ, κ and δ opioid agonists.

5 Summary

Injection studies in which opioid agonists are used to stimulate food intake are subject to many factors, including receptor selectivity, untoward side-effects, pharmacokinetics and site of action. In spite of such problems, it seems clear that central administration of selective agonists of the μ, δ and κ receptors can increase intake of food or palatable fluids, whereas antagonists of these receptors decrease consummatory behaviour. Systemic and ventricular routes of administration of opioids do not allow an examination of the specific neural structures mediating the effects of opioids on feeding. Studies with localized injections suggest that several areas of the brain may be involved and that, within certain areas, there may be a differential participation of μ, δ and κ receptors. During the past few years, μ, δ and κ receptors have been cloned and the distribution of messenger RNA for each of these receptors has been described (Evans et al., 1992; Bzdega et al., 1993; Meng et al., 1993; Zastawny et al., 1994). Including such biochemical tools with current pharmacological, neuroanatomical and behavioural methods may lead to a more lucid understanding of the role that opioids play in regulating ingestive behaviour.

Acknowledgements

Research in the authors' laboratories has been supported by NIDA grants DA05471 (BG), DA03999 (AL) and the Department of Veterans Affairs.

References

Akil, H., Watson, S. J., Young, E., Lewis, M. E. and Khachaturian, H. (1984). Endogenous opioids: biology and function. *Annu. Rev. Neurosci.* **7**, 223–255.

Badiani, A., Leone, P., Noel, M. B. and Stewart, J. (1995). Ventral tegmental area opioid mechanisms and modulation of ingestive behavior. *Brain Res.* **670**, 264–276.

Bakshi, V. P. and Kelley, A. E. (1993a). Striatal regulation of morphine-induced hyperphagia: an anatomical mapping study. *Psychopharmacology,* **111**, 207–214.

Bakshi, V. P. and Kelley, A. E. (1993b). Feeding induced by opioid stimulation of the ventral striatum: role of opiate receptor subtypes. *J. Pharmacol. Exp. Ther.* **265**, 1253–1260.

Berk, M. L. and Finkelstein, J. A. (1981). Afferent projections to the preoptic area and hypothalamic regions in the rat brain. *Neuroscience* **6**, 1601–1624.

Bertino, M., Abelson, M. L., Marglin, S. H., Neuman, R., Burkhardt, C. A. and Reid, L. D. (1988). A small dose of morphine increases intake of and preference for isotonic saline among rats. *Pharmacol. Biochem. Behav.* **29**, 617–623.

Bzdega, T., Chin, H., Kim, H., Jung, H. H., Kozak, C. A. and Klee, W. A. (1993). Regional expression and chromosomal localization of the δ opiate receptor gene. *Proc. Natl. Acad. Sci. USA* **90**, 9305–9309.

Carr, K. D., Aleman, D. O., Bak, T. H. and Simon, E. J. (1991). Effects of parabrachial opioid antagonism on stimulation-induced feeding. *Brain Res.* **545**, 283–286.

Chang, K. J., Rigdon, G. C., Howard, J. L. and McNutt, R. W. (1993). A novel, potent and selective nonpeptidic delta opioid receptor agonist BW373U86. *J. Pharmacol. Exp. Ther.* **267**, 852–857.

Clark, J. A., Liu, L., Price, M., Hersh, B., Edelson, M. and Pasternak, G. W. (1989). Kappa opiate receptor multiplicity: evidence for two U50 488H-sensitive κ_1 subtypes and a novel κ_3 subtype. *J. Pharmacol. Exp. Ther.* **251**, 461–468.

Cooper, S. J. (1983). Effects of opiate agonists and antagonists on fluid intake and saccharin choice in the rat. *Neuropharmacology,* **22**, 323–328.

Cooper, S. J. and Gilbert, D. B. (1984). Naloxone suppresses fluid consumption in tests of choice between sodium chloride solutions and water in male and female water-deprived rats. *Psychopharmacology,* **84**, 362–367.

Cooper, S. J., Moores, W. R., Jackson, A. and Barber, D. J. (1985). Effects of tifluadom on food consumption compared with chlordiazepoxide and kappa agonists in the rat. *Neuropharmacology,* **24**, 877–883.

Cooper, S. J., Jackson, A., Kirkham, T. C. and Turkish, S. (1988). Endorphins, opiates and food intake. In *Endorphins, Opiates and Behavioural Processes* (R. J. Rodgers and S. J. Cooper, eds.), pp. 143–186. John Wiley, New York.

Czirr, S. A. and Reid, L. D. (1986). Demonstrating morphine's potentiating effects on sucrose-intake. *Brain Res. Bull.* **17**, 639–642.

Devine, D. P., Leone, P., Pocock, D. and Wise, R. A. (1993). Differential involvement of ventral tegmental *mu*, *delta* and *kappa* opioid receptors in modulation of basal mesolimbic dopamine release: *in vivo* microdialysis studies. *J. Pharmacol. Exp. Ther.* **266**, 1236–1246.

Di Chiara, G., Acquas, E. and Carboni, E. (1992). Drug motivation and abuse: a neurobiological perspective. *Ann. N. Y. Acad. Sci.* **654**, 207–219.

Dykstra, L. A. (1990). Butorphanol, levallorphan, nalbuphine and nalorphine as antagonists in the squirrel monkey. *J. Pharmacol. Exp. Ther.* **254**, 245–252.

Evans, C. J., Keith, D. E., Jr., Morrison, H., Magendzo, K. and Edwards, R. H. (1992). Cloning of a delta opioid receptor by functional expression. *Science* **258**, 1952–1955.

Evans, K. R. and Vaccarino, F. J. (1990). Amphetamine- and morphine-induced feeding: evidence for involvement of reward mechanisms. *Neurosci. Biobehav. Rev.* **14**, 9–22.

Gmerek, D. E., Dykstra, L. A. and Woods, J. H. (1987). Kappa opioids in rhesus monkeys. III. Dependence associated with chronic administration. *J. Pharmacol. Exp. Ther.* **242**, 428–436.

Gold, R. M., Jones, A. P., Sawchenko, P. E. and Kapatos, G. (1977). Paraventricular area: critical focus of a longitudinal neurocircuitry mediating food intake. *Physiol. Behav.* **18**, 1111–1119.

Gosnell, B. A. (1987). Central structures involved in opioid-induced feeding. *Fed. Proc.* **46**, 163–167.

Gosnell, B. A. (1988). Involvement of μ opioid receptors in the amygdala in the control of feeding. *Neuropharmacology,* **27**, 319–326.

Gosnell, B. A. and Majchrzak, M. J. (1989). Centrally administered opioid peptides stimulate saccharin intake in nondeprived rats. *Pharmacol. Biochem. Behav.* **33**, 805–810.

Gosnell, B. A. and Majchrzak, M. J. (1990). Effects of a selective mu opioid receptor agonist and naloxone on the intake of sodium chloride solutions. *Psychopharmacology,* **100**, 66–71.

Gosnell, B. A. and Patel, C. K. (1993). Centrally administered μ- and δ-opioid agonists increase operant responding for saccharin. *Pharmacol. Biochem. Behav.* **45**, 979–982.

Gosnell, B. A., Levine, A. S. and Morley, J. E. (1983). *N*-allylnormetazocine (SKF-10 047): the induction of feeding by a putative sigma agonist. *Pharmacol. Biochem. Behav.* **19**, 737–742.

Gosnell, B. A., Levine, A. S., Morley, J. E. (1986a). The stimulation of food intake by selective agonists of mu, kappa and delta opioid receptors. *Life Sci.* **38**, 1081–1088.

Gosnell, B. A., Morley, J. E. and Levine, A. S. (1986b). Opioid-induced feeding: localization of sensitive brain sites. *Brain Res.* **369**, 177–184.

Gosnell, B. A., Majchrzak, M. J. and Krahn, D. D. (1990). Effects of preferential delta and kappa opioid receptor agonists on the intake of hypotonic saline. *Physiol. Behav.* **47**, 601–603.

Grandison, L. and Guidotti, A. (1977). Stimulation of food intake by muscimol and β endorphin. *Neuropharmacology,* **16**, 533–536.

Grossman, S. P. and Grossman, L. (1963). Food and water intake following lesions or electrical stimulation of the amygdala. *Am. J. Physiol.* **205**, 761–765.

Hamilton, M. E. and Bozarth, M. A. (1988). Feeding elicited by dynorphin (1–13) microinjections into the ventral tegmental area in rats. *Life Sci.* **43**, 941–946.

Herman, B. H., Leslie, F. and Goldstein, A. (1980). Behavioral effects and *in vivo* degradation of intraventricularly administered dynorphin-(1–13) and D-Ala^2-dynorphin-(1–11) in rats. *Life Sci.* **27**, 883–892.

Hermann, G. and Novin, D. (1980). Morphine inhibition of parabrachial taste units reversed by naloxone. *Brain Res. Bull.* **5** (supplement 4), 169–173.

Hernandez, L. and Hoebel, B. G. (1988). Food reward and cocaine increase extracellular dopamine in the nucleus accumbens as measured by microdialysis. *Life Sci.* **42**, 1705–1712.

Hughes, J., Smith, T. W., Kosterlitz, H. W., Fothergill, L. A., Morgan, A. and Morris, H. R. (1975). Identification of two related pentapeptides from the brain with potent opiate agonist activity. *Nature* **258**, 577–579.

Imura, H., Nakao, K., Yanaihara, N., Katsuura, G. and Nakamura, M. (1986). Potent action of leumorphin on consummatory behaviors in rats: comparison with other opioid peptides. *Neuroendocrinology* **44**, 142–148.

Jackson, A. and Cooper, S. J. (1985). Effects of κ opiate agonists on palatable food consumption in non-deprived rats, with and without food preloads. *Brain Res. Bull.* **15**, 391–396.

Jackson, H. C. and Sewell, R. D. E. (1984). The role of opioid receptor sub-types in tifluadom-induced feeding. *J. Pharm. Pharmacol.* **36**, 683–686.

Jackson, H. C. and Sewell, R. D. E. (1985). Are δ-opioid receptors involved in the regulation of food and water intake? *Neuropharmacology,* **24**, 885–888.

Jalowiec, J. E., Panksepp, J., Zolovick, A. J., Najam, N. and Herman, B. H. (1981). Opioid modulation of ingestive behavior. *Pharmacol. Biochem. Behav.* **15**, 477–484.

Jaw, S. P., Hoskins, B. and Ho, I. K. (1993). Opioid antagonists and butorphanol dependence. *Pharmacol. Biochem. Behav.* **44**, 497–500.

Jenck, F., Gratton, A. and Wise, R. A. (1987a). Opioid receptor subtypes associated with ventral tegmental facilitation of lateral hypothalamic brain stimulation reward. *Brain Res.* **423**, 34–38.

Jenck, F., Quirion, R. and Wise, R. A. (1987b). Opioid receptor subtypes associated with ventral tegmental facilitation and periaqueductal gray inhibition of feeding. *Brain Res.* **423**, 39–44.

Koch, J. E., Pasternak, G. W., Arjune, D. and Bodnar, R. J. (1992). Naloxone benzoylhydrazone, a κ$_3$ opioid agonist, stimulates food intake in rats. *Brain Res.* **581**, 311–314.

Krettek, J. E. and Price, J. L. (1978). Amygdaloid projections to subcortical structures within the basal forebrain and brainstem in the rat and cat. *J. Comp. Neurol.* **178**, 225–254.

Kumar, R., Mitchell, E. and Stolerman, I. P. (1971). Disturbed patterns of behaviour in morphine tolerant and abstinent rats. *Br. J. Pharmacol.* **42**, 473–484.

Leander, J. D. (1982). A κ opioid effect: increased urination in the rat. *J. Pharmacol. Exp. Ther.* **224**, 89–94.

Leander, J. D. (1983). Evidence that nalorphine, butorphanol and oxilorphan are partial agonists at a kappa-opioid receptor. *Eur. J. Pharmacol.* **86**, 467–470.

Leibowitz, S. F. and Hor, L. (1982). Endorphinergic and α-noradrenergic systems in the paraventricular nucleus: effects on eating behavior. *Peptides* **3**, 421–428.

Levine, A. S. and Morley, J. E. (1983). Butorphanol tartrate induces feeding in rats. *Life Sci.* **32**, 781–785.

Levine, A. S., Morley, J. E., Gosnell, B. A., Billington, C. J. and Bartness, T. J. (1985). Opioids and consummatory behavior. *Brain Res. Bull.* **14**, 663–672.

Levine, A. S., Grace, M., Billington, C. J. and Portoghese, P. S. (1990). Nor-binaltorphamine decreases deprivation and opioid-induced feeding. *Brain Res.* **534**, 60–64.

Levine, A. S., Grace, M. and Billington, C. J. (1991). β-Funaltrexamine (β-FNA) decreases deprivation and opioid-induced feeding. *Brain Res.* **562**, 281–284.

Levine, A. S., Grace, M., Portoghese, P. S. and Billington, C. J. (1994). The effect of selective opioid antagonists on butorphanol-induced feeding. *Brain Res.* **637**, 242–248.

Locke, K. W., Brown, D. R. and Holtzman, S. G. (1982). Effects of opiate antagonists and putative mu- and kappa-agonists on milk intake in rat and squirrel monkey. *Pharmacol. Biochem. Behav.* **17**, 1275–1279.

Lowy, M. T. and Yim, G. K. W. (1983). Stimulation of food intake following opiate agonists in rats but not hamsters. *Psychopharmacology*, **81**, 28–32.

Lynch, W. C. and Burns, G. (1990). Opioid effects on intake of sweet solutions depend both on prior drug experience and on prior ingestive experience. *Appetite* **15**, 23–32.

Majeed, N. H., Przewlocka, B., Wedzony, K., and Przewlocki, R. (1986). Stimulation of food intake following opioid microinjection into the nucleus accumbens septi in rats. *Peptides* **7**, 711–716.

Mansour, A., Khachaturian, H., Lewis, M. E., Akil, H. and Watson, S. J. (1987). Autoradiographic differentiation of mu, delta and kappa opioid receptors in the rat forebrain and midbrain. *J. Neurosci.* **7**, 2445–2464.

McLean, S. and Hoebel, B. G. (1983). Feeding induced by opiates injected into the paraventricular hypothalamus. *Peptides* **4**, 287–292.

Mark, G. P., Blander, D. S. and Hoebel, B. G. (1991). A conditioned stimulus decreases extracellular dopamine in the nucleus accumbens after the development of a learned taste aversion. *Brain Res.* **551**, 308–310.

Martin, W. R., Wikler, A., Eades, C. G. and Pescor, F. T. (1963). Tolerance to and physical dependence on morphine in rats. *Psychopharmacologia* **4**, 247–260.

Meng, F., Xie, G.-X., Thompson, R. C., Mansour, A., Goldstein, A., Watson, S. J. and Akil, H. (1993). Cloning and pharmacological characterization of a rat κ opioid receptor. *Proc. Natl. Acad. Sci. USA* **90**, 9954–9958.

Morley, J. E. and Levine, A. S. (1983). Involvement of dynorphin and the kappa opioid receptor in feeding. *Peptides* **4**, 797–800.

Morley, J. E., Levine, A. S., Grace, M. and Kniep, J. (1982). An investigation of the role of kappa opiate receptor agonists in the initiation of feeding. *Life Sci.* **31**, 2617–2626.

Morley, J. E., Levine, A. S., Grace, M., Kniep, J. and Zeugner, H. (1983a). The effect of the opioid-benzodiazephine, tifluadom, on ingestive behaviors. *Eur. J. Pharmacol.* **93**, 265–269.

Morley, J. E., Levine, A. S., Yim, G. K. and Lowy, M. T. (1983b). Opioid modulation of appetite. *Neurosci. Biobehav. Rev.* **7**, 281–305.

Morley, J. E., Levine, A. S., Kniep, J., Grace, M., Zeugner, H. and Shearman, G. T. (1985). The κ opioid receptor and food intake. *Eur. J. Pharmacol.* **112**, 17–25.

Moufid-Bellancourt, S. and Velley, L. (1994). Effects of morphine injection into the parabrachial area on saccharin preference: modulation by lateral hypothalamic neurons. *Pharmacol. Biochem. Behav.* **48**, 127–133.

Mucha R. F. and Iversen, S. D. (1986). Increased food intake after opioid microinjections into the nucleus accumbens and ventral tegmental area of rat. *Brain Res.* **397**, 314–224.

Nakano, Y., Oomura, Y., Lenard, L., Nishino, H., Aou, S., Yamamoto, T. and Aoyagi, K. (1986). Feeding-related activity of glucose- and morphine-sensitive neurons in the monkey amygdala. *Brain Res.* **399**, 167–172.

Nencini, P. and Stewart, J. (1990). Chronic administration of amphetamine increases food intake to morphine, but not to U-50 488H, microinjected into the ventral tegmental area in rats. *Brain Res.* **527**, 254–258.

Noel, M. B. and Wise, R. A. (1993). Ventral tegmental injections of morphine but not U-50 488H enhance feeding in food-deprived rats. *Brain Res.* **632**, 68–73.

Noel, M. B. and Wise, R. A. (1995). Ventral tegmental injections of a selective μ or δ opioid enhance feeding in food-deprived rats. *Brain Res.* **673**, 304–312.

Norgren, R. (1977). A synopsis of gustatory neuroanatomy. In *Olfaction and Taste*, (J. LeMagnen and P. MacLeod, eds.), vol. 6, pp. 225–232. Information Retrieval, Washington, D.C.

Oades, R. D. and Halliday, G. M. (1987). Ventral tegmental (A10) system: neurobiology. 1. Anatomy and connectivity. *Brain Res. Rev.* **12**, 117–165.

Pert, C. B. and Snyder, S. H. (1973). Opiate receptor: demonstration in nervous tissue. *Science* **179**, 1011–1014.

Picker, M. J. and Dykstra, L. A. (1989). Discriminative stimulus effects of mu and kappa opioids in the pigeon: analysis of the effects of full and partial mu and kappa agonists. *J. Pharmacol. Exp. Ther.* **249**, 557–566.

Picker, M. J., Negus, S. S. and Craft, R. M. (1990). Butorphanol's efficacy at mu and kappa opioid receptors: inferences based on the schedule-controlled behavior of nontolerant and morphine-tolerant rats and on the responding of rats under a drug discrimination procedure. *Pharmacol. Biochem. Behav.* **36**, 563–568.

Reid, L. D. (1985). Endogenous opioid peptides and regulation of drinking and feeding. *Am. J. Clin. Nutr.* **42**, 1099–1132.

Robert, J. J., Orosco, M., Rouch, C., Jacquot, C. and Cohen, Y. (1989). Effects of opiate agonists and an antagonist on food intake and brain neurotransmitters in normophagic and obese 'cafeteria' rats. *Pharmacol. Biochem. Behav.* **34**, 577–583.

Rudski, J. M., Schaal, D. W., Thompson, T., Cleary, J., Billington, C. J. and Levine, A. S. (1992). Effects of methadone on free feeding in satiated rats. *Pharmacol. Biochem. Behav.* **43**, 1033–1037.

Rudski, J. M., Billington, C. J. and Levine, A. S. (1994). Butorphanol increases food-reinforced operant responding in satiated rats. *Pharmacol. Biochem. Behav.* **49**, 843–847.

Rudski, J. M., Thomas, D., Billington, C. J. and Levine, A. S. (1995). Buprenorphine increases intake of freely available and operant-contingent food in satiated rats. *Pharmacol. Biochem. Behav.* **50**, 271–276.

Sanger, D. J. and McCarthy, P. S. (1980). Differential effects of morphine on food and water intake in food deprived and freely-feeding rats. *Psychopharmacology*, **72**, 103–106.

Sanger, D. J. and McCarthy, P. S. (1981). Increased food and water intake produced in rats by opiate receptor agonists. *Psychopharmacology*, **74**, 217–220.

Schaefer, G. J. and Holtzman, S. G. (1981). Morphine-like stimulus effects in the monkey: opioids with antagonist properties. *Pharmacol. Biochem. Behav.* **14**, 241–245.

Segall, M. A. and Margules, D. L. (1989). Central mediation of naloxone-induced anorexia in the ventral tegmental area. *Behav. Neurosci.* **103**, 857–864.

Self, D. W. and Stein, L. (1992). Receptor subtypes in opioid and stimulant reward. *Pharmacol. Toxicol.* **70**, 87–94.

Shannon, H. E. and Holtzman, S. G. (1977). Further evaluation of the discriminative effects of morphine in the rat. *J. Pharmacol. Exp. Ther.* **201**, 55–66.

Simon, E. J., Hiller, N. M. and Edelman, I. (1973). Stereospecific binding of the potent narcotic analgesic ^{3}H-etorphine to rat brain homogenate. *Proc. Natl. Acad. Sci. USA* **70**, 1947–1949.

Siviy, S. M. and Reid, L. D. (1983). Endorphinergic modulation of acceptability of putative reinforcers. *Appetite* **4**, 249–257.

Spanagel, R., Herz, A. and Shippenberg, T. S. (1990). The effects of opioid peptides on dopamine release in the nucleus accumbens: an *in vivo* microdialysis study. *J. Neurochem.* **55**, 1734–1740.

Spanagel, R., Almeida, O. F. X. and Shippenberg, T. S. (1994). Evidence that nor-binaltorphamine can function as an antagonist at multiple opioid receptor subtypes. *Eur. J. Pharmacol.* **264**, 157–162.

Stanley, B. G., Lanthier, D. and Leibowitz, S. F. (1989). Multiple brain sites sensitive to feeding stimulation by opioid agonists: a cannula-mapping study. *Pharmacol. Biochem. Behav.* **31**, 825–832.

Tepperman, F. S. and Hirst, M. (1982). Concerning the specificity of the hypothalamic opiate receptor responsible for food intake in the rat. *Pharmacol. Biochem. Behav.* **17**, 1141–1144.

Tepperman, F. S. and Hirst, M. (1983). Effect of intrahypothalamic injection of [D-Ala^2,D-Leu^5]enkephalin on feeding and temperature in the rat. *Eur. J. Pharmacol.* **96**, 243–249.

Tepperman, F. S., Hirst, M. and Gowdey, C. W. (1981). Hypothalamic injection of morphine: feeding and temperature responses. *Life Sci.* **28**, 2459–2467.

Thornhill, J. A. and Saunders, W. S. (1983). Acute stimulation of feeding with repeated injections of morphine sulphate to non-obese and fatty Zucker rats. *Prog. Neuropsychopharmacol. Biol. Psychiatry,* **7**, 477–485.

Thornhill, J. A. and Saunders, W. (1984). Ventromedial and lateral hypothalamic injections of naloxone or naltrexone suppress the acute food intake of food-deprived rats. *Appetite* **5**, 25–30.

Thornhill, J. A., Hirst, M. and Gowdey, C. W. (1976). Disruption of diurnal feeding patterns of rats by heroin. *Pharmacol. Biochem. Behav.* **4**, 129–135.

Thornhill, J. A., Hirst, M. and Gowdey, C. W. (1978). Tolerance and evidence of physical dependence to daily codeine injections in the rat. *Pharmacol. Biochem. Behav.* **9**, 433–438.

Ukai, M. and Holtzman, S. G. (1988). Effects of intrahypothalamic administration of opioid peptides selective for μ-, κ- and δ-receptors on different schedules of water intake in the rat. *Brain Res.* **459**, 275–281.

Walker, J. M., Katz, R. J. and Akil, H. (1980). Behavioral effects of dynorphin$_{1-13}$ in the mouse and rat: initial observations. *Peptides* **1**, 341–345.

Walker, J. M., Moises, H. C., Coy, D. H., Baldrighi, G. and Akil, H. (1982). Nonopiate effects of dynorphin and des-Tyr-dynorphin. *Science* **218**, 1136–1138.

White, J. M. and Holtzman, S. G. (1983). Further characterization of the three-choice morphine, cyclazocine and saline discrimination paradigm: opioids with agonist and antagonist properties. *J. Pharmacol. Exp. Ther.* **224**, 95–99.

Wise, R. A. (1987). The role of reward pathways in the development of drug dependence. *Pharmacol. Ther.* **35**, 227–263.

Wise, R. A. (1989). The brain and reward. In: *The Neuropharmacological Basis of Reward* (J. M. Liebman and S. J. Cooper, eds.), pp. 377–424. Oxford University Press, New York.

Woods, J. H. and Gmerek, D. E. (1985). Substitution and primary dependence studies in animals. *Drug Alcohol Depend.* **14**, 233–247.

Woods, J. S. and Leibowitz, S. F. (1985). Hypothalamic sites sensitive to morphine and naloxone: effects on feeding behavior. *Pharmacol. Biochem. Behav.* **23**, 431–438.

Yoshida, M., Yokoo, H., Mizoguchi, K., Kawahara, H., Tsuda, A., Nishikawa, T. and Tanaka, M. (1992). Eating and drinking cause increased dopamine release in the nucleus accumbens and ventral tegmental area in the rat: measurement by *in vivo* microdialysis. *Neurosci. Lett.* **139**, 73–76.

Young, E. A., Walker, J. M., Houghten, R. and Akil, H. (1987). The degradation of dynorphin A in brain tissue *in vivo* and *in vitro*. *Peptides* **8**, 701–707.

Zastawny, R. L., George, S. R., Nguyen, T., Cheng, R., Tsatsos, J., Briones-Urbina, R. and O'Dowd, B. F. (1994). Cloning, characterization, and distribution of a μ-opioid receptor in rat brain. *J. Neurochem.* **62**, 2099–2105.

8

Opioid Receptor Subtypes and Stimulation-Induced Feeding

KENNETH D. CARR

Millhauser Laboratories, Department of Psychiatry, New York University Medical Center, 550 First Avenue, New York, NY 10016, USA

1 Introduction

The brain opioid system is composed of three genetically distinct families of peptides whose cellular effects are mediated by μ, δ and κ receptors (for review see Simon and Hiller, 1994). *In vitro* binding and bioassay studies reveal the proenkephalin-derived enkephalin pentapeptides to be δ receptor-preferring, the pro-opiomelanocortin-derived β-endorphin to be δ and μ receptor-preferring, and the prodynorphin-derived peptides such as dynorphin A and B to be κ receptor-preferring ligands (for review see Corbett *et al.*, 1993). However, all opioid peptides cross-react with at least one non-preferred receptor type and the actual relationships between peptides and receptor types within physiological circuits remain to be elucidated. Opioid receptors are membrane bound, coupled to G proteins, and activate several effector systems (to inhibit adenylyl cyclase, decrease Ca^{++} conductance and increase K^+ conductance) (for review see North, 1993). Agonist binding with multiple opioid receptor types mediates both presynaptic and postsynaptic inhibition.

Based on the neuroanatomical distribution of opioid peptides and receptors (for review see Mansour *et al.*, 1988), a role in the regulation of feeding would be expected. High concentrations of peptides and/or receptors exist within hindbrain nuclei that mediate gustatory and visceral–metabolic functions (e.g. solitary, parabrachial and dorsal motor vagal nuclei), as well as within hypo-thalamic and limbic nuclei which are known to regulate ingestion (e.g. basolateral amygdala, bed nucleus of the stria terminalis, paraventricular,

DRUG RECEPTOR SUBTYPES AND INGESTIVE BEHAVIOUR
ISBN 0-12-187620-9

dorsomedial and ventromedial hypothalamic nuclei). Interestingly, the rat brain is relatively deficient in κ receptors, which predominate in many of the aforementioned brain regions (i.e. bed nucleus, paraventricular, dorsomedial and ventromedial hypothalamus). Opioid receptors within the 'final common pathway for incentive motivation' (believed to consist of ventral tegmental dopamine neurons that innervate nucleus accumbens (for review see Wise, 1982; Di Chiara and North, 1992; Koob, 1992)) would also be expected to modulate feeding.

To evaluate the involvement of opioid receptors in feeding, our laboratory has used electrical brain stimulation paradigms. Stimulation within the lateral hypothalamic medial forebrain bundle (ESLH), lateral or dorsolateral to the fornix, can elicit both feeding (i.e. stimulation-induced feeding; SIF) and, at higher stimulation frequencies, intracranial self-stimulation (ICSS). There is evidence that ESLH induces feeding by directly evoking incentive motivation, which can summate with the taste of food to reinforce ingestion. In a variant of the traditional SIF paradigm, it has been shown that rats will self-administer ESLH that is well below threshold for ICSS if palatable food is present and can be eaten during each train of brain stimulation (Coons and White, 1977). As the frequency of ESLH is increased, the palatability of the available food may be correspondingly decreased to yield the same net rewarding effect and maintain the animal's self-administration behaviour. As this trade-off is followed to its logical conclusion, an ESLH frequency is ultimately reached at which concurrent gustatory stimulation is no longer needed to maintain responding. That is, the incentive effect of ESLH has become sufficient to reinforce self-administration in the absence of food and SIF gives way to ICSS. Psychophysical studies of the interaction between gustatory stimulation and ESLH favour a convergence model, in which gustatory and electrical reward signals are conveyed by separate neural pathways that ultimately converge on a common integrator (Conover and Shizgal, 1994). However, it is premature to reject a series model, in which electrical and gustatory reward signals are carried by a common set of neurons in the lateral hypothalamus (LH).

The advantages of using brain stimulation paradigms to evaluate opioid mechanisms in feeding are several-fold:

1 The behaviour of the animal is under the control of the experimenter.
2 Treatment-related changes in SIF or ICSS can be quantified by measuring changes in the brain stimulation threshold for eliciting the criterion behavioural response.
3 Comparison of treatment effects on SIF and ICSS can help differentiate whether endogenous opioid mechanisms mediate the centrally evoked incentive motivational state or events that are specific to ingestion (e.g. orosensation, satiety).
4 Treatment effects that are specific to SIF cannot be attributed to general performance variables.

2   Stimulation-induced feeding and self-stimulation

2.1   Effects of non-selective opioid antagonists

In the behavioural studies to be described, a discrete trials method of limits is used to determine the minimum ESLH frequency required to elicit the criterion behavioural response. In SIF experiments, the criterion is 5 s of continuous eating of wet Purina chow mash at a latency no greater than 20 s from the onset of brain stimulation. In ICSS experiments, the criterion is 15 lever-presses per 1-min trial, where each lever-press produces a 1-s duration train of 0.1-ms cathodal pulses. In both cases, a complete test consists of 4–6 separate series of trials. On alternate series, brain stimulation frequency is systematically increased or decreased from one trial to the next. When frequencies are increased, threshold is defined as the first of two consecutive frequencies to sustain the criterion response. When frequencies are decreased, threshold is the last frequency to sustain the criterion before two consecutive failures. The threshold for a complete test is the mean of the 4–6 values obtained. In most experiments, tests of threshold are conducted before and after a treatment (e.g. drug administration).

When naloxone, which is a non-selective opioid antagonist, is administered systemically, the threshold for eliciting SIF is raised in a dose-related manner, while that for ICSS is unaffected (Carr and Simon, 1983a, 1984; Fig. 1). Since thresholds for SIF and ICSS are determined in the same animals, with the same electrodes, this result suggests that opioid receptors are specifically associated with feeding rather than eliciting brain stimulation. To discriminate whether the opioid receptors involved in SIF are located within the central nervous system (CNS) or peripheral tissues, the effects of systemically administered quaternary naloxone were investigated (Carr and Simon, 1983a). Quaternary naloxone is a polar compound that displays poor penetrability of the blood–brain barrier. Its peripheral antagonist potency is evidenced by its ability to block the inhibitory effect on SIF of loperamide, an opiate agonist that does not enter the brain (Carr and Simon, 1983b). Quaternary naloxone failed to affect the SIF threshold (Fig. 2). This result indicates that naloxone increases the threshold for SIF by blocking opioid receptors within the CNS.

The need to increase ESLH frequency after naloxone administration in order to sustain the criterion feeding response is comparable to the effect of reducing the palatability of available food. The possibility that naloxone increases the SIF threshold by reducing the perceived palatability of wet mash is supported by the pattern of threshold increase seen in a postinjection test. Naloxone characteristically has no effect on the first of four serially determined thresholds that comprise a test but reliably raises subsequently determined thresholds to progressively higher levels. This pattern occurs regardless of the interval between injection and the onset of testing (Carr and Simon, 1983a) and distinguishes naloxone from conventional appetite suppressants such as

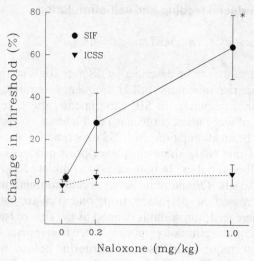

Fig. 1 Mean ± SEM percentage change in frequency thresholds for lateral hypothalamic stimulation-induced feeding (SIF) and self-stimulation (ICSS) following subcutaneous administration of naloxone. Repeated measurements were taken on four rats. *$P < 0.01$ compared with change following vehicle. Based, in part, on results reported by Carr and Simon (1983a), with kind permission from Elsevier Science Ltd, The Boulevard, Langford Lane, Kidlington OX5 1GB, UK.

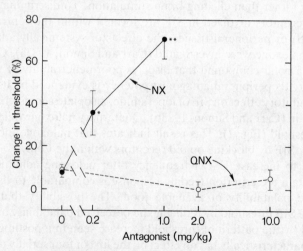

Fig. 2 Mean ± SEM percentage change in frequency thresholds for lateral hypothalamic stimulation-induced feeding following subcutaneous administration of naloxone (NX) and its quaternary analogue (QNX). Repeated measurements were taken on six rats. *$P < 0.05$, **$P < 0.1$ *vs* change following vehicle injection. From Carr and Simon (1983a), with permission of Elsevier Science Ltd, The Boulevard, Langford Lane, Kidlington OX5 1GB, UK.

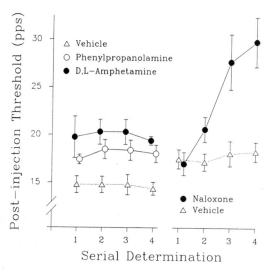

Serial Determination

Fig. 3 *Left*: Repeated measurements on four rats that received D,L-amphetamine (0.2 mg/kg), phenylpropanolamine (5.0 mg/kg) or vehicle, intraperitoneally, 20 min before testing frequency threshold for stimulation-induced feeding. *Right*: Repeated measurements on ten rats tested after subcutaneous administration of naloxone (1.0 mg/kg). In both cases, mean ± SEM thresholds are plotted as a function of the serial order in which they were obtained during a postinjection test (pps, pulses per second). Adapted from data in Carr *et al.* (1987, 1993).

phenylpropanolamine and amphetamine (Carr *et al.*, 1993; Fig. 3). These latter compounds increase the threshold from the outset of testing and do so to a uniform extent throughout the test, as would be expected of appetite suppressants. It would therefore seem that naloxone does not suppress appetite *per se*.

Instead, naloxone appears to interfere preferentially with the maintenance of feeding once initiated. Specifically, naloxone may diminish the incentive effect of food taste, which normally sustains eating. This interpretation is supported by findings obtained in a variety of other behavioural paradigms in which unconditioned taste reactivity, taste preference, palatability-induced hyperphagia and sucrose sham-feeding have been evaluated (Apfelbaum and Mandenoff, 1981; Rockwood and Reid, 1982; Lynch, 1986; Kirkham and Cooper, 1988; Parker *et al.*, 1992; Giraudo *et al.*, 1993). The hypothesis that naloxone inhibits SIF by interacting with gustatory rather than postingestive signals is supported by the finding that opening a gastric fistula does not diminish the inhibitory effect of naloxone on SIF (V. Papadouka, K. Carr, L. Leventhal and R. Bodnar, unpublished results).

2.2 Effects of antibodies to opioid peptides

In an attempt to identify the opioid peptide(s) that mediates SIF, specific antibodies directed against different opioid peptides were infused into the lateral ventricle (Carr *et al.*, 1987). Antibodies to dynorphin A_{1-13} increased

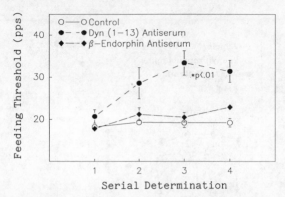

Fig. 4 Four determinations of the threshold for stimulation-induced feeding obtained in serial order within a postinjection test expressed as mean ± SEM pulses per second (pps). Repeated measurements were made on seven rats tested 2 h after lateral ventricular infusion of β-endorphin antiserum, dynorphin A_{1-13} antiserum or vehicle. Adapted from Carr *et al.* (1987).

SIF threshold while those to β-endorphin had no effect. Moreover, dynorphin antiserum produced the same pattern of progressively rising thresholds that had been produced by naloxone (Fig. 4) and had no effect on ICSS (Carr, 1990). These findings suggest that dynorphin A is the opioid peptide that normally sustains SIF. Moreover, the threshold-raising effect of naloxone may result from blockade of the receptors to which dynorphin A binds. When antisera specific for the biologically active 1–17 and 1–8 fragments of dynorphin A are infused into the lateral ventricle, both increase the SIF threshold (Fig. 5) (Carr and Bak, 1990). Thus, dynorphin A_{1-8}, which is more abundant in brain than A_{1-17} (Weber *et al.*, 1982) and less discriminating among opioid receptor types (Corbett *et al.*, 1993), may mediate SIF together with the more κ-preferring dynorphin A_{1-17}. These findings might lead us to expect κ receptor involvement in SIF but would not rule out other opioid receptor types.

2.3 Effects of receptor type-selective antagonists

To evaluate the involvement of multiple opioid receptor types in SIF, antagonists selective for μ, δ and κ receptors were infused into the lateral ventricle in separate groups of rats, and effects on thresholds for SIF and ICSS were determined (Papadouka and Carr, 1994). To evaluate μ receptor involvement, D-Tic-Cys-Tyr-D-Trp-Arg-Thr-Pen-Thr-NH_2 (TCTAP) was administered. This compound is a somatostatin analogue with virtually no residual somatostatin activity (Kazmierski *et al.*, 1988). TCTAP binds with high affinity to the μ opioid receptor and displays a μ/δ selectivity ratio of 1060 and a μ/somatostatin selectivity ratio of 28 613. Although competitive binding data are not available for TCTAP *vs* κ receptor-selective ligands, the μ/κ selectivity ratio for the

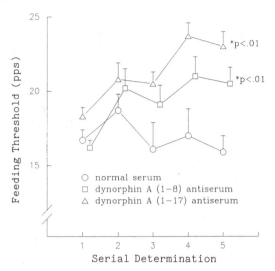

Serial Determination

Fig. 5 Five determinations of the threshold for stimulation-induced feeding obtained in serial order within a postinjection test expressed as mean ± SEM pulses per second (pps). Repeated measurements were made on ten rats tested 2 h after lateral ventricular infusion of antibodies to dynorphin A_{1-8}, dynorphin A_{1-17} and normal rabbit serum control. Adapted from Carr and Bak (1990).

closely related compound, CTOP, is greater than 1000 (Kosterlitz and Paterson, 1990). When infused into the lateral ventricle, TCTAP increased the SIF threshold while having no effect on ICSS threshold. This effect is similar to that produced by naloxone and more certainly indicates the involvement of μ receptors in SIF. To evaluate κ receptor involvement, nor-binaltorphamine (nor-BNI) was administered. This compound is a bivalent ligand derived from naltrexone (Portoghese *et al.*, 1987). Nor-BNI binds with high affinity to the κ receptor and displays a κ/μ selectivity ratio of 48 and a κ/δ selectivity ratio of 32 (Corbett *et al.*, 1993). When infused into the lateral ventricle, nor-BNI increased the SIF threshold while having no effect on ICSS threshold. This strongly suggests the involvement of κ receptors in SIF and is compatible with the threshold-increasing effect of dynorphin A antiserum. Finally, the involvement of δ receptors was evaluated by administering naltrindole (Portoghese *et al.*, 1988). This compound binds with reasonably high affinity to the δ receptor and displays a δ/μ binding selectivity ratio of 90 and a δ/κ ratio of 165 (Corbett *et al.*, 1993). Infused into the lateral ventricle, naltrindole had no effect on the SIF threshold, suggesting that δ receptors are not involved in SIF (Fig. 6).

The results of the study just described indicate that both μ and κ opioid receptors are involved in SIF and that the previously observed effect of naloxone may result from the antagonist effect of this non-selective compound at both μ and κ receptors. To support this possibility, most doses of TCTAP and nor-BNI produced a pattern of threshold increase reminiscent of naloxone

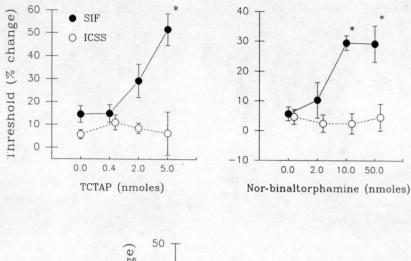

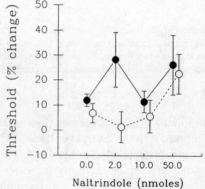

Fig. 6 Six separate groups of rats were used to determine effects of receptor type-selective opioid antagonists on the threshold for stimulation-induced feeding (SIF) and self-stimulation (ICSS). Thresholds obtained in postinjection tests are expressed as mean ± SEM percentage change in relation to preinjection means and plotted as a function of the intracerebroventricular dose administered. *Top left*: Effects of TCTAP (μ antagonist) on SIF ($n = 6$) and ICSS ($n = 4$). *$P < 0.01$. *Top right*: Effects of nor-binaltorphamine (κ antagonist) on SIF ($n = 4$) and ICSS ($n = 4$). *$P < 0.01$. *Bottom*: Effects of naltrindole (δ antagonist) on SIF ($n = 8$) and ICSS ($n = 4$). Adapted from Papadouka and Carr (1994), with kind permission of Elsevier Science Ltd.

insofar as the first determination of threshold postinjection was unaffected while later determinations were raised (Fig. 7).

2.4 Brain regional opioid binding during SIF

The conclusion that μ and κ but not δ receptors are involved in feeding agrees with results obtained in other feeding paradigms (Ukai and Holtzman, 1988; Arjune and Bodnar, 1990; Arjune et al., 1990; Levine et al., 1990, 1991;

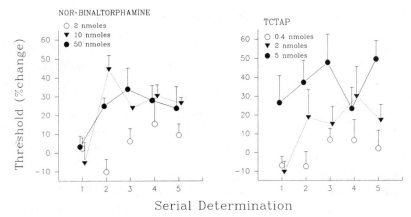

Serial Determination

Fig. 7 Mean ± SEM difference scores obtained by subtracting the percentage change in SIF threshold produced by vehicle from that produced by each dose of nor-binaltorphamine (nor-BNI) and TCTAP are plotted for each serial determination of threshold in postinjection tests. Separate groups containing four and six rats were used to test effects of nor-BNI and TCTAP, respectively. From Papadouka and Carr (1994), with kind permission of Elsevier Science Ltd.

Calcagnetti *et al.*, 1990). The sparing of ICSS by opioid antagonism, combined with evidence that opioid antagonism blocks gustatory reward, suggests that the critical opioid receptors may be located within structures innervated by the ascending gustatory pathway, whose outputs converge with those of the lateral hypothalamus. In an effort to localize the brain regions in which opioid peptides are released during SIF we conducted an *in vivo* autoradiographic study of opioid receptor binding in rats that engaged in SIF during intravenous injection of a tracer dose of [^{3}H]diprenorphine (Stein *et al.*, 1990). It was hypothesized that the radiolabelled compound, which is a non-selective opioid antagonist, would be competitively displaced from receptors by concurrently released opioid peptides. Consequently, sites in which opioid peptides bind with receptors during SIF would be distinguished by decreased radiolabelling compared with that in unstimulated control rats.

Binding was evaluated in more than 50 brain regions and the only region displaying decreased binding of [^{3}H]diprenorphine was the anterior cingulate cortex. Surprisingly, among nine brain regions with altered binding, eight displayed increases as a result of SIF. These regions included the lateral hypothalamus, medial septum, and basolateral and central nuclei of the amygdala. The meaning of increased binding is not clear but could reflect mobilization of cryptic receptors by SIF (e.g. via externalization or conformational changes).

Because the decreased binding in anterior cingulate represents the only change consistent with our hypothesis (i.e. reduced radiolabelling as a consequence of displacement by endogenously released peptide), a follow-up microinjection experiment was conducted (Carr and Wolinsky, 1994). While bilateral microinjection of naloxone did increase the SIF threshold, the effect was small and was not reproduced by TCTAP, nor-BNI or naltrindole. Since anterior cingulate comprises a large brain area with a diffuse distribution of opioid receptors, naloxone, which is highly lipophilic and rapidly diffuses away from the injection site (Schroeder *et al.*, 1991), may have been uniquely able to block receptors in a sufficient volume of tissue to affect behaviour. By the same token, naloxone may have diffused beyond the anterior cingulate to a remote site of action. Microinjection of agonists into anterior cingulate did however provide some support for μ receptor involvement in SIF; the μ agonist DAMGO reliably decreased the SIF threshold while the κ and δ agonists, U50 488 and DPDPE, respectively, had no effect.

The binding changes observed in the LH, central amygdala and basolateral amygdala are actually the most interesting from a functional and anatomical standpoint. Placement of the opioid mechanism(s) in any one of these structures would be more clearly compatible with the foregoing interpretation of the behavioural experiments. For example, LH neurons are directly and indirectly innervated by the ascending gustatory pathway (Norgren, 1976) and display inhibitory responses during ingestion that are blocked by naloxone (Oomura *et al.*, 1986); conveyance of opioid-mediated gustatory reward signals to LH neurons would be consistent with the 'series model' in which gustatory and electrical reward signals are carried by the same population of LH neurons. The central and basolateral amygdala both receive gustatory input: the central amygdala from the ascending gustatory pathway (Norgren, 1976) and the basolateral amygdala from ventral posteromedial thalamus and insular cortex (Turner and Herkenham, 1981; Saper, 1982). Cell body-specific lesions of these nuclei reduce preference and sham intake of sucrose solution (Siegel *et al.*, 1988; Touzani *et al.*, 1994). Importantly, microinjection of μ agonists, such as DAMGO and morphine, into amygdaloid sites stimulates feeding (Gosnell, 1988; Stanley *et al.*, 1989). These amygdaloid nuclei are of interest not only because of their possible involvement in gustatory reward and μ opioid facilitation of intake, but also because of their strong efferent connections with the LH and, in the case of the basolateral amygdala, the nucleus accumbens (Krettek and Price, 1978). Thus, opioid receptors in any one of these three regions could plausibly be involved in gustatory reward and influence the signals conveyed to the LH or a common reward integrator such as the nucleus accumbens.

3   Chronic food restriction and streptozotocin-induced diabetes

3.1   Effects on ICSS

Although the opioid antagonist treatments administered in the studies of SIF all failed to affect ICSS, it has been found that when rats are subject to chronic food restriction the ICSS threshold declines and that this decline can be

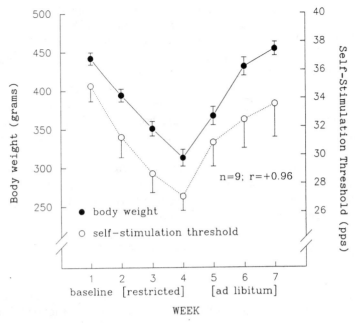

Fig. 8 Self-stimulation thresholds were monitored in nine rats throughout a 7-week experiment that included 1 week of baseline testing, 3 weeks of food restriction and 3 weeks of *ad libitum* refeeding. Weekly mean ± SEM bodyweights and self-stimulation thresholds are plotted separately as a function of experimental weeks. From Carr and Wolinsky (1993), with kind permission of Elsevier Science Ltd.

reversed by opioid antagonists (Carr and Wolinsky, 1993). This effect is interesting because it may be related to the enhanced incentive effect of food and food-related stimuli in hungry animals (Cabanac, 1971; Berridge, 1991). Investigations of the opioid mechanism underlying this phenomenon have revealed striking similarities to the opioid mechanism that mediates SIF and may therefore shed additional light on the function and location of multiple opioid receptor types that regulate ingestive behaviour.

When rats are placed on a regimen of chronic food restriction, with food access limited to a single 1-h period per day, ICSS threshold and bodyweight decline together. The decrease in ICSS threshold is present whether rats are tested before or after the daily meal (Abrahamsen *et al.*, 1995), and returns toward baseline only gradually following the reinstatement of *ad libitum* feeding (Fig. 8). A number of observations suggest that this phenomenon is related to the metabolic need state rather than the stress physiology associated with food restriction. For example: (1) stressors, such as inescapable foot-shock, and chronic varied stress generally inhibit ICSS (Zacharko and Anisman, 1991; Moreau *et al.*, 1992); (2) LH ICSS thresholds in food-restricted rats do not covary with plasma corticosterone levels, which are markedly increased before the daily meal and decline to the levels in animals fed *ad libitum* following the daily meal (Abrahamsen *et al.*, 1995); (3) ICSS in some electrode sites, such as the zona incerta, is not affected by food restriction (Carr and Wolinsky, 1993); and (4) streptozotocin-induced diabetes produces a similar decline in ICSS threshold (Carr, 1994).

When repeated measurements are taken on a group of rats under *ad libitum* and restricted access feeding conditions, intracerebroventricular infusions of naltrexone selectively increase ICSS threshold during food restriction (Carr and Wolinsky, 1993). Similarly, when rats rendered diabetic by streptozotocin are given naltrexone, the ICSS threshold returns to prediabetic values (Carr, 1994). These findings suggest that metabolic need states sensitize the reward system by triggering an opioid mechanism that is otherwise quiescent. Efforts to characterize this opioid mechanism further have been carried out primarily in food-restricted rats.

3.2   Effects of receptor type-selective antagonists and dynorphin antiserum

The same receptor-selective antagonists used to investigate SIF have been used to investigate the lowering of ICSS threshold by food restriction (Carr and Papadouka, 1994). For each antagonist, separate groups of *ad libitum* fed and food-restricted rats were used to conduct intracerebroventricular dose–response studies. In restricted rats, drugs were administered during the second and third weeks of the feeding regimen. Both the μ antagonist, TCTAP, and the κ antagonist, nor-BNI, selectively raised the ICSS threshold of food-restricted rats, while the δ antagonist, naltrindole, did not (Fig. 9). This finding suggests that both μ and κ receptors are involved in the facilitation of ICSS. Limited testing has also been carried out with antibodies to opioid peptides (Carr, 1990). The small but significant lowering of ICSS threshold produced by 24-h food deprivation was reversed by intracerebroventricular infusion of antibodies to dynorphin A_{1-13}. Similar antibody injections in the same animals under conditions of *ad libitum* feeding had no effect (Fig. 10).

4   Hypothesis: a common opioid mechanism mediates SIF and facilitates ICSS

There is an interesting parallel between the results of the SIF and ICSS studies outlined above. In both cases, opioid transmission has been inferred to promote responding by facilitating the incentive effect of a stimulus; in one case the stimulus is peripheral–gustatory and in the other central–electrical. Moreover, in both cases the opioid contribution to responding has been reduced by TCTAP, nor-BNI and antibodies to dynorphin A. This raises the possibility that palatable food taste and metabolic need may be separate triggers of a common opioid mechanism. If so, additional constraints would

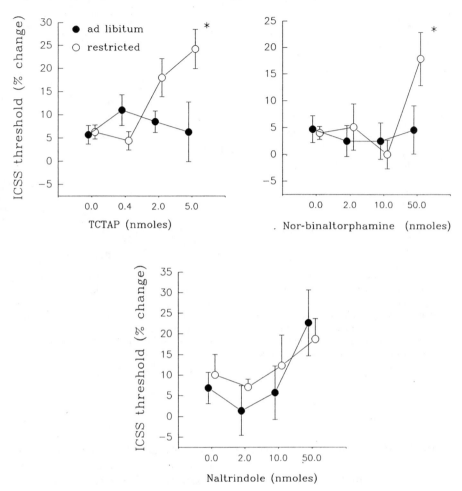

Fig. 9 Self-stimulation (ICSS) thresholds following vehicle and three receptor type-selective antagonists were determined in six separate groups ($n = 4$) of *ad libitum* fed and food-restricted rats and expressed as the percentage change from the preinjection value. Mean ± SEM changes in threshold are plotted above as a function of lateral ventricular dose of TCTAP (μ antagonist, top left; $^*P < 0.01$), nor-binaltorphamine (κ antagonist, top right; $^*P < 0.05$) and naltrindole (δ antagonist, bottom). From Carr and Papadouka (1994), with kind permission of Elsevier Science Ltd.

have to be placed on candidate opioid mechanisms. For example, the brain region(s) involved would not only receive gustatory inputs and convey outputs to the LH or a downstream reward integrator, but would also receive inputs relating to energy deficit or adiposity; the latter could include signals of hepatic vagal origin, neuronal glucoprivation or hormonal changes (e.g. increased corticosterone or decreased insulin levels). In addition, the opioid mechanism

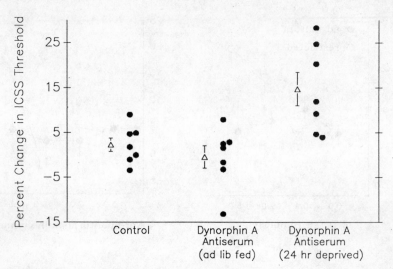

Fig. 10 Repeated measurements on seven rats whose stimulation frequency thresholds for self-stimulation (ICSS) were determined before and 2 h after lateral ventricular injection of vehicle or dynorphin A_{1-13} antiserum. The effect of dynorphin antiserum was tested under the baseline condition, where food and water had been available *ad libitum*, and the condition of 24-h food deprivation. Filled circles represent the percentage change in threshold on postinjection tests for individual animals. Hollow triangles represent the mean ± SEM percentage change. From Carr (1990), with kind permission of Elsevier Science Ltd.

would have to serve a modulatory rather than a mediating function in relation to incentive motivation; energy deficit, itself, could not be conceived as a rewarding event but instead as one that sensitizes the reward system to appropriate environmental stimuli (or electrical stimuli that supersede the normal afferent pathway but precede the point in the circuitry where opioid modulation occurs). A modulatory rather than a mediating role may actually be more consistent with analyses of the effects of opioid antagonists on ingestion. The maintenance of feeding does not always involve the opioid system. Rather, the opioid system appears to sustain feeding only to the extent that feeding is being driven by palatability. For example, there is a 1000-fold difference between the dose of naloxone required to reduce intake of chocolate chip cookies *vs* high-fibre chow (Giraudo *et al.*, 1993). This is compatible with the particular sensitivity of SIF to opioid antagonism. According to the model outlined above, SIF is reinforced by the net rewarding effect of ESLH and gustation. Thus, the palatability of a food is being selected from among its other sensory and postingestive properties, and combining with ESLH to reinforce feeding.

5 Brain regional opioid binding and peptide levels

5.1 Autoradiographic study of μ and κ binding in food-restricted rats

One approach to testing the hypothesis of a common opioid mechanism in SIF and ICSS would be to localize the brain opioid activity that accompanies food restriction and design follow-up microinjection experiments aimed at testing behavioural predictions. In an effort to localize brain opioid activity accompanying chronic food restriction, quantitative autoradiographic studies of μ and κ opioid binding and radioimmunoassay studies of prodynorphin-derived peptide levels have been conducted.

If chronic food restriction is accompanied by a change in tonic peptide release, compensatory changes might be expected to develop and be detectable at the level of the binding site. Although opioid receptors do not readily down-regulate, even in the face of chronic opiate narcotic exposure (e.g. Hollt et al., 1975), there have been previous reports that 72-h food deprivation reduces [^{3}H]naltrexone binding in the medial hypothalamus and medulla (Battistini et al., 1987), increases [^{3}H]naloxone binding in the midbrain (Tsujii et al., 1986a) and increases [^{3}H]dynorphin A$_{1-8}$ binding in the cortex, striatum and midbrain (Tsujii et al., 1986b). It therefore seemed that quantitative autoradiographic study of μ and κ binding in discrete regions of food-restricted rat brain could yield useful information. Rats were therefore subject to 2 weeks of food restriction and killed at meal-time on the final day. Binding was carried out on slide-mounted brain sections in vitro using [^{3}H]DAGO to label μ receptors and using [^{3}H]bremazocine, in the presence of excess DAGO and DPDPE to block μ and δ receptors, to label κ receptors. More than 50 brain regions, from medial prefrontal cortex to the nucleus solitarius, were analysed and only six structures displayed changes in binding (Wolinsky et al., 1994, 1995). μ binding was decreased in the basolateral–basomedial amygdala, parabrachial nucleus and habenula. κ binding was also decreased in the habenula but was increased in the bed nucleus of the stria terminalis, ventral pallidum, medial preoptic area and parabrachial nucleus (Table 1).

As alluded to above, the opioid activity that facilitates ICSS during food restriction need not cause adaptive changes in opioid binding. However, the observed changes do direct our attention to a number of structures for further consideration. Since saturating concentrations of ^{3}H-labelled ligands were used, the observed changes in binding are likely to reflect changes in receptor density, which are typically thought to occur as a compensatory response to changes in availability of endogenous ligand (Zukin and Tempel, 1986). The downregulation of μ receptors may therefore be indicative of an increase in tonic μ-ligand release; if receptors in the habenula, amygdala or parabrachial nucleus are involved in the facilitation of ICSS it would have to be concluded that receptor downregulation does not quite compensate for the increased release since a naltrexone–TCTAP-reversible behavioural effect is

Table 1 Effects of chronic food restriction on mu and kappa opioid binding in rat brain regions

Brain region	[³H]DAGO (fmol/mg tissue)		[³H]bremazocine (fmol/mg tissue)	
	Ad libitum	Restricted	*Ad libitum*	Restricted
Bed nucleus stria terminalis				
Medial anterior	39.0 ± 2.8	41.4 ± 7.6	28.5 ± 1.6	38.2 ± 1.6*
Laterodorsal	22.8 ± 0.8	27.5 ± 3.0	21.6 ± 1.4	29.1 ± 2.1*
Ventral	28.2 ± 0.8	32.5 ± 3.1	28.2 ± 1.1	43.1 ± 1.7*
Ventral pallidum	34.4 ± 1.1	38.4 ± 3.3	25.9 ± 0.7	36.0 ± 3.0*
Medial preoptic area	33.6 ± 1.7	36.8 ± 1.5	39.1 ± 1.9	62.3 ± 2.1*
Habenula				
Medial	53.2 ± 1.5	44.0 ± 7.3*	48.4 ± 5.1	35.1 ± 2.9*
Lateral	48.8 ± 1.0	42.1 ± 3.1*	28.8 ± 3.5	26.0 ± 2.0
Amygdala				
Basolateral	83.3 ± 2.8	72.2 ± 4.1*	34.6 ± 4.0	33.3 ± 2.9
Basomedial	43.0 ± 1.5	37.3 ± 1.4*	22.8 ± 1.6	21.8 ± 1.6
Parabrachial nucleus				
External lateral	273.7 ± 20.7	204.0 ± 18.0*	89.7 ± 4.7	107.5 ± 3.2*
External medial	211.5 ± 23.0	140.1 ± 8.0*	82.0 ± 14.0	89.4 ± 2.2

Values are expressed as mean ± SEM.
*$P < 0.05$.
Based on Wolinsky *et al.* (1994, 1995).

nevertheless expressed. The upregulation of κ receptors may be indicative of a suppression of tonic κ-ligand release, below basal levels; if receptors in the bed nucleus, ventral pallidum, medial preoptic area or parabrachial nucleus are involved in the facilitation of ICSS it might be presumed that stimulated release of a dynorphin peptide has a potentiated behavioural effect due to κ receptor supersensitivity.

Opioid receptors in the habenula, basolateral amygdala and parabrachial nucleus could all plausibly influence ICSS, given the evidence that these brain regions exert control over ICSS and/or impulse flow in the meso-accumbens dopamine pathway (Rolls, 1974; Nishikawa *et al.*, 1986; Ferssiwi *et al.*, 1987). In the context of the hypothesis that SIF and the potentiation of ICSS involve a common opioid mechanism, the basolateral amygdala, bed nucleus of the stria terminalis (BNST) and parabrachial nucleus (PBN) are of particular interest. Basolateral amygdala displays changes in opioid binding during both SIF and chronic food restriction, and possesses all the functional and anatomical characteristics required of a 'common opioid mechanism' (see above). BNST is a limbic forebrain terminus of the ascending gustatory pathway (Norgren, 1976) and has strong reciprocal connections with the LH as well as projections to the ventral tegmental area (VTA) (De Olmos *et al.*, 1985). The PBN, in addition to being the second-order gustatory relay nucleus (Norgren, 1976), has interconnections with LH neurons that control ICSS (Ferssiwi *et al.*, 1987), and is a site in which opiate agonist and antagonist microinjections affect feeding (Carr *et al.*, 1991; Moufid-Bellancourt and Velley, 1994).

5.2 Levels of prodynorphin-derived peptides in food-restricted and diabetic rats

In the light of the reversal of opioid effects in SIF and ICSS by dynorphin A antisera, plus the involvement of κ receptors in both behavioural phenomena, the effects of chronic food restriction on brain regional levels of prodynorphin-derived peptides were determined (Berman *et al.*, 1994). As in the autoradiographic study, rats had restricted access to food for 2 weeks and were killed at meal-time on the final day. Levels of immunoreactive dynorphin A_{1-17}, dynorphin A_{1-8} and dynorphin B_{1-13} were measured in 11 brain regions known to be involved in appetite, taste and reward. Of the 33 comparisons made (i.e. three peptides in 11 regions), food-restricted rats displayed seven significant changes: levels of A_{1-17} increased in dorsomedial, ventromedial and medial preoptic hypothalamic areas and decreased in the central amygdala; levels of A_{1-8} increased in the nucleus accumbens, BNST and LH (Figs 11–13). Interpretation of these results, and any effort to relate them to the binding changes discussed above, is limited by the absence of information as to whether altered peptide levels reflect cell body, fibre or extracellular content, and whether they are associated with changes in prodynorphin gene expression and/or post-translational processing. The results do, however, suggest that

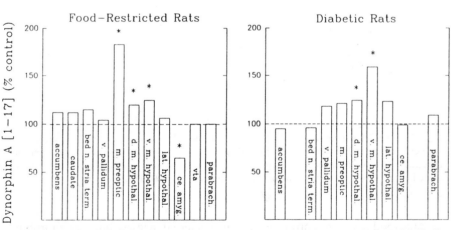

Fig. 11 Levels of immunoreactive dynorphin A_{1-17} in individual brain regions of chronically food-restricted rats ($n > 14$), streptozotocin-treated diabetic rats ($n > 8$) and corresponding control groups. Mean levels obtained in food-restricted and diabetic rats are expressed as a percentage of those in controls. Results are based on data in Berman *et al.* (1994, 1995).

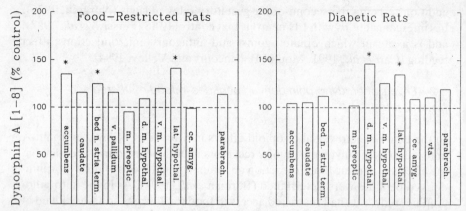

Fig. 12 Levels of immunoreactive dynorphin A$_{1-8}$ in individual brain regions of chronically food-restricted rats ($n > 14$), streptozotocin-treated diabetic rats ($n > 14$) and corresponding control groups. Mean levels obtained in food-restricted and diabetic rats are expressed as a percentage of those in controls. Results are based on data in Berman *et al.* (1994, 1995).

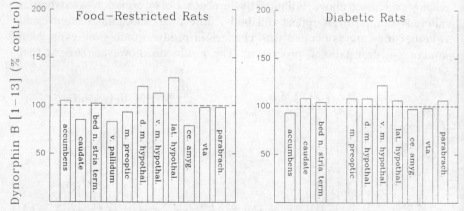

Fig. 13 Levels of immunoreactive dynorphin B$_{1-13}$ in individual brain regions of chronically food-restricted rats ($n > 7$), streptozotocin-treated diabetic rats ($n > 14$) and corresponding control groups. Mean levels obtained in food-restricted and diabetic rats are expressed as a percentage of those in controls. Results are based on data in Berman *et al.* (1994, 1995).

chronic food restriction produces region-specific changes within the dynorphin A domain and not the dynorphin B domain of the prodynorphin precursor, and that within any brain region the change is restricted to just one of the dynorphin A fragments. This could result from changes in post-translational processing that alter the balance between A_{1-8} and A_{1-17} within a particular brain region and, in turn, alter the subpopulation of opioid receptors stimulated, since A_{1-8} is less κ-preferring than A_{1-17}.

There are many behavioural and physiological changes that are produced by chronic food restriction and it cannot be assumed that all detected perturbations in the brain opioid system relate to feeding and/or the sensitization of reward. Because streptozotocin-induced diabetes represents another metabolic need state that is accompanied by increased appetite and an opioid-mediated facilitation of ICSS (Carr, 1994), levels of prodynorphin-derived peptides were measured in brain regions of rats that had been rendered diabetic for 2 weeks (Berman *et al.*, 1995). It was reasoned that changes in peptide levels that are similarly displayed by food-restricted and diabetic rats may be related to the facilitation of ICSS that is common to both. Of the 29 comparisons made in this study, four changes were observed; three of these were also seen in food-restricted rats. Diabetic and food-restricted rats both displayed increased levels of dynorphin A_{1-17} in the VMN and DMN, and increased levels of dynorphin A_{1-8} in the LH. All of these changes could plausibly relate to the observed facilitation of ICSS, and the latter two to observed changes in binding.

LH content of A_{1-8} derives from a combination of cell bodies and fibres. To the extent that increased levels reflect changes in the local utilization, the previously discussed change in binding that occurs during SIF, combined with the likelihood that the LH is a site of convergence between gustatory and electrical reward signals, makes LH itself a plausible locus for an opioid mechanism that mediates SIF and/or facilitates ICSS. There is, however, a substantial population of dynorphin A-containing cell bodies in the LH which project to several brain regions, including the central amygdala and PBN (Zardetto-Smith *et al.*, 1988)—regions in which binding changes during SIF and food restriction, respectively, were observed. For anatomical and functional reasons discussed above, an LH–central amygdala–LH and/or LH–PBN–LH opioid circuit could also plausibly regulate SIF and ICSS.

Increased dynorphin A peptide levels within the medial hypothalamus are also interesting. There is a long history of experimentation indicating that feeding and LH ICSS are co-regulated by a diversity of manipulations within the medial hypothalamus (Hernandez and Hoebel, 1989). Moreover, microinjection of dynorphin A_{1-13} into the medial hypothalamus has been shown to enhance feeding (Gosnell *et al.*, 1986), while injections of antibodies to prodynorphin-derived peptides diminish feeding (Schulz *et al.*, 1984). The changes in dynorphin A peptide levels observed in the DMN are particularly interesting, for several reasons. First, unlike the VMN, DMN contains a substantial population of dynorphin A cell bodies (Fallon and Leslie, 1986) and among the brain regions innervated by DMN cell bodies is the basolateral amygdala (Ter Horst and Luiten, 1986) in which binding changes have been documented during both SIF and chronic food restriction. In addition, DMN contains one of the highest densities of insulin receptors in brain (Corp et al., 1986) and accumulates high levels of radiolabelled insulin following intraventricular injection (Baskin et al., 1983). There is increasing evidence that plasma and cerebrospinal fluid insulin levels correlate with body adiposity, inform the brain of significant changes in bodyweight and are monitored by medial hypothalamic neurons that trigger compensatory changes in feeding and energy expenditure (Woods et al., 1985; Menendez and Atrens, 1991; McGowan et al., 1992). Since pre-meal insulin levels in food-restricted rats are as low as those of streptozotocin-treated diabetic rats (Y. Berman and K. D. Carr, unpublished results), it is possible that the hypoinsulinism of food restriction and diabetes facilitates feeding and ICSS via effects on medial hypothalamic insulin-sensitive neurons that synthesize or bind dynorphin A peptides.

6 Summary and conclusions

Results of the studies reviewed in this chapter suggest that the brain opioid system is involved in the facilitation of incentive motivational processes that bear on ingestive behaviour. More specifically, μ and κ receptors in combination with dynorphin A peptides appear to mediate this function. While it is premature to conclude that the opioid mechanisms triggered by palatable taste and metabolic need are one and the same, functional and pharmacological similarities between them have been noted. Efforts to localize and more fully characterize the opioid mechanisms activated during SIF and metabolic need states are still in progress.

Emergent from the results discussed are the rudiments of a model for a μ-κ opioid mechanism that can be engaged by both internal and external stimuli to facilitate the incentive motivating effects of food and thereby invigorate instrumental and consummatory responding. The mechanism has tentatively been placed within one or more of the brain regions that receive gustatory input, display opioid perturbations during SIF and/or metabolic need states, exert control over ICSS and/or feeding, and convey outputs to the LH or downstream elements in the reward system. Thus, the results obtained so far point to lateral hypothalamus, bed nucleus of the stria terminalis, basolateral amygdala, dorsomedial hypothalamus and parabrachial nucleus as candidate component structures of the opioid mechanism(s) of interest. Further development of this model awaits the results of additional biochemical, molecular biological and intracerebral microinjection studies.

Recent evidence that each of the major opioid receptor types may be further subdivided into multiple subtypes (see Simon and Hiller, 1994) adds another level of complexity to the problem under study. However, now that all of the major opioid receptors have been cloned and sequenced (Evans et al., 1992; Kieffer et al., 1992; Chen et al., 1993; Fukuda et al., 1993; Meng et al., 1993; Thompson et al., 1993; Yasuda et al., 1993), the number, distribution and cellular effects of distinct opioid receptor subtypes will become clearly defined. It is likely that molecular approaches, including *in vivo* administration of antisense oligodeoxynucleotides, will refine and extend our understanding of multiple opioid receptor types in the regulation of feeding.

Acknowledgements

The research reviewed in this chapter was supported by Grant DA03956 from NIDA.

References

Abrahamsen, G. C., Berman, Y. and Carr, K. D. (1995). Curve–shift analysis of self-stimulation in food-restricted rats: relationship between daily meal, plasma corticosterone and reward sensitization. *Brain Res.* **695**, 186–194.

Apfelbaum, M. and Mandenoff, A. (1981). Naltrexone suppresses hyperphagia induced in the rat by a highly palatable diet. *Pharmacol. Biochem. Behav.* **15**, 89–91.

Arjune, D. and Bodnar, R. J. (1990). Suppression of nocturnal, palatable and glucoprivic intake in rats by the κ opioid antagonist, nor-binaltorphamine. *Brain Res.* **534**, 313–316.

Arjune, D., Standifer, K. M., Pasternak, G. W. and Bodnar, R. J. (1990). Reduction by central β-funaltrexamine of food intake in rats under freely-feeding, deprivation and glucoprivic conditions. *Brain Res.* **535**, 101–109.

Baskin, D. G., Woods, S. C., West, D. B., van Houten, M., Posner, B. I., Dorsa, D. M. and Porte, D. (1983). Immunocytochemical detection of insulin in rat hypothalamus and its possible uptake from cerebrospinal fluid. *Endocrinology* **133**, 1818–1825.

Battistini, N., Giardino, L. and Calza, L. (1987). Opiate receptor autoradiography in fasting rats. *Int. J. Obes.* **11 (supplement 3)**, 17–21.

Berman, Y., Devi, L. and Carr, K. D. (1994). Effects of chronic food restriction on prodynorphin-derived peptides in rat brain regions. *Brain Res.* **664**, 49–53.

Berman, Y., Devi, L. and Carr, K. D. (1995). Effects of streptozotocin-induced diabetes on prodynorphin-derived peptides in rat brain regions. *Brain Res.* **685**, 129–134.

Berridge, K. C. (1991). Modulation of taste affect by hunger, caloric satiety and sensory-specific satiety in the rat. *Appetite* **16**, 103–120.

Cabanac, M. (1971). Physiological role of pleasure. *Science* **173**, 1103–1107.

Calcagnetti, D. J., Calcagnetti, R. L. and Fanselow, M. S. (1990). Centrally administered opioid antagonists, nor-binaltorphamine, 16-methyl cyprenorphine and MR2266, suppress intake of a sweet solution. *Pharmacol. Biochem. Behav.* **35**, 69–73.

Carr, K. D. (1990). Effects of antibodies to dynorphin A and β-endorphin on lateral hypothalamic self-stimulation in *ad libitum* fed and food-deprived rats. *Brain Res.* **534**, 8–14.

Carr, K. D. (1994). Streptozotocin-induced diabetes produces a naltrexone-reversible lowering of threshold for lateral hypothalamic self-stimulation. *Brain Res.* **664**, 211–214.

Carr, K. D. and Bak, T. H. (1990). Rostral and caudal ventricular infusion of antibodies to dynorphin A (1–17) and dynorphin A (1–8): effects on electrically-elicited feeding in the rat. *Brain Res.* **507**, 289–294.

Carr, K. D. and Papadouka, V. (1994). The role of multiple opioid receptors in the potentiation of reward by food restriction. *Brain Res.* **639**, 253–260.

Carr, K. D. and Simon, E. J. (1983a). Effects of naloxone and its quaternary analogue on stimulation-induced feeding. *Neuropharmacology* **22**, 127–130.

Carr, K. D. and Simon, E. J. (1983b). The role of opioids in feeding and reward elicited by lateral hypothalamic electrical stimulation. *Life Sci.* **33 (supplement I)**, 563–566.

Carr, K. D. and Simon, E. J. (1984). Potentiation of reward by hunger is opioid mediated. *Brain Res.* **297**, 369–373.

Carr, K. D. and Wolinsky, T. D. (1993). Chronic food restriction and weight loss produce opioid facilitation of perifornical hypothalamic self-stimulation. *Brain Res.* **607**, 141–148.

Carr, K. D. and Wolinsky, T. D. (1994). Regulation of feeding by multiple opioid receptors in cingulate cortex; follow-up to an *in vivo* autoradiographic study. *Neuropeptides*, **26**, 207–213.

Carr, K. D., Bak, T. H., Gioannini, T. L. and Simon, E. J. (1987). Antibodies to dynorphin A (1–13) but not β-endorphin inhibit electrically-elicited feeding in the rat. *Brain Res.* **422**, 384–388.

Carr, K. D., Aleman, D. O., Bak, T. H. and Simon, E. J. (1991). Effects of parabrachial opioid antagonism on stimulation-induced feeding. *Brain Res.* **545**, 283–286.

Carr, K. D., Papadouka, V. and Wolinsky, T. D. (1993). Norbinaltorphamine blocks the feeding but not the reinforcing effect of lateral hypothalamic electrical stimulation. *Psychopharmacology* **111**, 345–350.

Chen, Y., Mestek, A., Liu, J., Hurley, J. A. and Yu, L. (1993). Molecular cloning and functional expression of a μ-opioid receptor from rat brain. *Mol. Pharmacol.* **44**, 8–12.

Conover, K. L. and Shizgal, P. (1994). Competition and summation between rewarding effects of sucrose and lateral hypothalamic stimulation in the rat. *Behav. Neurosci.* **108**, 537–548.

Coons, E. E. and White, H. A. (1977). Tonic properties of orosensation and the modulation of intracranial self-stimulation: the CNS weighting of external and internal factors governing reward. *Ann. N.Y. Acad. Sci.* **290**, 158–179.

Corbett, A. D., Paterson, S. J. and Kosterlitz, H. W. (1993). In *Handbook of Experimental Pharmacology. Vol. 104: Opioids* (A. Herz, ed.), pp. 645–679. Springer, New York.

Corp, E. S., Woods, S. C., Porte, D., Dorsa, D. M., Figlewicz, D. P. and Baskin, D. G. (1986). Localization of ^{125}I-insulin binding sites in the rat hypothalamus by quantitative autoradiography. *Neurosci. Lett.* **70**, 17–22.

De Olmos, J., Alheid, G. F. and Beltramino, C. A. (1985). Amygdala. In *The Rat Nervous System* (G. Paxinos, ed.) pp. 223–334. Academic Press, New York.

Di Chiara, G. and North, A. R. (1992). Neurobiology of opiate abuse. *Trends Pharmacol. Sci.* **13**, 185–193.

Evans, C. J., Keith, D. E., Morrison, H., Magendzo, K. and Edwards, R. H. (1992). Cloning of a delta opioid receptor by functional expression. *Science* **258**, 1952–1955.

Fallon, J. H. and Leslie, F. M. (1986). Distribution of dynorphin and enkephalin peptides in the rat brain. *J. Comp. Neurol.* **249**, 293–336.

Ferssiwi, A., Cardo, B. and Velley, L. (1987). Electrical self-stimulation in the parabrachial area is depressed after ibotenic acid lesion of the lateral hypothalamus. *Behav. Brain Res.* **25**, 109–116.

Fukuda, K., Kato, S., Mori, K., Nishi, M. and Takeshima, H. (1993). Primary structures and expression from cDNAs of rat opioid receptor δ- and μ-subtypes. *FEBS Lett.* **327**, 311–314.

Giraudo, S. Q., Grace, M. K., Welch, C. C., Billington, C. J. and Levine, A. S. (1993). Naloxone's anorectic effect is dependent upon the relative palatability of food. *Pharmacol. Biochem. Behav.* **46**, 917–921.

Gosnell, B.A. (1988). Involvement of μ opioid receptors in the amygdala in the control of feeding. *Neuropharmacology* **27**, 319–326.

Gosnell, B. A., Morley, J. E. and Levine, A. S. (1986). Opioid-induced feeding: localization of sensitive brain sites. *Brain Res.* **369**, 177–184.

Hernandez, L. and Hoebel, B. G. (1989). Food intake and lateral hypothalamic self-stimulation covary after medial hypothalamic lesions or ventral midbrain 6-hydroxydopamine injections that cause obesity. *Behav. Neurosci.* **103**, 412–422.

Hollt, V., Dum, J., Blasig, J., Schubert, P. and Herz, A. (1975). Comparison of *in vivo* and *in vitro* parameters of opiate receptor binding in naive and tolerant/dependent rodents. *Life Sci.* **16**, 1823–1828.

Kazmierski, W., Wire, W. S., Lui, G. K., Knapp, R. J., Shook, J. E., Burks, T. F., Yamamura, H. I. and Hruby, V. J. (1988). Design and synthesis of somatostatin analogues with topographical properties that lead to highly potent and specific μ opioid receptor antagonists with greatly reduced binding at somatostatin receptors. *J. Med. Chem.* **31**, 2170–2178.

Kieffer, B. L., Befort, K., Gaveriaux-Ruff, C. and Hirth, C. G. (1992). The δ-opioid receptor: isolation of a cDNA by expression cloning and pharmacological characterization. *Proc. Natl. Acad. Sci.* **89**, 12 048–12 052.

Kirkham, T. C. and Cooper, S. J. (1988). Attenuation of sham feeding by naloxone is stereospecific: evidence for opioid mediation of orosensory reward. *Physiol. Behav.* **43**, 845–847.

Koob, G. F. (1992). Drugs of abuse: anatomy, pharmacology and function of reward pathways. *Trends Pharmacol. Sci.* **13**, 177–184.

Kosterlitz, H. W. and Paterson, S. J. (1990). D-Phe-Cys-Tyr-D-Trp-Orn-Thr-Pen-Thr-NH$_2$ is a highly selective μ-ligand with low *in vitro* antagonist activity. *Br. J. Pharmacol.* **99**, 291.

Krettek, J. E. and Price, J. L. (1978). Amygdaloid projections to subcortical structures within the basal forebrain and brainstem in the rat and cat. *J. Comp. Neurol.* **178**, 225–254.

Levine, A. S., Grace, M., Billington, C. J. and Portoghese, P. S. (1990). Norbinaltorphamine decreases deprivation and opioid-induced feeding. *Brain Res.* **534**, 60–64.

Levine, A. S., Grace, M. and Billington, C. J. (1991) β-Funaltrexamine (β-FNA) decreases deprivation and opioid-induced feeding. *Brain Res.* **562**, 281–284.

Lynch, W. C. (1986). Opiate blockade inhibits saccharin intake and blocks normal preference acquisition. *Pharmacol. Biochem. Behav.* **24**, 833–836.

McGowan, M. K., Andrews, K. M. and Grossman, S. P. (1992). Chronic intrahypothalamic infusions of insulin or insulin antibodies alter body weight and food intake in the rat. *Physiol. Behav.* **51**, 753–766.

Mansour, A., Khachaturian, H., Lewis, M. E., Akil, H. and Watson, S. J. (1988). Anatomy of CNS opioid receptors. *Trends Neurosci.* **11**, 308–314.

Menendez, J. A. and Atrens, D. M. (1991). Insulin and the paraventricular hypothalamus: modulation of energy balance. *Brain Res.* **555**, 193–201.

Meng, F., Xie, G. X., Thompson, R. C., Mansour, A., Goldstein, A., Watson, S. J. and Akil, H. (1993). Cloning and pharmacological characterization of a rat kappa opioid receptor. *Proc. Natl. Acad. Sci.* **90**, 9954–9958.

Moreau, J. L., Jenck, F. and Martin, J. R. (1992). Antidepressant treatment prevents chronic unpredictable mild stress-induced anhedonia as assessed by ventral tegmental self-stimulation behavior in rats. *Eur. Neuropsychopharmacol.* **2**, 43–49.

Moufid-Bellancourt, S. and Velley, L. (1994). Effects of morphine injection into the parabrachial area on saccharin preference: modulation by lateral hypothalamic neurons. *Pharmacol. Biochem. Behav.* **48**, 127–133.

Nishikawa, T., Fage, D. and Scatton, B. (1986). Evidence for, and nature of, the tonic inhibitory influence of habenulointerpeduncular pathways upon cerebral dopaminergic transmission in the rat. *Brain Res.* **373**, 324–336.

Norgren, R. (1976). Taste pathways to hypothalamus and amygdala. *J. Comp. Neurol.* **166**, 17–30.

North, R. A. (1993). In *Handbook of Experimental Pharmacology. Vol. 104: Opioids* (Herz, A., ed.), pp. 773–797. Springer, New York.

Oomura, Y., Nishino, H., Aou, S. and Lenard, L. (1986). Opiate mechanism in reward-related responses during operant feeding behavior of the monkey. *Brain Res.* **365**, 335–339.

Papadouka, V. and Carr, K. D. (1994). The role of multiple opioid receptors in the maintenance of stimulation-induced feeding. *Brain Res.* **639**, 42–48.

Parker, L. A., Maier, S., Rennie, M. and Crebolder, J. (1992). Morphine- and naltrexone-induced modification of palatability: analysis by the taste reactivity test. *Behav. Neurosci.* **106**, 999–1010.

Portoghese, P. S., Lipkowski, A. W. and Takemori, A. E. (1987). Binaltorphimine and nor-binaltorphamine, potent and selective κ-opioid receptor antagonists. *Life Sci.* **4**, 1287–1292.

Portoghese, P. S., Sultana, M. and Takemori, A. E. (1988). Naltrindole, a highly selective and potent non-peptide δ opioid receptor antagonist. *Eur. J. Pharmacol.* **146**, 185–186.

Rockwood, G. A. and Reid, L. D. (1982). Naloxone modifies sugar-water intake in rats drinking with open gastric fistulas. *Physiol. Behav.* **29**, 1175–1178.

Rolls, E. T. (1974). The neural basis of brain stimulation reward. *Prog. Neurobiol.* **3**, 71–160.

Saper, C. B. (1982). Convergence of autonomic and limbic connections in the insular cortex of the rat. *J. Comp. Neurol.* **210**, 163–173.

Schulz, R., Wilhelm, A. and Dirlich, G. (1984). Intracerebral injection of different antibodies against endogenous opioids suggest α-neoendorphin participation in control of feeding behavior. *Naunyn Schmiedebergs Arch. Pharmacol.* **320**, 222–226.

Schroeder, R. L., Weinger, M. B., Vakassian, L. and Koob, G. F. (1991). Methylnaloxonium diffuses out of the rat brain more slowly than naloxone after direct intracerebral injection. *Neurosci. Lett.* **121**, 173–177.

Siegel, A., Joyner, K. and Smith, G. P. (1988). Effect of bilateral ibotenic acid lesions in the basolateral amygdala on the sham feeding response to sucrose in the rat. *Physiol. Behav.* **42**, 231–235.

Simon, E. J. and Hiller, J. M. (1994). Opioid peptides and opioid receptors. In *Basic Neurochemistry: Molecular, Cellular, and Medical Aspects* (G. J. Siegel *et al.*, eds), 5th edn, pp. 321–339. Raven Press, New York.

Stanley, B. G., Lanthier, D. and Leibowitz, S. F. (1989). Multiple brain sites sensitive to feeding stimulation by opioid agonists: a cannula-mapping study. *Pharmacol. Biochem. Behav.* **31**, 825–832.

Stein, E. A., Carr, K. D. and Simon, E. J. (1990). Brain stimulation-induced feeding alters regional opioid receptor binding in the rat: an *in vivo* autoradiographic study. *Brain Res.* **533**, 213–222.

Ter Horst, G. J. and Luiten, P. G. M. (1986). The projections of the dorsomedial hypothalamic nucleus in the rat. *Brain Res. Bull.* **16**, 231–248.

Thompson, R. C., Mansour, A., Akil, H. and Watson, S. J. (1993). Cloning and pharmacological characterization of a rat μ opioid receptor. *Neuron* **11**, 903–913.

Touzani, K., Taghzouti, K. and Velley, L. (1994). Amygdaloid central nucleus participates in gustatory reinforcement processes. *Soc. Neurosci. Abstr.* **20**, 366.

Tsujii, S., Nakai, Y., Fukata, J., Koh, T., Takahashi, H., Usui, T. and Imura, H. (1986a). Effects of food deprivation and high fat diet on opioid receptor binding in rat brain. *Neurosci. Lett.* **72**, 169–173.

Tsujii, S., Nakai, Y., Koh, T., Takhashi, H., Usui, T., Ikeda, H., Matsuo, T. and Imura, H. (1986b). Effect of food deprivation on opioid receptor binding in the brain of lean and fatty Zucker rats. *Brain Res.* **399**, 200–203.

Turner, B. and Herkenham, M. (1981). An autoradiographic study of thalamo-amygaloid connections in the rat. *Anat. Rec.* **199**, 260A.

Ukai, M. and Holtzman, S. G. (1988). Effects of β-funaltrexamine on ingestive behaviors in the rat. *Eur. J. Pharmacol.* **153**, 161–165.

Weber, E., Evans, C. J. and Barchas, J. D. (1982). Predominance of the amino-terminal octapeptide fragment of dynorphin in rat brain regions. *Nature* **299**, 77–79.

Wise, R. A. (1982). Common neural basis for brain stimulation reward, drug reward, and food reward. In *The Neural Basis of Feeding and Reward* (B.G. Hoebel and D. Novin, eds), pp. 445–454. Haer Institute, Brunswick, Maine.

Wolinsky, T. D., Carr, K. D., Hiller, J. M. and Simon, E. J. (1994). Effects of chronic food restriction on mu and kappa opioid binding in rat forebrain: a quantitative autoradiographic study. *Brain Res.* **656**, 274–280.

Wolinsky, T. D., Carr, K. D., Hiller, J. M. and Simon, E. J. (1995). Chronic food restriction alters mu and kappa opioid receptor binding in the parabrachial nucleus of the rat: A quantitative autoradiographic study. *Brain Res.* (In press).

Woods, S. C., Porte, D., Bobbioni, E., Ionescu, E., Sauter, J. F., Rohner-Jeanrenaud, F. R. and Jeanrenaud, B. (1985). Insulin: its relationship to the central nervous system and to the control of food intake and body weight. *Am. J. Clin. Nutr.* **42**, 1063–1071.

Yasuda, K., Raynor, K., Kong, H., Breder, C. D., Takeda, J., Reisine, T. and Bell, G. I. (1993). Cloning and functional comparison of κ and δ opioid receptors from mouse brain. *Proc. Natl. Acad. Sci.* **90**, 6736–6740.

Zacharko, R. M. and Anisman, H. (1991). Stressor-induced anhedonia in the mesocorticolimbic system. *Neurosci. Biobehav. Rev.* **15**, 391–405.

Zardetto-Smith, A. M., Moga, M. M., Magnuson, D. J. and Gray, T. S. (1988). Lateral hypothalamic dynorphinergic efferents to the amygdala and brainstem in the rat. *Peptides* **9**, 1121–1127.

Zukin, R. S. and Tempel, A. (1986). Neurochemical correlates of opiate receptor regulation. *Biochem. Pharmacol.* **35**, 1623–1627.

9

Sensitization to the Ingestive Effects of Opioids

PAOLO NENCINI

Institute of Medical Pharmacology, University of Rome 'La
Sapienza', P. le A. Moro 5, 00185 Rome, Italy

1 Introduction

The effects of opioid drugs on feeding behaviour cannot be described as strong.
In fact, they are generally weak and apparently unpredictable. They can vary
between activation of feeding behaviour on one hand and its suppression on the
other. In some experimental conditions, opioids may leave feeding behaviour
unaffected, unless given in large doses when they may exert a feeding
suppressant effect. However, these apparently conflicting effects are not
entirely unpredictable, because they depend largely on the internal state of the
animal. A state of satiation, for instance, can facilitate the prophagic effect of
opioids, whereas hunger may reveal an anorectic effect (for comprehensive
reviews see Morley et al., 1983; Cooper et al., 1985, 1988; Cooper and
Kirkham, 1993). Hence, the feeding response to opioids seems to differ from
analgesia, respiratory depression and other robust pharmacological effects,
which occur reliably with little dependence on the specific conditions of the
experimental procedure.

However, when the effects of drugs are considered in a human setting, even
an apparently weak pharmacological effect may have important implications.
For example, the addictive potential of morphine and its congeners is less
strong than is commonly thought, since addiction develops in only a small
proportion of people who try them. The efficacy with which opioids produce
addiction can easily be reduced in humans, since addictiveness depends on the
presence of a number of 'soft determinants' (for example, peers, family or
particular environmental settings) which interact with the particular characteristics of the individual involved (Falk and Feingold, 1987).

The sensitivity of drug-taking behaviour to both internal and external factors
is only one of the reasons for considering this behaviour as relevant to an
analysis of the effects of opioids on feeding behaviour. The commonplace

DRUG RECEPTOR SUBTYPES AND INGESTIVE BEHAVIOUR
ISBN 0-12-187620-9

observation that people who are inordinately fond of a particular kind of food are 'addicted' to it may be more than a cliché. It should not surprise us to read, for example, that 'The motivation produced by morphine and food is isomorphic', as the title of a study showing that the motivational effects of morphine can substitute for food in food-deprived animals contends (Nader and van der Kooy, 1994). We now have good reason to believe that commonalties exist between the neurobiological processes underlying drug-taking and feeding behaviours.

Yet, some 15 years ago, when the first studies on the prophagic effects of opioids appeared, it would have seemed utterly unfounded to consider the motivational effects produced by morphine and food as isomorphic. Even though, at an early stage, an increase in food palatability was proposed to account for the prophagic actions of opioids (for a review see Morley *et al.*, 1983), this opioid effect was attributed mainly to the prevention of the decline of pleasantness of food produced by the process of satiety (Fantino *et al.*, 1986) (for discussion see Cooper *et al.*, 1988). This interpretation fitted well with the view that food intake is controlled by plasma levels of nutrients (including glucose, free fatty acids and amino-acids) through the activation of central integrators located in the so-called hypothalamic centres of appetite (lateral hypothalamus) and satiation (ventromedial hypothalamus) (see, for example, Morley and Levine, 1983; Bray, 1985). Accordingly, microinjections of β-endorphin into the ventromedial and paraventricular hypothalamic nuclei were found to elicit feeding responses in satiated rats. Pharmacological evidence, obtained with receptor-specific agonists and antagonists, then confirmed that opioidergic transmission in the hypothalamus plays a role in the activation of feeding responses (for reviews see Morley *et al.*, 1983; Leibowitz, 1986; Cooper *et al.*, 1988). Since metabolic requirements can control feeding behaviour but cannot control addictive behaviour, the mechanisms responsible for the stimulation of feeding behaviour produced by opioids should be different from those involved in their addictive effects.

In agreement with the view that the prophagic effects of opioids are connected with metabolic mechanisms of feeding control, the first clinical application of these experimental observations was the attempt to reduce bodyweight in obese patients by giving the opioid antagonist naltrexone (Atkinson *et al.*, 1985; Malcolm *et al.*, 1985). However, clinical trials have not demonstrated the efficacy of naltrexone in reducing bodyweight (Atkinson *et al.*, 1985; Malcolm *et al.*, 1985). Meanwhile, the idea that the prophagic and addictive effects of opioids have some substrates in common has progressively gained recognition. Nowadays, there is growing awareness that the 'hedonic' value of food is an important substrate of drug action (see, for example, Cooper, 1994).

This chapter will review the more recent literature that supports the view that the prophagic and addictive properties of opioids have motivational mechanisms in common. I shall place particular emphasis on the sensitization process that can modify these properties. An important consequence of this change of perspective has been to shift interest from the role of the opioid system in obesity to its role in the pathogenesis of ingestive disorders and, notably, of bulimia. This is a welcome shift because 'with reference to eating disorders, our understanding of CNS pathophysiology has lagged behind the advances made in understanding many other psychiatric disorders' (Kaye *et al.*, 1990).

2 Feeding behaviour and the 'motive circuit'

Hunger is far from being the sole reason for eating and, even in a fully satiated subject, feeding can be elicited by presenting a palatable food. By definition, palatable food is a rewarding stimulus and, once tried, an individual is likely to be more motivated to obtain it. In other words, pleasant taste confers positive reinforcing properties on foods, making the amount of food ingested to some extent independent of the individual's metabolic requirements.

The neural network that releases appetitive behaviour in response to food, as well as to drug presentation, is an integral part of the so-called 'motive circuit' (Kalivas *et al.*, 1993) and has been the subject of extensive study for the past decade. As is well known, the mesolimbic dopaminergic system, deeply inserted into the 'motive circuit', is thought to have an important role in elaborating rewarding stimuli. Thus, either lever-pressing for food or exposure to stimuli associated with food, increases dopamine release in the nucleus accumbens (Hernandez and Hoebel, 1988; Blackburn *et al.*, 1989; McCullough and Salamone, 1992). The same effect has been produced through exposure to addictive drugs, such as opioids and psychomotor stimulants (Di Chiara and Imperato, 1988). Therefore, not only do palatable foods and addictive drugs share the label of positive reinforcers due to their ability to activate appetitive behaviours, but they also share the ability to activate the same motivational circuit.

This commonality of effects and mechanisms may be viewed as the mere result of a sensorimotor gating process that organizes appropriate motor responses to adequate stimuli, whether they be food, a receptive female, or drugs (Salamone, 1992). Accordingly, the prophagic and addictive properties of opioids share motivational mechanisms that may consist of a common hedonic evaluation of diverse motivational stimuli. Such a model probably suffers from oversimplification because it fails to account for a possible interaction between these diverse motivational stimuli. For instance, activation of the dopaminergic mesolimbic system by pharmacological stimuli might enhance food palatability. Morphine is a good example of this interaction. Behavioural studies agree with the conclusion that morphine increases the consumption of a preferred food. Cooper and Kirkham (1990) demonstrated that it increased the time rats spent in eating biscuits, without increasing the time they spent in eating the standard food pellets. Gosnell *et al.* (1990)

showed that morphine increased carbohydrate intake in carbohydrate-preferring rats and increased fat intake in fat-preferring animals. Gosnell and Patel (1993) have also shown that intracerebroventricular administration of the selective μ opioid peptide [D-Ala^2,N-Me-Phe^4,Gly-ol^5]-enkephalin (DAMGO) or of the selective δ opioid peptide [D-Thr^2]-leucine-enkephalin-Thr (DTLET) increased operant responding for saccharin. These results suggest that morphine and its analogues increase food intake by enhancing the activity of reward pathways in the brain. Accordingly, it has been shown repeatedly that the microinjection of morphine or other μ opioid agonists into the ventral tegmental area or into the nucleus accumbens and ventromedial striatum elicits a hyperphagic response in non-food-deprived rats (Majeed *et al.*, 1986; Mucha and Iversen, 1986; Evans and Vaccarino, 1990; Nencini and Stewart, 1990; Bakshi and Kelley, 1993a,b, 1994; Noel and Wise, 1993). The finding that the administration of naloxone into the ventral tegmental area inhibits the intake of palatable food further supports the view that opioid mechanisms affecting the mesolimbic dopaminergic system regulate the consumption of palatable food (Segall and Margules, 1989). Since animals self-administer morphine and opioid peptides, which are active at μ and δ opioid receptors, directly into the ventral tegmental area (Bozarth and Wise, 1981; Devine and Wise, 1994), this area must also be an important site for the rewarding effect of the drugs. Finally, administration of morphine into the ventral tegmental area produces dopamine release at the nucleus accumbens (Leone *et al.*, 1991), probably by inhibiting inhibitory γ-aminobutyric acid (GABA)ergic interneurons (Kalivas and Stewart, 1991; Johnson and North, 1992; Devine *et al.*, 1993).

For these reasons, activation of the mesolimbic dopaminergic system is one of the ways in which morphine stimulates feeding behaviour. If this interpretation is correct, then drugs that activate this system should also stimulate food intake. This conclusion is supported by evidence that microinjecting amphetamine into the nucleus accumbens also increases food intake in the rat (Evans and Vaccarino, 1986, 1990). Thus, when its action is experimentally restricted to the mesolimbic dopaminergic system, even a prototypical anorectic drug such as amphetamine becomes an orexigenic drug.

Note, however, that this system does not always contribute to the activation of feeding behaviour produced by opioid drugs. The κ opioid agonist U-50 488H, for example, when administered systemically, strongly stimulates feeding (for a review see Cooper *et al.*, 1988). However, when it is micro-injected into the ventral tegmental area and into other areas of the mesolimbic dopaminergic system it is devoid of prophagic actions (Nencini and Stewart, 1990; Bakshi and Kelley, 1993a; Noel and Wise, 1993). This is not surprising, because, in contrast to μ opioids, U-50 448H is not self-administered, produces a conditioned place aversion and reduces locomotor activity (Tang and Collins, 1985; Cooper, 1991). In addition, it inhibits dopamine release in the mesolimbic dopaminergic system (Di Chiara and Imperato, 1988b), probably through direct modulation of dopaminergic perikarya located in the ventral tegmental area (Pickel *et al.*, 1993). Accordingly, intracerebroventricular administration of U-50 488H does not increase saccharin preference in non-deprived rats (Gosnell and Majchrzak, 1989). Likewise, the dynorphin A analogue DAKLI (Tyr-Gly-Gly-Phe-Leu-Arg-Arg-Ke-Arg-Pro-Arg-Leu-Arg-Gly-5-amino-pentylamide) does not affect operant responding to saccharin (Gosnell and Patel, 1993). The microanalysis of feeding behaviour shows that U-50 488H does not increase the initial rate of food ingestion, a measure thought to reflect palatability. In contrast, U-50 488H delays the termination of the first bout of feeding, reduces interbout intervals and increases the number of bouts per meal. All these effects suggest an inhibition of the satiation process (Jackson and Cooper, 1986; Badiani and Stewart, 1993; Stewart and Badiani, 1993b).

The absence of any prophagic effect of U-50 488H, when injected into areas belonging to the mesolimbic dopaminergic system, demonstrates that when a pharmacological stimulus elicits feeding by activating the mesolimbic dopaminergic system it should also be capable of releasing other appetitive behaviours. Accordingly, morphine and amphetamine increase food palatability, and induce self-administration and conditioned place-preference. In contrast, a drug, such as U-50 488H, which is not self-administered and induces conditioned place-aversion, does not activate feeding behaviour when injected into the mesolimbic dopaminergic system. Whether there is any connection between the aversive properties of U-50 488H and its ability to delay satiation, and whether this odd association reflects some peculiar physiological role of the κ opioid system, remains unclear.

3 Sensitization of motivated behaviour

An important attribute of the behavioural effects of drugs mediated mainly by the mesolimbic dopaminergic system is that they become progressively augmented when the drug is given chronically but intermittently. In pharmacological terms, this sensitization appears as a shift to the left in the dose–response curve of the drug. The most thoroughly explored example of behavioural sensitization is the increased locomotor response produced by chronic intermittent administration of some psychotropic drugs, including psychomotor stimulants and opioid agonists active at μ receptors. Several recent reviews provide a comprehensive discussion of drug-induced sensitization of motor activity (see, for instance, Kalivas and Stewart, 1991; Kalivas *et al.*, 1993; Robinson and Berridge, 1993; Stewart and Badiani, 1993a; Wise and Leeb, 1993). For the purposes of the present chapter, a few of the attributes of this phenomenon deserve to be stressed.

First, apart from the effects of systemic administration, sensitization can also be produced by direct injection of the drug into specific areas of the mesolimbic dopaminergic system, most notably the regions of the dopaminergic cell bodies (i.e. the ventral tegmental area and substantia nigra). Second, cross-sensitization can occur between the effects of psychomotor stimulants and μ opioids, although dopaminergic mechanisms seem to be more important than opioidergic mechanisms for the development of sensitization. Third, sensitization is produced *only* by intermittent exposure to the drug, since continuous exposure mainly produces tolerance. Why this happens is still unclear, but the fact that intermittence in drug administration is a crucial requirement for behavioural sensitization has some interesting consequences. The inter-drug interval, for instance, can be extended by several days without impeding the development of sensitization. In addition, once sensitization is established, it seems to persist almost indefinitely, as shown by the enhanced response to drug administration even months after termination of the sensitizing cycle of drug administration.

Although locomotion is typically an investigatory activity that puts the subject in contact with elements of its environment, caution must be exercised in extending findings from the study of spontaneous locomotion to motivated behaviours. In other words, investigatory wandering around differs from appetitive locomotion. As has been correctly observed '. . .a dopamine-dependent increase in locomotor activity may not generalize to reinforcement-related behaviour' (Phillips *et al.*, 1994). These doubts are strengthened by evidence that locomotor sensitization, at least that to psychomotor stimulants, is associated with the appearance and progressive enhancement of non-finalized, fragmented and repetitive behaviours (i.e. stereotyped responses), which of course compete with motivated behaviours (for a review see Robinson and Becker, 1986).

However, under experimental contingencies in which behaviour is sustained by the presentation of an addictive drug, it is easy to demonstrate that drugs which produce locomotion sensitization also cause sensitization to their motivational effects. Notably, non-contingent adminstration of psychomotor stimulants, such as cocaine, metamphetamine and amphetamine, facilitates the later acquisition of their self-administration (Woolverton *et al.*, 1984; Piazza *et al.*, 1989; Horger *et al.*, 1990). In addition, amphetamine, cocaine and morphine pretreatment enhances the efficacy of environmental stimuli conditioned to these drugs in a paradigm of conditioned place preference (Lett, 1989). The latter study also provides strong evidence in favour of cross-sensitization between the motivational effects of drugs belonging to different pharmacological classes. Animals pretreated with amphetamine showed an enhanced place preference for morphine and vice versa (Lett, 1989). Finally, microinjecting drugs directly into specific areas of the mesolimbic dopaminergic system leads to sensitization and cross-sensitization for motivated behaviours. For instance, repeated intra-accumbens injection of μ opioid agonists enhances the amphetamine-mediated increase in responding for conditioned reward (Cunningham and Kelley, 1992).

Locomotion and reinforcement-related behaviours therefore resemble one another in the way they increase in intensity in response to chronic but intermittent exposure to some psychoactive drugs. Incidentally, it is remarkable that, although so much research has been done on locomotion sensitization, relatively little has been carried out on sensitization to the motivational effects of these drugs. This bias may have arisen because of the observation that progressive augmentation, or sensitization, of behavioural hyperactivity is elicited by repeated administration of psychostimulants in both humans and experimental animals. This 'has led to the suggestion that understanding the neural mechanisms of sensitization in rodents may provide insight into the neural substrates of both drug-induced and idiopathic psychosis' (Kalivas and Stewart, 1991). Only recently has it become clear that drug-induced behavioural sensitization is relevant to other kinds of human psychopathology, categorized as impulsive disorders, which include drug or food craving (Fahy and Eisler, 1993; Bakshi and Kelley, 1994; Carr and Papadouka, 1994). Because the mesolimbic dopaminergic system plays an important role in activating the approaching behaviour to food, and because opioids facilitate this activation, it is not surprising to discover that sensitization develops to the prophagic effects of opioids.

4 Chronic administration of opioids and feeding behaviour

Relatively few studies have addressed the question of what happens to the prophagic effects of opioids when these drugs are administered chronically. Unfortunately, in some of these studies opioids have been injected in high daily doses (as high as 25 mg/kg morphine intraperitoneally; Morley *et al.*, 1982, 1985) or even infused using minipumps for several days (Gosnell and Krahn, 1993a). At these levels of exposure, opioids are likely to produce physical dependence, a condition that has a complex influence on feeding behaviour. Although the sickness and anorexia typical of the withdrawal syndrome come immediately to mind, in morphine-tolerant rats morphine also increases motor activity, temperature and metabolic rate (Martin *et al.*, 1963; Kumar *et al.*, 1971; Clark, 1979). The loss of weight resulting from these increases may, in turn, stimulate regulatory feeding behaviour, making it difficult to isolate the effects of chronic opioid treatments that are related to feeding maintained by the 'hedonic' properties of food (i.e. palatability). Thus, from an experimental point of view, it is helpful that, in satiated rats, morphine is able to stimulate food intake at doses as low as 1–2 mg/kg intraperitoneally (Sanger and McCarthy, 1981; Nencini, 1988; Gosnell and Krahn, 1993a), which are most unlikely to cause physical dependence when administered daily. In contrast, at these doses, an intermittent schedule of administration would probably eventually induce sensitization in the prophagic response. Therefore, I shall consider here only studies that adopted this schedule of administration. The animals were maintained under experimental conditions that differed according to the level of satiation, to the kind of food presented and to the schedule of access to food.

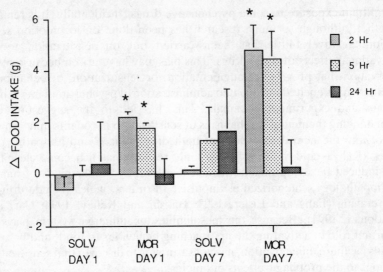

Fig. 1 Time course of the effects of daily injections of morphine (MOR) (1 mg/kg sub-cutaneously) on food intake at 2, 5 and 24 h in male Sprague–Dawley rats maintained in conditions of free access to food. Data are expressed as the difference in grams of food with respect to the last baseline day (solvent injection). Each bar represents the mean ± SEM of six data. SOLV, solvent. $P < 0.05$ vs baseline (Student's paired t test).

Taking into account these methodological constraints, studies are consistent in suggesting that the prophagic effect produced by the acute administration of opioids is not abated following chronic exposure to them (Levine *et al.*, 1985). In other words, tolerance does not develop to the prophagic effects of opioids. For instance, in rats maintained under conditions of free access to food, stimulation of spontaneous feeding produced by the κ opioid agonist U-50 488H remained stable throughout 5 weeks of daily intraperitoneal administration (Nencini *et al.*, 1988). Chronic administration of other opioids has yielded similar results, or sometimes even an increased feeding response. After a small dose (1 mg/kg subcutaneously), morphine typically elicits a progressive daily enhancement of the feeding response at 2 and 5 h, but not at 24 h (Fig. 1). Note, however, that this enhancement does not necessarily result from a sensitization of the drug's prophagic effect. Because morphine has both orexigenic and anorectic effects, we cannot rule out the possibility that the apparent sensitization to the prophagic effects might actually be the result of tolerance to the drug's feeding-suppressant effects (Leshem, 1988; Wolgin and Benson, 1991). This suggestion is supported by other evidence that repeated administration causes a reduction in the magnitude and duration of the opioid depressant effect on feeding (Morley *et al.*, 1982). Whatever contribution tolerance to the anorectic effects of opioids makes to the increment of the stimulation of food intake, ample recent evidence now indicates that sensitization does develop to their prophagic effects.

5 Sensitization to the prophagic effects of κ opioids

The first evidence for this sensitization comes from studies focused on the mechanism of tolerance to the anorectic effects of amphetamines. Because amphetamines and κ opioids showed opposite effects on food intake, we reasoned that the mechanisms responsible for the anorectic effects of amphetamines may include inhibition of κ opioid-mediated facilitation of feeding behaviour (Nencini et al., 1988). A persistent drug-induced inhibition of a physiological function can elicit an adaptive process that counters the effect of the drug. This process leads to tolerance to the effect of the drug and, in absence of the drug, to an unopposed compensatory reaction (rebound effect). The adaptive process can also lead to sensitization to drugs mimicking the inhibited physiological function. For instance, chronic exposure to β-blockers or clonidine enhances the sensitivity to sympathomimetic drugs (Gerber and Nies, 1990). Thus, if amphetamine administration inhibits κ opioid-mediated facilitation of feeding behaviour, and if this inhibition persists, we would expect it to augment the sensitivity to the prophagic effect of a κ opioid agonist.

Confirming our working hypothesis, the results showed that, in rats maintained under conditions of free feeding, chronic intermittent administration of moderate doses of cathinone, a naturally occurring amphetamine-like compound, or of amphetamine, significantly increased the feeding response to systemic administration of U-50 488H (Nencini, 1988; Nencini et al., 1988). This increased sensitivity to the κ opioid agonist was associated with a reduced inhibition of feeding produced by the psychomotor stimulant, which persisted for at least 2 weeks after discontinuation of treatment with the psychomotor stimulant (Nencini, 1988).

Extending this line of research, Badiani and Stewart (1993) analysed the microstructure of the feeding response to U-50 488H after seven daily injections of D-amphetamine (3 mg/kg). They showed that the κ opioid agonist increased the size and length of the first meal. This effect was further enhanced in amphetamine-pretreated animals. Since amphetamine exposure left the antidipsic effect of U-50 488H unmodified, sensitization to the prophagic effect of the drug seemed not to depend on a non-specific behavioural activation. Finally, the lack of an increase in the initial rate of ingestion ruled out the possibility that the interaction between amphetamines and U-50 488H made the food more palatable. Previous experiments from the same laboratory had also shown that ten daily 20-min sessions of restraint augmented the prophagic response to U-50 488H (Badiani and Stewart, 1992), a finding consistent with the possible cross-sensitization between stress and amphetamine (Kalivas and Stewart, 1991). Badiani and Stewart's studies support the findings, previously discussed, that κ opioid-mediated feeding behaviour is probably due not to the activation of rewarding mechanisms but to a delay of satiation.

Further support for this conclusion comes from a study showing that either under basal conditions or after 10 daily intraperitoneal injections of 3 mg/kg

D-amphetamine, U-50 488H microinjected into the ventral tegmental area had no prophagic effect (Nencini and Stewart, 1990). Nevertheless, the same animals appeared to be sensitized to the prophagic action of the κ opioid agonist when the drug was injected systemically (Nencini and Stewart, 1990).

In conclusion, chronic intermittent exposure to amphetamines clearly leads to an augmentation of κ opioid activation of feeding behaviour. This sensitization process does not seem to involve the mesolimbic dopaminergic system. The contrary would have been puzzling, considering that U-50 488H has inhibitory effects on this system and that repeated administration of psychomotor stimulants probably causes the inhibition to decline in strength. This is suggested by a report showing that 9 days of metamphetamine treatment attenuates the inhibitory effect of dynorphin on dopamine release in the rat nucleus accumbens (Yokoo et al., 1992).

The complexity of the interaction between psychomotor stimulants and κ opioids is stressed by a study that measured food intake in freely-fed rats treated daily with amphetamine in combination with U-50 488H (Nencini and Valeri, 1994). Under these experimental conditions U-50 488H, at the dose of 4 mg/kg, increased food intake during the first 2 h and reduced it in the following 3 h. Amphetamine, at a dose of 3 mg/kg intraperitoneally, had roughly the opposite effect, completely suppressing food intake during the first 2 h and reactivating it in the ensuing 3 h. As expected, this reactivating phase progressively increased with daily amphetamine administration. Interestingly enough, when the two drugs were given in combination, amphetamine prevented feeding stimulation produced by U-50 488H during the first 2 h, whereas the κ opioid inhibited the hyperphagic phase that rats showed between 2 and 5 h after amphetamine administration. In consequence, food intake was remarkably suppressed throughout the 5 h of observation. Tolerance did not develop to the first 2 h suppression of feeding, whereas the late hyperphagic phase slowly recovered across the 9 days of combined treatment. Since U-50 488H treatment did not affect the hyperdipsic response to amphetamine, it is unlikely that the suppression of food intake was due to a behavioural impairment produced by interaction between amphetamine and U-50 488H.

The inhibitory effect of U-50 488H on the late hyperphagic response to amphetamine is reminiscent of the recent finding that sensitization to the motor effect of cocaine is prevented by administration of the κ opioid agonist U-69 593 (Heidbreder et al., 1993). It is also consistent with evidence that, in general, κ opioids inhibit the behavioural effects of psychomotor stimulants (Ohno et al., 1989; Spealman and Bergman, 1992; Ukai et al., 1992a,b). If we consider that κ opioids prevent firing of the dopamine cells of the substantia nigra (Walker et al., 1987; Thompson and Walker, 1990) and prevent dopamine release from striata (Mulder et al., 1991) and the nucleus accumbens (Di Chiara and Imperato, 1988a,b), the most parsimonious explanation for the results obtained by Nencini and Valeri (1994) is that U-50 488H prevents the prophagic effects of amphetamine, by inhibiting dopaminergic mechanisms facilitating feeding behaviour. However, this interpretation does not account for the enhanced sensitivity to the prophagic effect of U-50 488H during chronic amphetamine treatment. As suggested above, a persistent amphetamine-mediated inhibition of κ opioid activity may be responsible for this sensitization. Although we have no direct evidence of such a mechanism, circumstantial evidence indicates that psychomotor stimulants upregulate κ opioid mechanisms. Methamphetamine and cocaine produce an increase in the striatal and mesolimbic content of dynorphin, the putative endogenous ligand of κ opiate receptors (Hanson et al., 1988, 1991; Smiley et al., 1990). Likewise, chronic treatment with dopaminergic drugs markedly increases striatal dynorphin messenger RNA (Gerfen et al., 1990). As already suggested, this increase may be due to a reduced use of the opioid peptide (Smiley et al., 1990). In conditions of prolonged inhibition of its release, accumulation of the transmitter is usually associated with sensitization of the effector. Unfortunately, no studies have yet shown that amphetamine-induced sensitization of the prophagic effects of U-50 488H is related to changes of κ opioid receptor sensitivity in discrete regions of the brain. Although we found that 5 weeks of cathinone administration changed neither the affinity nor the number of κ opioid receptors in the whole rat brain (Nencini et al., 1988), these findings do not rule out the possibility that these changes actually develop in circumscribed brain regions.

In summary, κ opioid and catecholaminergic systems exert reciprocal control. Chronic amphetamine administration may cause adaptive modifications in this control, resulting in an enhanced sensitivity to prophagic stimuli.

In the interaction of amphetamine with the κ opioid system on feeding behaviour an important problem remains to be solved. It consists of determining which neurotransmitter released by amphetamine is responsible for interaction of the drug with the κ opioid system, a direct action of amphetamine on this system having been excluded. Some peripheral effects of U-50 488H may be mediated by noradrenaline, because the administration of dapiprazole, a selective α-adrenergic antagonist, blocked its diuretic action. Yet, dapiprazole did not affect the ingestive response to κ opioid (Nencini et al., 1992). As previously outlined, ample evidence shows that stimulation of κ receptors depresses dopaminergic activity in brain areas where amphetamine is able to activate prophagic mechanisms (for instance, the nucleus accumbens). In spite of this, haloperidol and U-50 488H seem to have roughly opposite effects on the ingestive response to daily amphetamine administration (Nencini and Valeri, 1994). Haloperidol speeds up augmentation of the late hyperphagic response to amphetamine, but slows the development of its hyperdipsic effect, whereas the κ opioid drug slows the first response and leaves the second unchanged.

Of course, this is too little evidence to exclude a role for the dopaminergic system in the interaction between amphetamine and the κ opioid system. Considering the growing evidence that expression of D_2 agonist activity requires some intrinsic D_1 agonist action (Clark and White, 1987; Plaznik *et al.*, 1989; Eilam *et al.*, 1992), blocking D_2 receptors alone, as haloperidol does, may not be sufficient to prevent sensitization to the ingestive effects of amphetamine and κ opioids. Some support for this objection has recently been provided by a study focused on the role of D_1 and D_2 dopaminergic receptors in the hyperdipsia produced by chronic administration of amphetamine (Nencini *et al.*, 1994b). When given in combination, agonists at the D_2 (quinpirole) and D_1 (SKF-38 393) receptors both facilitated and reinstated amphetamine-induced hyperdipsia. In contrast, quinpirole or SKF-38 393, given alone, slowed the development of amphetamine-induced hyperdipsia. This finding raises the question of whether the peculiar interaction of U-50 488H and amphetamine on feeding behaviour requires the concurrent involvement of D_1 and D_2 dopaminergic receptors.

6 Sensitization to the prophagic effects of μ opioids

6.1 Spontaneous feeding

The same schedule of amphetamine administration that increases the prophagic response to U-50 488H also enhances the feeding activation elicited by systemic administration of subanalgesic doses of morphine (2 mg/kg intraperitoneally) (Nencini, 1988). In these experimental conditions, however, amphetamine does not augment the feeding activation elicited by diazepam. Amphetamine might, therefore, selectively sensitize the opioidergic mechanisms controlling feeding behaviour. Despite its common functional expression, this 'selective' sensitization involves mechanisms that differ according to the opioid receptor class implicated. As already mentioned, U-50 488H, microinjected into the ventral tegmental area, does not affect food intake either in basal conditions or after chronic intermittent administration of amphetamine. In contrast, morphine microinjected into the same area causes rats to respond by increasing their food intake and this response was further augmented in amphetamine-pretreated subjects (Nencini and Stewart, 1990).

Thus, the mesolimbic dopaminergic system is instrumental in the expression of amphetamine-mediated sensitization to the prophagic effects of morphine. Chronic administration of amphetamine heightens activity responses to morphine microinjected into the ventral tegmental area (Stewart and Vezina, 1987) and more recent studies have also found that in a drug-discrimination paradigm, microinjection of morphine into the same brain area causes amphetamine-trained rats to respond on the drug lever (Druhan *et al.*, 1993). The commonalties in the site and mechanism of morphine and amphetamine action on feeding behaviour suggest that these two drugs interact to augment the subjective pleasurable effects of food.

However, an enhancement of 'pleasure' is only one of the possible interpretations of the increased prophagic effect of morphine induced by amphetamine. A recent study by Badiani and co-workers (1995) offers a different perspective. First of all, they showed that the increase of feeding produced by the microinjection of the selective μ opioid peptide DAMGO into the ventral tegmental area was enhanced by a cycle of daily systemic injections of amphetamine. They then analysed this sensitization further and provided evidence that the augmented behaviour was oriented not only towards food, but also towards gnawable objects, such as pieces of balsa wood, or a drinking tube. In contrast, when the appetitive component of feeding behaviour was studied by making powdered or highly palatable food available at the end of a tunnel, pharmacological treatment apparently failed to influence either the latency to eat or the total food intake.

In conclusion, it appears that a μ opioid-induced increase in dopamine transmission in the mesolimbic system enhances the salience of available incentive stimuli, whatever 'hedonic' or regulatory values they have. Thus, when food is the only incentive stimulus available, food intake increases, because its salience also increases; but when multiple stimuli are available, drug treatment increases their salience non-selectively so that the subject moves from one stimulus to another, thereby yielding fragmented behaviour.

Recently, in the frame of 'an incentive-sensitization theory of addiction', Robinson and Berridge (1993) suggested that chronic administration of psychotropic drugs, such as psychomotor stimulants and μ opioids, brings about an increase in the salience of motivational stimuli without changing their rewarding properties. As they put it, in these conditions, 'sensitization of the neural systems responsible for incentive salience (for 'wanting') can occur independently of changes in neural systems that mediate the subjective pleasurable effects of drugs (drug 'liking')' (p. 247). Although this theory has been developed to provide a comprehensive explanation of the natural history of drug addiction, and in particular of its relapsing episodes, it helps to shift the focus of interest from 'pleasure' to incentive salience, also in sensitization to the prophagic effects of opioids. If the 'irrationality of the [addictive] behaviour is due to an increasing dissociation between the incentive properties of drugs (incentive salience) and their subjective pleasurable effects' (p. 267), we may be tempted to look at bulimic behaviour as the result of a similar dissociation process. The study of Badiani and co-workers (1995) seems to provide interesting experimental support for the 'incentive-sensitization theory' in the field of ingestive behaviour.

6.2   Operant responding for food

In a recent study we evaluated the influence of chronic daily amphetamine administration on the effects of morphine on lever-pressing for food in fasted and in satiated rats (Nencini et al., 1994a). Being a reliable model for the study of appetitively motivated behaviour, we thought that instrumental lever-pressing for food would also be a useful model to test the hypothesis that the

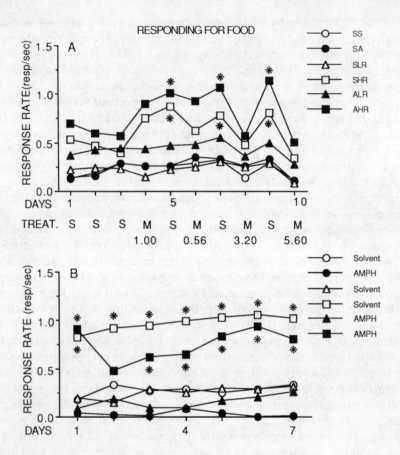

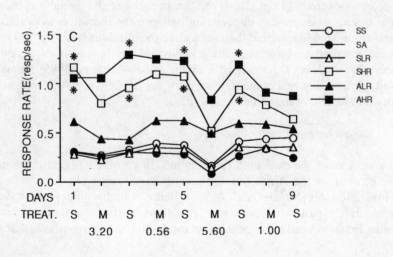

increased feeding response to morphine produced by chronic amphetamine reflects an incremental motivation for food. In this study, motivation for food was manipulated by maintaining rats either in a condition of free-feeding, when access to food was allowed by an FR-5 schedule of reinforcement, or in a condition of mild food restriction (bodyweight maintained constant), when the schedule of reinforcement was incremented up to FR-20. After a period of operant training, the animals received 9 days of amphetamine (5 mg/kg intraperitoneally) in free-feeding conditions. When responding was reinstated, it appeared that amphetamine had significantly enhanced baseline response rates, but only in food-restricted rats. The effects of morphine on operant responding remained unchanged. In contrast, a further 7-day cycle of amphetamine administration (1 mg/kg intraperitoneally) contingent to operant sessions (10 min beforehand) completely prevented the suppressant effects of the highest dose of morphine (5.6 mg/kg) on responding in food-restricted rats. Animals were then moved to a condition of free-feeding and the 2-h food intake was measured after administration of vehicle or a range of morphine doses. Rats with a history of amphetamine administration and food restriction appeared to be more sensitive to the prophagic effects of morphine. However, this interaction between amphetamine and morphine was not detected in satiated rats.

Thus, a history of food restriction and amphetamine administration seem to produce a long-lasting increase in sensitivity to the prophagic effects of morphine. Since food restriction enhances the behavioural effects of amphetamine (Campbell and Fibiger, 1971), it is not surprising that a history of amphetamine administration and food restriction converges in enhancing the sensitivity to the prophagic effects of morphine.

Although the above study was designed only to investigate the interaction between amphetamine and food restriction across different schedules of food presentation, the raw data indicated a remarkable increase in the intra-group dispersion of values when fasted rats received the first dose of morphine (1 mg/kg intraperitoneally) (Fig. 2). Notably, some rats showed a remarkable increase in the response rate, which persisted when saline was injected before the operant session and also resisted the suppressant effects of amphetamine (1

Fig. 2 Mean response rates of lever-pressing for food (45-mg Noyes pellets) during daily 15-min sessions. Solvent (S) or drugs were injected 10 min before the session. The reinforcement schedule was FR20 in food-restricted and FR5 in satiated rats. (A) Reinstatement of responding and dose–response curve for morphine (M) after 9 days of daily amphetamine (5 mg/kg intraperitoneally) in conditions of free access to food. (B) Effects of amphetamine (AMPH) (1 mg/kg intraperitoneally 10 min before session; closed symbols) on response rates. (C) Results obtained by replicating the morphine dose–response curve after amphetamine administration. *$P < 0.05$ vs respective low-responder groups (Tukey's test). SS, satiated controls; SA, satiated amphetamine-treated animals; SLR, fasted low-responder controls; SHR, fasted high-responder controls; ALR, fasted amphetamine-treated low responders; AHR, fasted amphetamine-treated high responders. Values in abscissa of panels A and C indicate intraperitoneally injected doses of morphine (mg/kg).

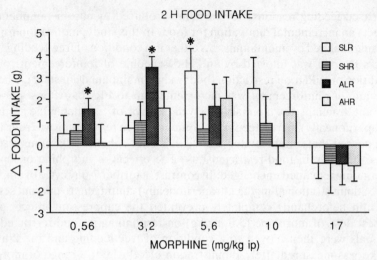

Fig. 3 Mean ± SEM of 2-h food intake of freely feeding rats with a history of food restriction. Data are expressed as the difference between grams of food eaten on the morphine day and the mean eaten on the two previous solvent days. SLR, fasted low-responder controls; SHR, fasted high-responder controls; ALR, fasted amphetamine-treated low responders; AHR, fasted amphetamine-treated high responders. *$P < 0.05$ *vs* solvent day (Student's paired t test).

mg/kg intraperitoneally). The response rates of the remaining fasted rats differed little from those of satiated rats. Yet, when free-feeding conditions were reinstated, under the influence of morphine these non-responder fasted rats became the most voracious eaters (Fig. 3). Thus, animals that apparently could not adapt to the demanding condition of obtaining most of the daily food intake by lever-pressing in a limited period of time (15 min) were those that appeared more 'sensitized' to the prophagic effects of morphine when they had free access to food.

That morphine interacted with food restriction to affect the response rates in some rats but not in others is consistent with the evidence of large individual differences in the behavioural response to psychotropic drugs. Since Demellweek and Goudie (1983) observed that in 'all of our studies on amphetamine tolerance we have noted large differences in tolerance acquisition between different subjects' and recommended that a 'complete account of psychostimulant tolerance will have to explain such large individual differences between subjects', research has extended year by year the list of drug effects liable to interindividual differences. Among these effects are also ingestive responses. In particular, studies in animals show clear evidence of interindividual differences in the propensity to develop hyperdipsia following chronic intermittent amphetamine administration (Mittleman and Valenstein, 1985; Camanni and Nencini, 1994; Nencini and Fraioli, 1994). In addition, individual differences in sugar intake have been found to predict the locomotor response to acute and repeated amphetamine administration (Sills and Vaccarino, 1994). Finally, a recent report has noted that only in some experimental subjects does food restriction produce opioid facilitation of perifornical hypothalamic self-stimulation (Carr and Wolinsky, 1993).

7 Food restriction and sensitization to the prophagic effects of opioids

The results of the experiment shown in Figs 2 and 3 suggest that food deprivation parallels amphetamine administration in producing long-lasting increased sensitivity to the effects of opioids on ingestion of food. This is not surprising, as the effects of fasting on the μ opioid system closely resemble those of chronic intermittent amphetamine administration. For instance, in self-administration and place-preference procedures, food restriction enhances (sensitizes) the stimulus properties of μ opioids (Meisch and Kliner, 1979; Gaiardi et al., 1987). More importantly, food restriction has been found to increase reward by activating opioid mechanisms (Carr and Simon, 1984; Carr and Wolinsky, 1993; Carr and Papadouka, 1994).

Food restriction therefore seems to enhance the motivationally arousing properties of diverse stimuli, by facilitating opioid mechanisms. Since amphetamine produces similar motivational effects, it would be interesting to assess at what point in the motivational process food restriction and the effects of amphetamine converge. The anorectic action of amphetamine produces a non-regulatory suppression of feeding, which might have stimulus properties similar to those of food restriction. This speculation is supported by a study in which rats, trained to discriminate 3 h (satiation condition) from 22 h (fasted condition) of food deprivation, mainly responded on the deprivation lever when they received amphetamine injections (Corwin et al., 1990). Hence, a non-regulatory reduction of food intake could be the stimulus that augments the opioid control of ingestive behaviour and, in turn, an increased reactivity to opioids might be the mechanism that translates non-regulatory reduction of feeding into increased motivation for food (the so-called positive allaesthesia; Cabanac, 1971).

We have already mentioned that, in spite of profound differences in the way in which μ and κ opioids activate feeding behaviour, amphetamine sensitizes both these activating processes. The same intriguing lack of selectivity occurs when the sensitizing stimulus is fasting. Rats deprived of food and transiently maintained at 75–80% of bodyweight during development show an increased sensitivity to the prophagic effect of butorphanol during the period after reinstatement of free-feeding and recovery of normal bodyweight (Hagan and Moss, 1991). Recently, Specker and co-workers (1994) not only confirmed this finding, but also showed that the same modalities of food deprivation produced an earlier acquisition of cocaine self-administration, although differences from control animals were not statistically significant. The prophagic effects of butorphanol are considered to be mediated mainly by κ opioid receptors (Levine *et al*., 1994), but κ receptor stimulation inhibits the behavioural effects of cocaine, which in contrast seem to be positively mediated by μ and δ opioid receptors (Menkens *et al*., 1992; Spealman and Bergman, 1992).

Similar non-selective effects have been observed in a study examining the influence of a history of food restriction on perifornical lateral hypothalamic self-stimulation. Because the highly selective μ opioid antagonist, TCTAP, and the κ opioid antagonist, nor-binaltorphamine, prevented the facilitation of self-stimulation (Carr and Papadouka, 1994), food restriction presumably facilitated self-stimulation by activating both μ and κ opioid mechanisms. For the reasons discussed above, the μ and κ receptors mediating this facilitation are unlikely to be located at the same brain sites. The investigators suggested ascending gustatory pathways as the site of the κ opioid-mediated effect.

Besides having a similar influence on the behavioural effects of opioids, food restriction and chronic exposure to psychomotor stimulants have similar influences at the molecular level. We reviewed above the studies that have given evidence of profound changes induced by chronic administration of psychomotor stimulants on the striatal dynorphinergic system. In rats, voluntary exercise (22.5 h per day) under food restriction (1.5 h per day) produces a significant loss of bodyweight which is associated with an increase in supraoptic hypothalamic content of dynorphin A, the putative endogenous ligand of κ opioid receptors, and with an increased β-endorphin content in plasma and in the arcuate hypothalamic nucleus (Aravich *et al*., 1993). These increases persist under resting-fed conditions. As already outlined, in conditions of prolonged inhibition of its release, accumulation of the transmitter is usually associated with sensitization of the effector. Accordingly, in rats, food deprivation has been reported to increase dynorphin A binding in the cortex, midbrain and striatum (Tsujii *et al*., 1986). It would be interesting to know whether this is the mechanism responsible for the increased sensitivity to the prophagic effects of κ opioids that is produced by either fasting or amphetamine administration.

8   Sensitization to the prophagic effects of opioids as a model of ingestive disorders

In summary, chronic exposure to amphetamine or to fasting episodes seems to converge in sensitizing experimental subjects to the prophagic effects of opioids. If these effects are translated into the realm of human psychopathology, ingestive disorders are the most promising field of investigation. For instance, the natural history of bulimia often includes episodes of food restriction and fasting, which later develop into binge eating and purging. Accordingly, 'restrained eating may be a predisposing factor for the development of bulimia nervosa' (Pike *et al*., 1990). The fact that, in experimental conditions, restrained eating sensitizes opioid-mediated prophagic mechanisms is most interesting, since a role has been proposed for the opioid system in the pathogenesis of bulimia and anorexia nervosa. In particular, women with bulimia apparently have reduced β-endorphin levels in the cerebrospinal fluid (Brewerton et al., 1992). In addition, naltrexone reportedly alleviates binge eating in bulimic patients (Kennedy and Goldbloom, 1991).

Apparently, chronic exposure to amphetamines is equivalent to fasting episodes in sensitizing opioid-mediated prophagic mechanisms. Bulimic episodes are known to be an integral part of the psychomotor-stimulant abstinence syndrome. The cluster of symptoms characterizing the late phase of the post-cocaine crash syndrome, for instance, includes hyperphagia (Gawin and Kleber, 1986). Because this abstinence symptom could be mediated by opioid mechanisms made supersensitive by chronic exposure to the psychomotor stimulant, it would be interesting to test the efficacy of opioid antagonists in preventing the post-cocaine hyperphagic overshoot. In the past few years the concept that the opioid system is involved in the development of psychomotor stimulant addiction has gained credit. Accordingly, partial agonists (e.g. buprenorphine) or antagonists (e.g. naltrexone) of the opioid system have been used to prevent the relapse of cocaine-taking behaviour (Kosten et al., 1989; Gawin, 1991; Foltin and Fischman, 1994). Unfortunately, no study has yet evaluated the effects of these pharmacological treatments on the feeding behaviour of cocaine addicts. Studies addressed to this specific point would be most useful because they would challenge in a clinical setting the hypothesis that psychomotor stimulants result in sensitization to the prophagic effects of opioids. They would also provide information about the role of bulimic episodes in the relapse of cocaine-taking behaviour.

Nevertheless, the intrusion of episodes of eating disorder into a history of drug abuse may be more than a pharmacological accident. Lacey and Evans (1986) identified among bulimic patients a subgroup with increased rates of impulsive behaviour related not to food but, in some cases, to drug-taking. This subgroup varies in size from 9% to 55% (Gwirtsman, 1993), and apparently these patients have a worse outcome. The observation that binge-eaters are more likely to have a drug addict among their first-degree relatives implies that family history plays a role in this association (Bulik, 1987; Zelitch Yanovski et al., 1993). In some patients food and addictive drugs may therefore be stimuli that have a similar, pathological, salience. For these patients, taking too much food or taking drugs may simply depend on contingencies that make one of the two behaviours more likely to be reinforced. This parsimonious interpretation of the association between bulimia and drug-taking based on behavioural economic theories (Bickel et al., 1993) may have some alternatives. Fasting episodes, as well as episodic drug-taking, could reproduce the intermittence of drug exposure, which causes behavioural sensitization under experimental conditions. Acting on an individual's vulnerability, they may produce a stable increase in the salience of reinforcing stimuli such as food or addictive drugs. In an oversimplification of Robinson and Berridge's (1993) theory of incentive sensitization, we would suggest that bulimia and drug addiction result from a common process of behavioural sensitization. In this respect, some of the experimental events reviewed here may have more than face validity with regard to the pathophysiology of ingestive disorders. In particular, the enhanced sensitivity to the prophagic effects of opioids may model a more general role of opioid mechanisms in the development of feeding and drug-taking disorders.

References

Aravich, P. F., Rieg, T. S., Lauterio, T. J. and Doerries, L. E. (1993). β-Endorphin and dynorphin abnormalities in rats subjected to exercise and restricted feeding: relationship to anorexia nervosa? *Brain Res.* **622**, 1–8.

Atkinson, R. L., Berke, L. K., Drake, C. R., Bibbs, M. L., Williams, F. L. and Kaiser, D. L. (1985). Effects of long-term therapy with naltrexone on body weight in obesity. *Clin. Pharmacol. Ther.* **38**, 419–422.

Badiani, A. and Stewart, J. (1992). Chronic restraint stress enhances the prophagic effect of the κ-agonist U-50 488H. *Soc. Neurosci. Abstr.* **18**, 1429.

Badiani, A. and Stewart, J. (1993). Enhancement of the prophagic but not of the antidipsogenic effect of U-50 488H after chronic amphetamine. *Pharmacol. Biochem. Behav.* **44**, 77–86.

Badiani, A., Leone, P., Noel, M. B. and Stewart, J. (1995). Ventral tegmental area opioid mechanisms and modulation of ingestive behavior. *Brain Res.* **670**, 264–276.

Bakshi, V. P. and Kelley, A. E. (1993a). Feeding induced by opioid stimulation of the ventral striatum: role of opiate receptor subtypes. *J. Pharmacol. Exp. Ther.* **265**, 1253–1260.

Bakshi, V. P. and Kelley, A. E. (1993b). Striatal regulation of morphine-induced hyperphagia: an anatomical mapping study. *Psychopharmacology* **111**, 207–214.

Bakshi, V. P. and Kelley, A. E. (1994). Sensitization and conditioning of feeding following multiple morphine microinjections into the nucleus accumbens. *Brain Res.* **648**, 342–346.

Bickel, W. K., DeGrandpre, R. J. and Higgins, S. T. (1993). Behavioral economics: a novel experimental approach to the study of drug dependence. *Drug Alcohol Depend.* **33**, 173–192.

Blackburn, J. R., Phillips, A. G., Jakubovic, A. and Fibiger, H. C. (1989). Dopamine and preparatory behavior: II. A neurochemical analysis. *Behav. Neurosci.* **103**, 15–23.

Bozarth, M. A. and Wise, R. A. (1981). Intracranial self-administration of morphine into the ventral tegmental area in rats. *Life Sci.* **28**, 551–555.

Bray, G. A. (1985). Autonomic and endocrine factors in the regulation of food intake. *Brain Res. Bull.* **14**, 505–510.

Brewerton, T. D., Lydiard, R. B., Laraia, M. T., Shook, J. E. and Ballenger, J. C. (1992). CSF β-endorphin and dynorphin in bulimia nervosa. *Am. J. Psychiatry* **149**, 1086–1090.

Bulik, C. M. (1987). Drug and alcohol abuse by bulimic women and their families. *Am. J. Psychiatry* **144**, 1604–1606.

Cabanac, M. (1971). Physiological role of pleasure. *Science* **173**, 1103–1107.

Camanni, S. and Nencini, P. (1994). Physiological and environmental aspects of drinking stimulated by chronic exposure to amphetamine in rats. *Gen. Pharmacol.* **25**, 7–13.

Campbell, B. A. and Fibiger, H. C. (1971). Potentiation of amphetamine-induced arousal by starvation. *Nature* **233**, 424–425.

Carr, K. D. and Simon, E. J. (1984). Potentiation of reward by hunger is opioid mediated. *Brain Res.* **297**, 369–373.

Carr, K. D. and Papadouka, V. (1994). The role of multiple opioid receptors in the potentiation of reward by food restriction. *Brain Res.* **639**, 253–260.

Carr, K. D. and Wolinsky, T. D. (1993). Chronic food restriction and weight loss produce opioid facilitation of perifornical hypothalamic self-stimulation. *Brain Res.* **607**, 141–148.

Clark, W. (1979). Influence of opioids on central thermoregulatory mechanisms. *Pharmacol. Biochem. Behav.* **10**, 609–613.

Clark, D. and White, F. J. (1987). Review: D_1 dopamine receptor—the search for a function: a critical evaluation of the D_1/D_2 dopamine receptor classification and its functional implications. *Synapse* **1**, 347–388.

Cooper, S. J. (1991). Interactions between endogenous opioids and dopamine: implications for reward and aversion. In *The Mesolimbic Dopamine System: From Motivation to Action* (P. Willner and J. Scheel-Kruger, eds), pp. 331–366. J. Wiley, Chichester, UK.

Cooper, S. J. (1994). Behavioral pharmacology of taste hedonics: a model for studying natural rewards and its relevance to the study of drug abuse. In *Strategies for Studying Brain Disorders. Vol. 1: Depressive, Anxiety and Drug Abuse Disorders* (T. Palomo and T. Archer, eds), pp. 391–410. Editorial Complutense and Ferrand Press, Madrid and London.

Cooper, S. J. and Kirkham, T. C. (1990). Basic mechanisms of opioids' effects on eating and drinking. In *Opioids, Bulimia, and Alcohol Abuse and Alcoholism* (L. D. Reid, ed.), pp. 91–110. Springer, Berlin.

Cooper, S. J. and Kirkham, T. C. (1993). Opioid mechanisms in the control of food consumption and taste preferences. In *Opioids* (A. Herz, H. Akil and E. J. Simon, eds), Part II, pp. 239–262. Springer, Berlin.

Cooper, S. J., Jackson, A. and Kirkham, T. C. (1985). Endorphins and food intake: κ opioid receptor agonists and hyperphagia. *Pharmacol. Biochem. Behav.* **23**, 889–901.

Cooper, S. J., Jackson, A., Kirkham, T. C. and Turkish, S. (1988). Endorphins, opiates and food intake. In *Endorphins, Opiates and Behavioural Processes* (R. J. Rodgers and S. J. Cooper, eds), pp. 143–186. J. Wiley, Chichester, UK.

Corwin, R. L., Woolverton, W. L. and Schuster, C. R. (1990). Effects of cholecystokinin, D-amphetamine and fenfluramine in rats trained to discriminate 3 from 22 hr of food deprivation. *J. Pharmacol. Exp. Ther.* **253**, 720–728.

Cunningham, C. L. and Kelley, A. E. (1992). Evidence for opiate–dopamine cross-sensitization in the nucleus accumbens: studies of conditioned reward. *Brain Res. Bull.* **29**, 675–680.

Demellweek, C. and Goudie, A. J. (1983). Behavioural tolerance to amphetamine and other psychostimulants; the case for considering behavioural mechanisms. *Psychopharmacology* **80**, 287–307.

Devine, D. P. and Wise, R. A. (1994). Self-administration of morphine, DAMGO and DPDPE into the ventral tegmental area of rats. *J. Neurosci.* **14**, 1978–1984.

Devine, D. P., Leone, P. and Wise, R. A. (1993). Mesolimbic dopamine neurotransmission is increased by administration of mu-opioid receptor antagonists. *Eur. J. Pharmacol.* **243**, 55–64.

Di Chiara, G. and Imperato, A. (1988a). Opposite effects of μ and κ opiate agonists on dopamine release in the nucleus accumbens and in the dorsal caudate of freely moving rats. *J. Pharmacol. Exp. Ther.* **244**, 1067–1080.

Di Chiara, G. and Imperato, A. (1988b). Drugs abused by humans preferentially increase synaptic dopamine concentrations in the mesolimbic system of freely moving rats. *Proc. Natl. Acad. Sci.* **85**, 5274–5278.

Druhan, J. P., Deschamps, S.-E. and Stewart, J. (1993). D-amphetamine-like stimulus properties are produced by morphine injections into the ventral tegmental area but not into the nucleus accumbens. *Behav. Brain Res.* **59**, 41–51.

Eilam, D., Talangbayan, H., Canaran, G. and Szechtman, H. (1992). Dopaminergic control of locomotion, mouthing, snout contact, and grooming: opposing roles of D_1 and D_2 receptors. *Psychopharmacology* **106**, 447–454.

Evans, K. R. and Vaccarino, F. J. (1986). Intra-nucleus accumbens amphetamine: dose-dependent effects on food intake. *Pharmacol. Biochem. Behav.* **25**, 1149–1151.

Evans, K. R. and Vaccarino, F. J. (1990). Amphetamine- and morphine-induced feeding: evidence for involvement of reward mechanisms. *Neurosci. Biobehav. Rev.* **14**, 9–22.

Fahy, T. and Eisler, I. (1993). Impulsivity and eating disorders. *Br. J. Psychiatry* **162**, 193–197.

Falk, J. L. and Feingold, D. A. (1987). Environmental and cultural factors in the behavioral action of drugs. In *Psychopharmacology: The Third Generation of Progress* (H. U. Meltzer, ed.), pp. 1503–1510. Raven Press, New York. 1987.

Fantino, M., Hosotte, J. and Apfelbaum, M. (1986). An opioid antagonist, naltrexone, reduces preference for sucrose in humans. *Am. J. Physiol.* **251**, R91–R96.

Foltin, R. W. and Fischman, M. W. (1994). Effects of buprenorphine on the self-administration of cocaine by humans. *Behav. Pharmacol.* **5**, 79–89.

Gaiardi, M., Bartoletti, M., Bacchi, A., Gubellini, C. and Babbini, M. (1987). Increased sensitivity to the stimulus properties of morphine in food deprived rats. *Pharmacol. Biochem. Behav.* **26**, 719–723.

Gawin, F. H. (1991). Cocaine addiction: psychology and neurophysiology. *Science* **251**, 1580–1586.

Gawin, F. H. and Kleber, H. D. (1986). Abstinence symptomatology and psychiatric diagnosis in cocaine abusers. *Arch. Gen. Psychiatry* **43**, 107–113.

Gerber, J. G. and Nies, A. S. (1990). Antihypertensive agents and the drug therapy of hypertension. In *Goodman and Gilman's The Pharmacological Basis of Therapeutics* (A. Goodman Gilman, T. W. Rall, A. S. Nies and P. Taylor, eds), 8th edn, pp. 784–813. Pergamon Press, New York.

Gerfen, C. R., Engber, T. M., Mahan, L. C., Susel, Z., Chase, T. N., Monsma, F. J. Jr and Sibley, D. R. (1990). D_1 and D_2 dopamine receptor-regulated gene expression of striatonigral and striatopallidal neurons. *Science* **250**, 1429–1431.

Gosnell, B. A. and Krahn, D. D. (1993a). The effects of continuous morphine infusion on diet selection and body weight. *Physiol. Behav.* **54**, 853–859.

Gosnell, B. A. and Krahn, D. D. (1993b). Morphine-induced feeding: a comparison of the Lewis and Fischer 344 inbred rat strains. *Pharmacol. Biochem. Behav.* **44**, 919–924.

Gosnell, B. A. and Majchrzak, M. J. (1989). Centrally administered opioid peptides stimulate saccharin intake in nondeprived rats. *Pharmacol. Biochem. Behav.* **33**, 805–810.

Gosnell, B. A. and Patel, C. K. (1993). Centrally administered mu- and delta-opioid agonists increase operant responding for saccharin. *Pharmacol. Biochem. Behav.* **45**, 979–982.

Gosnell, B. A., Krahn, D. D. and Majchrzak, M. J. (1990). The effects of morphine on diet selection are dependent upon baseline diet preferences. *Pharmacol. Biochem. Behav.* **37**, 207–212.

Gwirtsman, H. E. (1993). Bulimic disorders: pharmacotherapeutic and biological studies. *Psychopharmacol. Bull.* **29**, 109–114.

Hagan, M. M. and Moss, D. E. (1991). An animal model of bulimia nervosa: opioid sensitivity to fasting episodes. *Pharmacol. Biochem. Behav.* **39**, 421–422.

Hanson, G. R., Merchant, K. M., Letter, A. A., Bush, L. and Gibb, J. W. (1988). Characterization of methamphetamine effects on the striatal–nigral dynorphin system. *Eur. J. Pharmacol.* **155**, 11–18.

Hanson, G. R., Singh, N., Bush, L. and Gibb, J. W. (1991). Response of extrapyramidal and limbic neuropeptides to fenfluramine administration: comparison with methamphetamine. *J. Pharmacol. Exp. Ther.* **259**, 1197–1202.

Heidbreder, Ch. A., Goldberg, S. R. and Shippenberg, T. S. (1993). The kappa-opioid receptor agonist U-69 593 attenuates cocaine-induced behavioral sensitization in the rat. *Brain Res.* **616**, 335–338.

Hernandez, L. and Hoebel, B. G. (1988). Food reward and cocaine increase extracellular dopamine in the nucleus accumbens as measured by microdialysis. *Life Sci.* **42**, 1705–1712.

Horger, B. A., Shelton, K. and Schenk, S. (1990). Preexposure sensitizes rats to the rewarding effects of cocaine. *Pharmacol. Biochem. Behav.* **37**, 707–711.

Jackson, A. and Cooper, S. J. (1986). An observational analysis of the effect of the selective kappa opioid agonist, U-50 488H, on feeding and related behaviours in the rat. *Psychopharmacology* **90**, 217–221.

Johnson, S. W. and North, R. A. (1992). Opioids excite dopamine neurons by hyperpolarization of local interneurons. *J. Neurosci.* **12**, 483–488.

Kalivas, P. W. and Stewart, J. (1991). Dopamine transmission in the initiation and expression of drug- and stress-induced sensitization of motor activity. *Brain Res. Rev.* **16**, 223–244.

Kalivas, P. W., Sorg, B. A. and Hooks, M. S. (1993). The pharmacology and neural circuitry of sensitization to psychostimulants. *Behav. Pharmacol.* **4**, 315–334.

Kaye, W. H., Berrettini, W., Gwirtsman, H. and George, D. T. (1990). Altered cerebrospinal fluid neuropeptide Y and peptide YY immunoreactivity in anorexia and bulimia nervosa. *Arch. Gen. Psychiatry* **47**, 548–556.

Kennedy, S. H. and Goldbloom, D. S. (1991). Current perspectives on drug therapies for anorexia nervosa and bulimia nervosa. *Drugs* **41**, 367–377.

Kosten, T. R., Kleber, H. D. and Morgan, C. (1989). Role of opioid antagonists in treating intravenous cocaine abuse. *Life Sci.* **44**, 887–892.

Kumar, R., Mitchell, E. and Stolerman, I. P. (1971). Disturbed patterns of behavior in morphine tolerant and abstinent rats. *Br. J. Pharmacol.* **42**, 473–484.

Lacey, J. H. and Evans, C. D. H. (1986). The impulsivist: a multi-impulsive personality disorder. *Br. J. Addict.* **81**, 641–649.

Leibowitz, S. F. (1986). Brain monoamines and peptides: role in the control of eating behavior. *FASEB J.* **45**, 1396–1403.

Leone, P., Pocock, D. and Wise, R. A. (1991). Morphine–dopamine interaction: ventral tegmental morphine increases nucleus accumbens dopamine release. *Pharmacol. Biochem. Behav.* **39**, 469–472.

Leshem, M. (1988). Morphine induces delayed anorexia in rats. *Psychopharmacology* **94**, 254–258.

Lett, B. T. (1989). Repeated exposures intensify rather than diminish the rewarding effects of amphetamine, morphine and cocaine. *Psychopharmacology* **98**, 357–362.

Levine, A. S., Morley, J. E., Gosnell, B. A., Billington, C. J. and Bartness, T. J. (1985). Opioids and consummatory behavior. *Brain Res. Bull.* **14**, 663–672.

Levine, A. S., Grace, M., Portoghese, P. S. and Billington, C. J. (1994). The effects of selective opioid antagonists on butorphanol-induced feeding. *Brain Res.* **637**, 242–248.

McCullough, L. D. and Salamone, J. D. (1992). Involvement of nucleus accumbens dopamine in the motor activity induced by periodic food presentation: a microdialysis and behavioral study. *Brain Res.* **592**, 29–36.

Majeed, N. H., Przewlocka, B., Wedzony, K. and Przewlocki, R. (1986). Stimulation of food intake following opioid microinjection into the nucleus accumbens septi in rats. *Peptides* **7**, 711–716.

Malcolm, R., O'Neil, P. M., Sexauer, J. D., Currey, H. S. and Carrol, C. (1985). A controlled trial of naltrexone in obese humans. *Int. J. Obes.* **9**, 347–353.

Martin, W. R., Wikler, A., Eades, C. G. and Pescor, F. T. (1963). Tolerance to and physical dependence on morphine in rats. *Psychopharmacologia (Berl.)* **4**, 247–260.

Meisch, R. A. and Kliner, D. J. (1979). Etonitazene as a reinforcer for rats: increased etonitazene-reinforced behavior due to food deprivation. *Psychopharmacology* **63**, 97–98.

Menkens, K., Bilsky, E. J., Wild, K. D., Portoghese, P. S., Reid, L. D. and Porrec, F. (1992). Cocaine place preference is blocked by the delta-opioid receptor antagonist, naltrindole. *Eur. J. Pharmacol.* **219**, 345–346.

Mittleman, G. and Valenstein, E. S. (1985). Individual differences in non-regulatory ingestive behavior and catecholamine systems. *Brain Res.* **348**, 112–117.

Morley, J. E. and Levine, A. S. (1983). The central control of appetite. *Lancet* **i**, 398–401.

Morley, J. E., Levine, A. S., Grace, M. and Kneip, J. (1982). An investigation of the role of κ opiate receptors in the initiation of feeding. *Life Sci.* **31**, 2617–2626.

Morley, J. E., Levine, A. S., Yim, G. K. and Lowy, M. T. (1983). Opioid modulation of appetite. *Neurosci. Biobehav. Rev.* **7**, 281–305.

Morley, J. E., Levine, A. S., Kneip, J., Grace, M., Zeugner, H. and Shearman, G. T. (1985). The κ opioid receptor and food intake. *Eur. J. Pharmacol.* **112**, 17–25.

Mucha, R. F. and Iversen, S. D. (1986). Increased food intake after opioid microinjections into nucleus accumbens and ventral tegmental area of rat. *Brain Res.* **397**, 214–224.

Mulder, A. H., Burger, D. M., Wardeh, G., Hogenboom, F. and Frankhuyzen, A. L. (1991). Pharmacological profile of various agonists at kappa-, mu- and delta-opioid receptors mediating presynaptic inhibition of neurotransmitter release in the rat brain. *Br. J. Pharmacol.* **102**, 518–522.

Nader, K. and van der Kooy, D. (1994). The motivation produced by morphine and food is isomorphic: approaches to specific motivational stimuli are learned. *Psychobiology* **22**, 68–76.

Nencini, P. (1988). The role of opiate mechanisms in the development of tolerance to the anorectic effects of amphetamine. *Pharmacol. Biochem. Behav.* **30**, 755–764.

Nencini, P. and Fraioli, S. (1994). Environment-specific reinstatement of amphetamine-mediated hyperdipsia by morphine and (−)-norpseudoephedrine. *Pharmacol. Biochem. Behav.* **47**, 339–343.

Nencini, P. and Stewart, J. (1990). Chronic systemic administration of amphetamine increases food intake to morphine, but not to U-50 488H, microinjected into the ventral tegmental area in rats. *Brain Res.* **527**, 254–258.

Nencini, P. and Valeri, P. (1994). The role of opioid mechanisms in the anorectic effects of stimulants: U-50 488H enhances amphetamine inhibition of free feeding in rats. *Pharmacol. Biochem. Behav.* **48**, 63–68.

Nencini, P., Johanson, C. E. and Schuster, C. R. (1988). Sensitization to κ opioid mechanisms associated with tolerance to the anorectic effect of cathinone. *J. Pharmacol. Exp. Ther.* **245**, 147–154.

Nencini, P., Valeri, P. and Pimpinella, G. (1992). The alpha-1-blocker dapiprazole inhibits diuresis but not drinking and feeding induced by U-50 488H. *Brain Res. Bull.* **29**, 401–405.

Nencini, P., Perrella, D., Fraioli, S. and Paroli, E. (1994a). Morphine produces a persistent enhancement of operant responding for food in rats: the role of fasting and amphetamine administration. *Behav. Pharmacol.* **5**, 33.

Nencini, P., Fraioli, S. and Perrella, D. (1994b). The role of dopaminergic D_1 and D_2 receptors in the development of amphetamine hyperdipsia. *Soc. Neurosci. Abstr.* **20**, 585.

Noel, M. B. and Wise, R. A. (1993). Ventral tegmental injections of morphine but not U-50 488H enhance feeding in food-deprived rats. *Brain Res.* **632**, 68–73.

Ohno, M., Yamamoto, T. and Ueki, S. (1989). Inhibitory effect of a selective κ receptor agonist, U-50 488H, on methamphetamine-elicited ipsilateral circling behavior in rats with unilateral nigral lesions. *Psychopharmacology* **97**, 219–221.

Phillips, G. D., Robbins, T. W. and Everitt, B. J. (1994). Mesoaccumbens dopamine–opiate interactions in the control over behaviour by a conditioned reinforcer. *Psychopharmacology* **114**, 345–359.

Piazza, P. V., Deminière, J. M., Le Moal, M. and Simon, H. (1989). Factors that predict individual vulnerability to amphetamine self-administration. *Science* **245**, 1511–1513.

Pickel, V. M., Chan, J. and Sesack, S. R. (1993). Cellular substrates for interactions between dynorphin terminals and dopamine dendrites in rat ventral tegmental area and substantia nigra. *Brain Res.* **602**, 275–289.

Pirke, K. M., Tuschl, R. J., Spyra, B., Laessle, R. G., Schweiger, U., Broocks, A., Sambauer, S. and Zitzelsberger, G. (1990). Endocrine findings in restrained eaters. *Physiol. Behav.* **47**, 903–906.

Plaznik, A., Stefanski, R. and Kostowski, W. (1989). Interaction between accumbens D_1 and D_2 receptors regulating rat locomotor activity. *Psychopharmacology* **99**, 558–562.

Robinson, T. E. and Becker, J. B. (1986). Enduring changes in brain and behavior produced by chronic amphetamine administration: a review and evaluation of animal models of amphetamine psychosis. *Brain Res. Rev.* **11**, 157–198.

Robinson, T. E. and Berridge, K. C. (1993). The neural basis of drug craving: an incentive-sensitization theory of addiction. *Brain Res. Rev.* **18**, 247–291.

Salamone, J. D. (1992). Complex motor and sensorimotor functions of striatal and accumbens dopamine: involvement in instrumental behavior processes. *Psychopharmacology* **107**, 160–174.

Sanger, D. J. and McCarthy, P. S. (1981). Increased food and water intake produced in rats by opiate receptor agonists. *Psychopharmacology* **74**, 217–220.

Segall, M. A. and Margules, D. L. (1989). Central mediation of naloxone-induced anorexia in the ventral tegmental area. *Behav. Neurosci.* **103**, 857–864.

Sills, T. L. and Vaccarino, F. J. (1994). Individual differences in sugar intake predict the locomotor response to acute and repeated amphetamine administration. *Psychopharmacology* **116**, 1–8.

Smiley, P. C., Johnson, M., Bush, L., Gibb, J. W. and Hanson, G. R. (1990). Effects of cocaine on extrapyramidal and limbic dynorphin systems. *J. Pharmacol. Exp. Ther.* **253**, 938–943.

Spealman, R. D. and Bergman, J. (1992). Modulation of the discriminative stimulus effects on cocaine by μ and κ opioids. *J. Pharmacol. Exp. Ther.* **261**, 607–615.

Specker, S. M., Lac, S. T. and Carroll, M. E. (1994). Food deprivation history and cocaine self-administration: an animal model of binge eating. *Pharmacol. Biochem. Behav.* **48**, 1025–1029.

Stewart, J. and Badiani, A. (1993a). Tolerance and sensitization to the behavioral effects of drugs. *Behav. Pharmacol.* **4**, 289–312.

Stewart, J. and Badiani, A. (1993b). The kappa-agonist, U-50 488H, increases the intake of sucrose solutions at high concentrations: evidence for effect on satiation. *Soc. Neurosci. Abstr.* **19**, 1819.

Stewart, J. and Vezina, P. (1987). Environment-specific enhancement of the hyperactivity induced by systemic or intra-VTA morphine injections in rats pre-exposed to amphetamine. *Psychobiology* **15**, 144–153.

Tang, A. H. and Collins, R. J. (1985). Behavioral effects of a novel κ opioid analgesic, U-50 488, in rats and rhesus monkeys. *Psychopharmacology* **85**, 309–314.

Thompson, L. A. and Walker, J. M. (1990). Inhibitory effects of the κ opiate U-50 488H in the substantia nigra pars reticulata. *Brain Res.* **517**, 81–87.

Tsujii, S., Nakai, Y., Koh, T., Takahashi, H., Usui, T., Ikeda, H., Matsuo, T. and Imura, H. (1986). Effect of food deprivation on opioid receptor binding in the brain of lean and fatty Zucker rats. *Brain Res.* **399**, 200–203.

Ukai, M., Kamiya, T., Toyoshi, T. and Kameyana, T. (1992a). Systemic administration of dynorphin A(1–13) markedly inhibits different behavioural responses induced by cocaine in the mouse. *Neuropharmacology* **31**, 843–849.

Ukai, M., Toyoshi, T. and Kameyana, T. (1992b). Multidimensional behavioral analyses show dynorphin A-(1–13) modulation of methamphetamine-induced behaviors in mice. *Eur. J. Pharmacol.* **222**, 7–12.

Walker, J. M., Thompson, L. A., Frascella, J. and Friederich, M. W. (1987). Opposite effects of μ and κ opiates on the firing-rate of dopamine cells in the substantia nigra of the rat. *Eur. J. Pharmacol.* **134**, 53–59.

Wise, R. A. and Leeb, K. (1993). Psychomotor stimulant sensitization: a unitary phenomenon? *Behav. Pharmacol.* **4**, 339–350.

Wolgin, D. L. and Benson, H. D. (1991). Role of associative and nonassociative mechanisms in tolerance to morphine 'anorexia'. *Pharmacol. Biochem. Behav.* **39**, 279–286.

Woolverton, W. L., Cervo, L. and Johanson, C. E. (1984). Effects of repeated methamphetamine administration on methamphetamine self-administration in rhesus monkeys. *Pharmacol. Biochem. Behav.* **21**, 737–741.

Yokoo, H., Yamada, S., Yoshida, M., Tanaka, M. and Nishi, S. (1992). Attenuation of the inhibitory effect of dynorphin on dopamine release in the rat nucleus accumbens by repeated treatment with methamphetamine. *Eur. J. Pharmacol.* **222**, 43–47.

Zelitch Yanovski, S., Nelson, J. E., Dubbert, B. K. and Spitzer, R. L. (1993). Association of binge eating disorder and psychiatric comorbidity in obese subjects. *Am. J. Psychiatry* **150**, 1472–1479.

10

Dopamine–Opioid Mechanisms in Ingestion

FRANCO J. VACCARINO

Departments of Psychology and Psychiatry, University of Toronto, 100 St George Street, Toronto, Ontario M5S 1A1, Canada

1 Introduction

This chapter focuses on the stimulatory effects of opiate and dopaminergic drugs on ingestive behaviour, and on the relationship between the opiate and dopaminergic substrates mediating these ingestive effects. Moreover, because dopamine–opioid interactions have been studied largely in the context of the mesolimbic system, much of the work discussed here will emphasize mesolimbic dopamine–opiate mechanisms.

2 Psychomotor stimulant and opiate-induced feeding

2.1 Dopamine-induced feeding

Like other psychomotor stimulants, amphetamine has traditionally been thought to be anorexigenic. However, several studies have found increased food intake following amphetamine treatment (Holtzman, 1974; Dobrzanski and Doggett, 1976; Blundell and Latham, 1978; Winn et al., 1982; Evans and Vaccarino, 1987). Since the facilitatory effects of amphetamine on feeding in rats have been observed with low doses (i.e. <1.0 mg/kg; Winn et al., 1982), while anorectic effects are typically observed with higher doses (i.e. >1.0 mg/kg; Winn et al., 1982), dose may be a critical factor in determining the degree to which excitatory feeding effects are found. It is interesting to note that the optimal feeding-stimulatory doses at amphetamine are typically lower than those required to produce general behavioural activation (e.g. Evans and Vaccarino, 1986, 1990).

The specific brain site at which amphetamine acts may also be important in determining the effects of this drug on feeding. While hypothalamic dopaminergic mechanisms appear to mediate the anorexic effects of dopamine

DRUG RECEPTOR SUBTYPES AND INGESTIVE BEHAVIOUR
ISBN 0-12-187620-9

agonists, including amphetamine (Leibowitz, 1980; Cooper *et al.*, 1990; Parada *et al.*, 1990; Capuano *et al.*, 1992; Al-Naser and Cooper, 1994), increased feeding has been found following amphetamine administration into the caudate (Winn *et al.*, 1982), a terminal region of the nigrostriatal dopamine pathway, and the nucleus accumbens (Evans and Vaccarino, 1986, 1990; Colle and Wise, 1988; Sills *et al.*, 1993; Vaccarino, 1994), a terminal region of the mesolimbic dopaminergic pathway. Further, central and peripheral administration of other dopamine agonists have also been shown to produce increased food intake (Eichler and Antelman, 1977; Hernandez *et al.*, 1983; Evans and Eikelboom, 1987). Consistent with the notion of an excitatory role for dopamine in feeding, interference with central dopaminergic transmission can reduce food intake (Ungerstedt, 1971; Xenakis and Sclafani, 1981; Rowland and Stricker, 1982; Redgrave *et al.*, 1984; Kelley and Gauthier, 1987; Fletcher and Davies, 1990a,b; Duong and Weingarten, 1993). Taken together, these findings provide support for an excitatory role for dopamine in feeding and further indicate that the striatum and nucleus accumbens are important sites of action in this regard.

Support for the involvement of dopamine in feeding is also found in studies using microdialysis techniques. Radhakishun *et al.* (1988) found that initiation of feeding in food-deprived rats was associated with a concomitant rise in the levels of dopamine and its metabolites, which did not return to baseline until after feeding had stopped. It has also been reported that bar-pressing for food reward is associated with increased dopaminergic activity in the nucleus accumbens (Hernandez and Hoebel, 1988). These authors also reported that increased dopaminergic activity in the nucleus accumbens was associated with the actions of amphetamine, as well as medial forebrain bundle (MFB) stimulation, all conditions that are known to be rewarding (Vaccarino *et al.*, 1989). More recent microdialysis studies, as well as studies utilizing *in vivo* electrochemical detection techniques, have confirmed that increased dopaminergic activity in the nucleus accumbens is associated with feeding (Yoshida *et al.*, 1992; Phillips *et al.*, 1993; Westerink *et al.*, 1994). Interestingly, it has been found that there is increased dopamine release in both the mesolimbic dopaminergic cell body region (ventral tegmental area) (Yoshida *et al.*, 1992) and in the nucleus accumbens, and that increased dopaminergic activity in the nucleus accumbens is also associated with the increased behavioural activation observed during food presentation (McCullough and Salamone, 1992).

2.2   Opiate-induced feeding

Unlike amphetamine and dopaminergic agonists, which are perhaps best known for their anorexigenic rather than feeding-stimulatory effects, opiates are well known for their stimulatory role in feeding, The first evidence that morphine produced increased food intake was provided by Flowers and co-workers (1929). Since then, opiate agonists have been shown to induce feeding over a range of doses, administration sites and feeding conditions, and in such diverse species as mice, sheep, monkeys, cats, rabbits and wolves (Morley *et al.*, 1983; Levine *et al.*, 1985). Opiate antagonists reduce baseline feeding as well as feeding induced by a variety of pharmacological and non-pharmacological manipulations (King *et al.*, 1979; Simone *et al.*, 1985; Jenck *et al.*, 1986; Kirkham, 1990; Levine *et al.*, 1990; Fletcher, 1991; Gulati *et al.*, 1992; Hawkins *et al.*, 1992). A number of hypothalamic and extrahypothalamic sites have been implicated in opiate feeding mechanisms. In an effort to maintain a focus on opioid–dopaminergic mechanisms, the following discussion will emphasize opiate feeding effects associated with actions on the mesolimbic dopaminergic system.

3   Dopamine–opiate interactions and feeding: key involvement of reward mechanisms

3.1   Mesolimbic function and reward

Arguably the most studied aspect of dopamine–opiate interactions deals with the role of dopaminergic and opioid systems in reward processes. In this regard, the mesolimbic system plays a prominent role. It is now well established that the mesolimbic dopaminergic system is a critical substrate for the rewarding properties of psychostimulants such as cocaine and amphetamine (see Wise and Bozarth, 1987; Vaccarino *et al.*, 1989). More specifically, the ability of these drugs to increase dopamine transmission in mesolimbic terminal regions is considered a key mechanism for their well-known rewarding properties.

3.1.1   Dopamine-dependent and -independent opiate reward
The importance of mesolimbic dopamine in drug reward has been extended to account for the rewarding properties of opiates such as morphine and heroin. Indeed, there is now considerable evidence showing that a component of opiate reward relies on the ability of opiates to activate mesolimbic dopaminergic neurons indirectly through actions in the ventral tegmental area (VTA) (Bozarth and Wise, 1981a,b, 1983; Britt and Wise, 1983; for reviews see also Wise and Bozarth, 1987; Vaccarino *et al.*, 1989). Essentially this evidence shows that the rewarding effects of opiate drugs are dependent on intact dopaminergic function.

It is important to note, however, that there is also evidence for a dopamine-independent opiate reward signal (Ettenberg *et al.*, 1982; Koob *et al.*, 1987). Studies supporting this notion have shown that rats are still capable of experiencing opiate reward following interference with dopaminergic function. Of special interest is the fact that, in addition to being a key site for dopaminergic reward-relevant actions, the nucleus accumbens is also a site for dopamine-independent reward-relevant opiate receptors (Kalivas *et al.*, 1983;

Vaccarino *et al.*, 1985). The key factor distinguishing dopamine-dependent and -independent opiate reward appears to be the site of opiate action. Opiate actions in the VTA produce rewarding effects that rely on the integrity of mesolimbic dopaminergic activity, while opiate actions in the nucleus accumbens produce rewarding effects that do not require the integrity of dopaminergic neurons for their expression. These results indicate that both the VTA and nucleus accumbens are important structures to consider in the context of dopaminergic–opiate interactions, and that the nucleus accumbens is an important output structure for opiate and dopaminergic reward. The origins of the reward-relevant opioid innervation in the VTA and nucleus accumbens is unknown.

3.2 Evidence for involvement of reward processes in opiate and dopamine-derived feeding

3.2.1 Neurochemical anatomy
Taken in the context of the dopamine–opiate reward literature, the feeding effects associated with the mesolimbic system may reflect actions on reward systems that are applied in the feeding context. Certainly, the anatomical and pharmacological literature indicate a strong overlap between the neurochemical anatomy of reward and feeding (associated with opiate or dopaminergic drugs). That is, the VTA and nucleus accumbens are critical sites of action for both opiate-induced feeding and reward, and the nucleus accumbens is a critical site of action for the rewarding and feeding effects of amphetamine of dopaminergic agonists (Roberts *et al.*, 1977; Wise, 1978; Lyness *et al.*, 1979; Morley *et al.*, 1982; Olds, 1982; Roberts and Koob, 1982; Bozarth and Wise, 1983; Britt and Wise, 1983; Goeders *et al.*, 1984; Vaccarino *et al.*, 1985; Cador *et al.*, 1986; Mucha and Iverson, 1986; Corrigall and Vaccarino, 1988; Evans and Vaccarino, 1990; Pal and Thombre, 1993). The pharmacological and neurochemical literature further suggests that increased dopamine release in the nucleus accumbens is a key mechanism for psychostimulant-induced feeding or reward, as well as opiate-induced feeding or reward derived from the VTA (see references above). As in the case of opiate-induced reward, opiate-induced feeding or reward derived from the nucleus accumbens may not require dopaminergic activity (although it may be that dopaminergic input to the nucleus accumbens modulates opiate-induced feeding or reward derived from the nucleus accumbens (Koob *et al.*, 1987; Evans and Vaccarino, 1990; Vaccarino *et al.*, 1995).

3.2.2 Sensitization
Additional neurochemical and pharmacological evidence suggesting that opiate-induced feeding is associated with reward processes comes from studies showing that chronic amphetamine treatment enhances the feeding response to

intra-VTA morphine administration (Nencini and Stewart, 1990). Chronic intermittent administration of amphetamine is thought to sensitize dopaminergic behaviours via its actions on mesolimbic dopaminergic neurons (Robinson and Becker, 1986). The fact that morphine-induced feeding derived from the VTA is enhanced in rats sensitized to the effects of amphetamine is consistent with the notion that dopaminergic reward mechanisms are an output for VTA-derived opioid feeding effects.

3.2.3 Behavioural analysis

Further support for the notion that the dopaminergic and opiate actions underlying feeding behaviour are associated with reward processes comes from the behavioural analysis of feeding effects. For example, the fact that dopaminergic receptor blockade is particularly effective at reducing intake of palatable solutions (Levine et al., 1982; Sclafini et al., 1982; Geary and Smith, 1985; Schneider et al., 1986; Evans and Vaccarino, 1990), and taste-elicited drinking is depressed more than deprivation-induced drinking following neuroleptic treatment (Sclafani et al., 1982), implicates food-reward processes in these effects. Consistent with this, dopamine agonists selectively increase the intake of palatable foods in rats (Evans and Vaccarino, 1990). Furthermore, some authors have found that neuroleptic-induced reductions in feeding are more likely to be observed following repeated testing (Wise and Raptis, 1986), suggesting that neuroleptic treatment may attenuate the rewarding properties of food intake (i.e. induce a state of anhedonia) (Wise and Raptis, 1986), which in turn results in an extinction of eating over time. These findings are consistent with the notion that dopamine is acting on food reward mechanisms.

Behavioural analysis also supports a role for reward processes in feeding induced by opioid systems. For example, opioid antagonists selectively block the preference for highly palatable foods, while μ and δ opioid agonists increase the intake of saccharin-sweetened solution (relative to water or less sweetened solutions) (Cooper et al., 1988; Gosnell and Majchrzak, 1989). Based on behavioural analysis of aversive and hedonic reactions to taste, Doyle and colleagues (1993) found that morphine-induced feeding was associated with hedonic taste reactions. Aversive reactions were unchanged (Doyle et al., 1993).

3.2.4 Individual differences

Recently, it has been demonstrated that the marked individual differences in the baseline sugar preference and intake of rats are dopamine dependent (Sills et al., 1993). Administration of amphetamine into the nucleus accumbens was found to increase sugar intake in low sugar feeders, but had little effect on high sugar feeders. Intra-nucleus accumbens treatment with a dopamine antagonist attenuated the increased feeding induced by amphetamine in low feeders, as well as the naturally increased intake in high feeders (Sills et al., 1993). These results were taken to suggest that individual differences in baseline dopaminergic activity in the nucleus accumbens can account for individual differences in sugar preference and intake.

In view of the central role played by the mesolimbic system in reward processes, and the fact that opioid and dopaminergic manipulations induce hedonically relevant feeding effects, the mesolimbic dopaminergic system is a good candidate system for mediating food reward processes associated with dopaminergic and opioid actions. The similarity in the hedonic profile of opioid and dopaminergic feeding effects further suggests that, in addition to being the substrate for dopamine-relevant food reward, the mesolimbic dopaminergic system may also be an important substrate for food reward processes associated with opioid actions. This is consistent with the fact that dopamine antagonists attenuate opioid-induced feeding (Morley *et al.*, 1982).

4 Nucleus accumbens opiate and dopaminergic actions mediate distinct feeding effects

As discussed above, opioid and dopaminergic reward are functionally dissociable at the level of the nucleus accumbens. In view of this, it is reasonable to expect that opiate and dopaminergic effects on feeding are behaviourally dissociable. Indeed, although there is considerable overlap in the behavioural (particularly hedonic) characteristics of feeding associated with opioid and dopaminergic manipulations, it is important to note that there are also differences. For example, while much of the evidence seems to suggest that dopaminergic food reward processes are selective for sweet taste, opiate food reward appears to be more general (Evans and Vaccarino, 1990; Gosnell *et al.*, 1990). That is, although feeding induced by dopaminergic activation is largely directed at carbohydrate-containing and sweet-tasting foods, feeding induced by opiate treatments is directed at whatever food is most preferred in a given situation, irrespective of the basis for the preference (Evans and Vaccarino, 1990; Gosnell *et al.*, 1990). For example, while both morphine and amphetamine (at low doses) selectively increased sugar intake in animals given a choice of sugar and chow, only morphine (not amphetamine) increases protein intake in protein-preferring protein-deprived rats (Evans and Vaccarino 1990).

The differences between amphetamine- and opiate-induced feeding have been replicated following intra-nucleus accumbens morphine and amphetamine treatment (Evans and Vaccarino, 1990). Moreover, although dopaminergic antagonists are effective at attenuating the effects of amphetamine on food choice and intake, they have, at best, weak effects on morphine-induced feeding and food choices (Evans and Vaccarino, 1990). These results are consistent with the reward literature indicating that, while opiate reward derived from the VTA is dependent on dopaminergic activity, opiate actions in the nucleus accumbens may not require the actions of dopamine (Ettenberg *et al.*, 1982; Kalivas *et al.*, 1983; Vaccarino *et al.*, 1985; Koob *et al.*, 1987). Thus, opioid and dopaminergic input to the nucleus accumbens may represent the convergence of two related, but different, reward signals.

The differences found between opiate- and amphetamine-induced feeding derived from the nucleus accumbens provide clues regarding the nature of the difference between nucleus accumbens and dopaminergic reward. The dopamine-dependent feeding effects of amphetamine in the nucleus accumbens (and probably the VTA-derived feeding effects of opiates) are more narrow than those associated with nucleus accumbens opiate effects. Amphetamine appears to increase the receptivity of the animals to sweet and carbohydrate-rich reinforcers. Thus, the expressions of dopamine's rewarding effects in the context of feeding may be limited to the presence of a narrow range of reinforcers. This further suggests that conventional reward paradigms that utilize chow or water as reinforcers may not be optimal for accessing dopamine-specific reward systems.

In contrast to the effects of amphetamine in the nucleus accumbens, the dopamine-independent opiate feeding effects derived from the nucleus accumbens are more general. That is, opiate actions in the nucleus accumbens appear to increase the intake of the most preferred food regardless of the basis for the preference (i.e. nutrient-specific hunger, taste or individual differences in preference). It may be that, depending on the particular situation or need state of the animal, either opiate or dopaminergic systems in the nucleus accumbens are engaged. For example, in a situation of serious food deprivation, where the animal cannot afford the luxury of responding only to sweet carbohydrate reinforcers, opioid actions in the nucleus accumbens may be engaged. In contrast, a situation requiring a quick energy source (not necessarily hunger related) may engage dopaminergic actions.

4.1 Functional antagonism between nucleus accumbens dopaminergic and opioid signals

The fact that opiate and dopaminergic effects on feeding rely on common (i.e. VTA) as well as dissociable (i.e. nucleus accumbens) neurochemical mechanisms presents a confusing picture regarding substrates underlying dopamine–opiate interactions. In terms of functional coupling of opiate and dopaminergic signals, the VTA presents the most straightforward mechanism. With respect to VTA opiate actions, mesolimbic dopaminergic neurons appear to be an output pathway for feeding and reward functions. With respect to the nucleus accumbens, however, it appears that opiate and dopaminergic activity do not serve a mutually complementary function. In fact, the opposite may be true.

Of special interest here are the paradoxical effects of chronic dopamine blockade on opiate-induced behavioural effects. It has been found that chronic interference with dopamine transmission produces supersensitivity to the rewarding and locomotor activating effects of systemic and nucleus accumbens opiates (Stinus et al., 1985, 1986, 1989). The fact that interference with

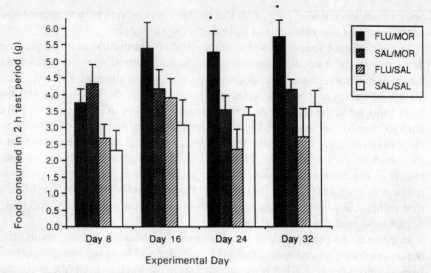

Fig. 1 Effects of chronic flupenthixol (FLU) treatment on acute morphine (MOR)-induced feeding on test days 8, 16, 24 and 32. Control treatment is indicated by saline (SAL). Four groups tested were: chronic flupenthixol plus morphine treatment on test days (FLU/MOR); flupenthixol control plus morphine treatment on test days (SAL/MOR); chronic flupenthixol plus saline treatment on test days (FLU/SAL); flupenthixol control plus saline treatment on test days (SAL/SAL). $*P < 0.05$ vs control.

Table 1 Mean ± SEM bodyweight at each feeding test day for each drug condition

Drug condition	Feeding test day			
	Day 8	Day 16	Day 24	Day 32
Saline plus saline	316.8 ± 8.09	368.8 ± 7.48	398.2 ± 8.63	435.8 ± 8.21
Saline plus morphine	309.6 ± 12.58	369.0 ± 7.64	442.8 ± 45.44	427.2 ± 9.18
Flupenthixol plus saline	315.0 ± 6.81	354.8 ± 7.04	379.4 ± 7.49	380.6 ± 11.87
Flupenthixol plus morphine	321.8 ± 8.84	361.6 ± 5.46	386.6 ± 7.80	407.0 ± 8.41

mesolimbic dopaminergic activity can enhance nucleus accumbens opiate functions suggests that dopaminergic and opiate action in the nucleus accumbens are functionally antagonistic. This opposing relationship between dopaminergic and opiate actions in the nucleus accumbens is in contradiction to the permissive role of dopamine for VTA opiate function.

Recently, Vaccarino et al. (1995) have extended these result to opiate-induced feeding and found that chronic treatment with a neuroleptic increases the feeding-stimulatory effects of morphine (Fig. 1). These effects were specific to feeding and appeared to be unrelated to weight, since there were no significant differences in weight between groups (Table 1). Although this study was based on systemic drug treatments, the nucleus accumbens is the most likely site for this opiate–dopamine interaction (Stinus *et al.*, 1985, 1986, 1989). Thus, in contrast to a positive functional link between opioid and dopaminergic actions in the VTA (as discussed earlier in this chapter), the exaggerated opiate response following chronic dopamine blockade suggests the presence of opioid actions in the nucleus accumbens, which may be antagonized endogenously by dopaminergic actions (Stinus *et al.*, 1985, 1986, 1989; Vaccarino *et al.*, 1995). This antagonistic relationship between opioid and dopaminergic actions in the nucleus accumbens may have important implications for mechanisms underlying the previously discussed difference in the feeding effects associated with opiate and dopaminergic actions.

Acknowledgements

The author thanks Veronica Franco for help in the preparation of this manuscript, and the Medical Research Council (Canada) for support.

References

Al-Naser, H. A. and Cooper, S. J. (1994). A-68 930, a novel, potent dopamine D_1 receptor agonist: a microstructural analysis of its effects on feeding and other behaviour in the rat. *Behav. Pharmacol.* **5**, 210–218.

Blundell, J. E. and Latham, C. J. (1978). Pharmacological manipulation feeding behaviour: possible influences of serotonin and dopamine on food intake. In *Central Mechanisms of Anorectic Drugs* (S. Garattini and R. Semanin, eds), pp. 83–109, Raven Press, New York.

Bozarth, M. A. and Wise, R. A. (1981a). Heroin reward is dependent on a dopaminergic substrate. *Life Sci.* **29**, 1881–1886.

Bozarth, M. A. and Wise, R. A. (1981b). Intracranial self-adminstration of morphine into the ventral tegmental areas. *Life Sci.* **28**, 551–555.

Bozarth, M. A. and Wise, R. A. (1983). Neural substrates of opiate reinforcement. *Life Sci.* **29**, 1881–1886.

Britt, M. D. and Wise, R. A. (1983). Ventral tegmental site of opiate reward: antagonism by a hydrophilic opiate receptor blocker. *Brain Res.* **258**, 105–108.

Cador, M., Kelley, A. E., LeMoal, M. and Stinus, L. (1986). Ventral tegmental area infusion of substance P, neurotensin and enkephalin: differential effects on feeding behaviour. *Neuroscience* **18**, 567–573.

Capuano, C. A., Leibowitz, S. F. and Barr, G. A. (1992). The pharmaco-ontogeny of the perifornical lateral hypothalamic β_2-adrenergic and dopaminergic receptor systems mediating epinephrine- and dopamine-induced suppression of feeding in the rat. *Brain Res.* **70**, 1–7.

Colle, L. M. and Wise, R. A. (1988). Facilitory and inhibitory effects of nucleus accumbens AMPH on feeding. *Ann. N.Y. Acad. Sci.* **537**, 491–492.

Cooper, S. J., Jackson, A., Kirkham, T. C. and Turkish, S. (1988). Endorphins, opiates and food intake. In *Endorphins, Opiates, and Behavioral Processes* (R. J. Rodgers and S. J. Cooper, eds), pp. 143–186. Wiley, New York.

Cooper, S. J., Francis, J. and Rusk, I. N. (1990). The anorectic effects of SK&F 38 393, a selective dopamine D_1 receptor agonist: a microstructural analysis of feeding and related behaviour. *Psychopharmacology* **100**, 182–187.

Corrigall, W. A. and Vaccarino, F. J. (1988). Antagonist treatment in nucleus accumbens or periaqueductal grey affects heroin self-adminstration. *Pharmacol. Biochem. Behav.* **30**, 443–450.

Dobrzanski, S. and Doggett, N. S. (1976). The effects of (+)-amphetamine and fenfluramine on feeding in starved and satiated mice. *Psychopharmacologia* **48**, 283–286.

Doyle, T. G., Berridge, K. C. and Gosnell, B. A. (1993). Morphine enhances hedonic taste palatability in rats. *Pharmacol. Biochem. Behav.* **46**, 745–749.

Duong, A. and Weingarten, H. P. (1993). Dopamine antagonists act on central, but not peripheral, receptors to inhibit sham and real feeding. *Physiol. Behav.* **54**, 449–454.

Eichler, A. J. and Antelman, S. M. (1977). Apomorphine: feeding or anorexia depending on internal state. *Commun. Psychopharmacol.* **1**, 533–540.

Ettenberg, A., Pettie, H., Bloom, F. E. and Koob, G. F. (1982). Heroin cocaine intravenous self-administration in rats. *Psychopharmacology* **78**, 204–209.

Evans, K. R. and Eikelbloom, R. E. (1987). Feeding induced by ventricular bromocriptine and (+)-amphetamine: a possible excitatory role for dopamine in eating behaviour. *Behav. Neurosci.* **101**, 591–593.

Evans, K. R. and Vaccarino, F. J. (1986). Intra-nucleus accumbens amphetamine: dose-dependent effects on food intake. *Pharmacol. Biochem. Behav.* **25**, 1149–1151.

Evans, K. R. and Vaccarino, F. J. (1987). Effects of D- and L-amphetamine on food intake: evidence for a dopaminergic substrate. *Pharmacol. Biochem. Behav.* **27**, 649–652.

Evans, K. R. and Vaccarino, F. J. (1990). Amphetamine- and morphine-induced feeding: evidence for involvement of reward mechanisms. *Neurosci. Biobeh. Rev.* **14**, 9–22.

Fletcher, P. J. (1991). Opiate antagonists inhibit feeding induced by 8-OH-DPAT: possible mediation in the nucleus accumbens. *Brain Res.* **560**, 260–267.

Fletcher, P. J. and Davies, M. (1990a). The involvement of 5-hydroxytryptaminergic and dopaminergic mechanisms in the eating induced by buspirone, gepirone and ipsapirone. *Br. J. Pharmacol.* **99**, 519–525.

Fletcher, P. J. and Davies, M. (1990b). A pharmacological analysis of the eating response induced by 8-OH-DPAT injected into the dorsal raphe nucleus reveals the involvement of a dopaminergic mechanism. *Psychopharmacology* **100**, 188–194.

Flowers, S. H., Dunham, E. S. and Barbour, H. G. (1929). Addition edema and withdrawal edema in morphinized rats. *Proc. Soc. Exp. Biol. Med.* **26**, 572–574.

Geary, N. and Smith, G. P. (1985). Pimozide decreases the positive reinforcing effect of sham fed sucrose in the rat. *Pharmacol. Biochem. Behav.* **22**, 787–790.

Goeders, N. E., Lane, J. D. and Smith, J. E. (1984). Self-administration of methionine enkephalin into the nucleus accumbens. *Pharmacol. Biochem. Behav.* **20**, 451–455.

Gosnell, B. A. and Majchrzak, M. J. (1989). Centrally administered opioid peptides stimulate saccharin intake in nondeprived rats. *Pharmacol. Biochem. Behav.* **33**, 805–810.

Gosnell, B. A., Krahn, D. D. and Majchrzak, M. J. (1990). The effects of morphine on diet selection are dependent upon baseline diet preferences. *Pharmacol. Biochem. Behav.* **37**, 207–212.

Gulati, K., Ray, A. and Sharma, K. K. (1992). Effects of acute or chronic opioid agonists and their modulation by diurnal rhythmicity and satiety states on food intake in rats. *Ind. J. Exp. Biol.* **30**, 185–189.

Hawkins, M. F., Cubic, B., Baumeister, A. A. and Barton, C. (1992). Microinjection of opioid antagonists into the substantia nigra reduces stress-induced eating in rats. *Brain Res.* **584**, 261–275.

Hernandez, L. and Hoebel, B. G. (1988). Food reward and cocaine increases extracellular dopamine in the nucleus accumbens as measured by microdialysis. *Life Sci.* **42**, 1705–1712.

Hernandez, L., Parada, M. and Hoebel, B. G. (1983). Amphetamine-induced hyperphagia and obesity caused by intraventricular or lateral hypothalamic injections in rats. *J. Pharmacol. Exp. Ther.* **227**, 524–530.

Holtzman, S. G. (1974). Behavioural effects of separate and combined administration of naloxone and D-amphetamine. *J. Pharmacol. Exp. Ther.* **189**, 51–60.

Jenck, R., Gratton, A. and Wise, R. A. (1986). Effects of pimozide and naloxone on latency or hypothalamically induced feeding. *Brain Res.* **375**, 329–337.

Kalivas, P. W., Widerlov, E., Stanley, D., Breese, G. and Prange, A. J. (1983). Enkephalin action on the mesolimbic system: a dopamine-independent increase in locomotor activity. *J. Pharmacol. Exp. Ther.* **227**, 229–237.

Kelley, A. E. and Gauthier, A. (1987). Differential effects on spontaneous motor behaviour, feeding and oral stereotypy following amphetamine microinjection into anatomically defined subregions of rat striatum. *Soc. Neurosci. Abstr.* **13**(1), 31.

King, B. M., Castellanos, F. X., Kastin, A. J., Berzas, M. C., Mauk, M. D., Olson, G. A. and Olson, R. D. (1979). Naloxone-induced suppression of food intake in normal and hypothalamic obese rats. *Pharmacol. Biochem. Behav.* **11**, 729–732.

Kirkham, T. C. (1990). Enhanced anorectic potency of naloxone in rats sham feeding 30% sucrose: reversal by repeated naloxone administration. *Physiol. Behav.* **47**, 419–426.

Koob, G. F., Vaccarino, F. J., Amalric, M. and Bloom, F. E. (1987). Positive reinforcement properties of drugs: search for neural substrates. In *Brain Reward Systems and Abuse* (J. Engel, L. Oreland, D. H. Ingvar, B. Pernow, S. Rossner and L. A. Pellborn, eds), pp. 35–50. Raven Press, New York.

Leibowitz, S. F. (1980). Neurochemical systems of the hypothalamus. Control of feeding and drinking behaviour and water–electrolyte excretion. In *Handbook of the Hypothalamus* (P. J. Morgane and J. Panksepp, eds), vol. 3, pp. 299–437. Dekker, New York.

Levine, A. S., Murray, S. S., Kneip, J., Grace, M. and Morley, J. E. (1982). Flavour enhances the antidipsogenic effect of naloxone. *Physiol. Behav.* **28**, 23–25.

Levine, A. S., Morley, J. E., Gosnell, B. A., Billington, C. J. and Bartness, T. J. (1985). Opioids and consummatory behaviour. *Brain Res. Bull.* **14**, 663–672.

Levine, A. S., Grace, M. and Billington, C. J. (1990). The effect of centrally administered naloxone on deprivation and drug-induced feeding. *Pharmacol. Biochem. Behav.* **36**, 409–412.

Lyness, W. H., Friedle, N. M. and Moore, K. E. (1979). Destruction of dopaminergic nerve terminals in nucleus accumbens: effect on D-amphetamine self-administration. *Pharmacol. Biochem. Behav.* **11**, 553–556.

McCullough, L. D. and Salamone, J. D. (1992). Involvement of nucleus accumbens dopamine in the motor activity activity induced by periodic food presentation: a microdialysis and behavioral study. *Brain Res.* **592**, 29–36.

Morley, J. E., Levine, A. S., Grace, M. and Kneip, J. (1982). Dynorphin-(1–13), dopamine and feeding in rats. *Pharmacol. Biochem. Behav.* **16**, 701–705.

Morley, J. E., Levine, A. S., Yim, G. K. W. and Lowy, M. T. (1982). Opioid modulation of appetite. *Neurosci. Biobehav. Rev.* **7**, 281–305.

Mucha, R. F. and Iversen, S. D. (1986). Increased food intake after opioid microinjections into the nucleus accumbens and ventral tegmental area of rat. *Brain Res.* **397**, 214–224.

Nencini, P. and Stewart, J. (1990). Chronic systemic administration of amphetamine increases food intake to morphine, but not to U50-488H, microinjected into the ventral tegmental area in rats. *Brain Res.* **527**, 254–258.

Olds, M. E. (1982). Reinforcing effects of morphine in the nucleus accumbens. *Brain Res.* **237**, 429–440.

Pal, G. K. and Thombre, D. P. (1993). Modulation of feeding and drinking by dopamine in caudate and accumbens nuclei in rats. *Ind. J. Exp. Biol.* **31**, 750–754.

Parada, M. A., Hernandez, L., Puig de Parada, M., Paez, X. and Hoebel, B. G. (1990). Dopamine in the lateral hypothalamus may be involved in the inhibition of loco-motion related to food and water seeking. *Brain Res. Bull.* **25**, 961–968.

Phillips, A. G., Atkinson, L. J., Blackburn, J. R. and Blaha, C. D. (1993). Increased extracellular dopamine in the nucleus accumbens of the rat elicited by a conditional stimulus for food: an electrochemical study. *Can. J. Physiol. Pharmacol.* **71**, 387–393.

Radhakishun, F. S., VanRee, J. M. and Westerink, B. H. C. (1988). Scheduled eating increases dopamine release in the nucleus accumbens of food-deprived rats as assessed with on-line brain dialysis. *Neurosci. Lett.* **85**, 351–356.

Redgrave, P., Dean, P. and Taha, E. B. (1984). Feeding induced by injection of muscimol into the substantia nigra of rats: unaffected by haloperidol but abolished by large lesions of the superior colliculus. *Neuroscience* **13**, 77–85.

Roberts, D. C. S. and Koob, G. F. (1982). Disruption of cocaine self-administration following 6-OHDA lesions of the VTA in rats. *Pharmacol. Biochem. Behav.* **17**, 901–904.

Roberts, D. C. S., Corcoran, M. E. and Fibiger, H. C. (1977). On the role of ascending catechoaminergic systems in intravenous self-administration of cocaine. *Pharmacol. Biochem. Behav.* **6**, 615–620.

Robinson, T. E. and Becker, J. B. (1986). Enduring changes in brain and behavior produced by chronic amphetamine adminstration: a review and evaluation of animal models of amphetamine psychosis. *Brain Res. Rev.* **11**, 157–198.

Rowland, N. and Stricker, E. M. (1982). Effects of dopamine-depleting brain lesions on experimental hyperphagia in rats. *Physiol. Behav.* **28**, 271–277.

Schneider, L. H., Gibbs, J. and Smith, G. D. (1986). D-2 selective receptor antagonists suppress sucrose sham feeding in the rat. *Brain Res. Bull.* **17**, 605–611.

Sclafani, A., Aravich, P. F. and Xenakis, S. (1982). Dopaminergic and endorphinergic mediation of a sweet reward. In *The Neural Basis of Feeding and Rewards* (B. G. Hoebel and D. Novin, eds), pp. 507–515. Haer Institute, Brunswick, ME.

Sills, T. L., Baird, J. P. and Vaccarino, F. J. (1993). Individual differences in the feeding effects of amphetamine: role of nucleus accumbens dopamine and circadian factors. *Psychopharmacology* **112**, 211–218.

Simone, D. A., Bodnar, R. J., Goldman, E. J. and Pasternak, G. W. (1985). Involvement of opioid receptor subtypes in rat feeding behaviour. *Life Sci.* **38**, 829–833.

Stinus, L., Winnock, M. and Kelly, A. E. (1985). Chronic neuroleptic treatment and mesolimbic dopamine denervation induce behavioural supersensitivity to opiates. *Psychopharmacology* **85**, 323–328.

Stinus, L., Nadaud, D., Jauregui, J. and Kelly, A. E. (1986). Chronic treatment with five different neuroleptics elicits behavioral supersensitivity to opiate infusion into the nucleus accumbens. *Biol. Psychiatry* **21**, 34–48.

Stinus, L., Nadaud, D., Deminiere, J. M., Jauregui, J., Hand, T. T. and Le Moal, M. (1989). Chronic flupentixol treatment potentiates the reinforcing properties of systemic heroin administration. *Biol. Psychiatry* **26**, 363–371.

Ungerstedt, U. (1971). Adipsia and aphagia after 6-hydroxydopamine induced de-generation of the nigrostriatal dopamine system. *Acta Physiol. Scand. Suppl.* **367**, 95–122.

Vaccarino, F. J. (1994). Nucleus accumbens dopamine–CCK interactions in psycho-stimulant reward and related behaviors. *Neurosci. Biobehav. Rev.* **18**, 207–214.

Vaccarino, F. J., Bloom, F. E. and Koob, G. F. (1985). Blockade of nucleus accumbens opiate receptors attenuates intravenous heroin reward in the rat. *Psychopharmacology* **86**, 37–42.

Vaccarino, F. J., Schiff, B. B. and Glickman, S. E. (1989). A biological view of reinforcement. In *Contemporary Learning Theories* (S. B. Klein and R. R. Mowrer, eds), pp. 111–142. Lawrence Erlbaum, Hillsdale, NJ.

Vaccarino, F. J., Mogil, J. S. and Stinus, L. (1995). Chronic dopamine antagonism facilitates opiate-induced feeding. *J. Psychiatry Neurosci.* **20**(3), 210–214.

Westerink, B. H. C., Teisman, A. and de Vries, J. B. (1994). Increase in dopamine release from the nucleus accumbens in response to feeding: a model to study interactions between drugs and naturally activated dopaminergic neurons in the rat brain. *Naunyn Schmiedebergs Arch. Pharmacol.* **349**, 230–235.

Winn, P., Williams, S. F. and Herberg, L. J. (1982). Feeding stimulated by very low doses of D-amphetamine administered systematically or by microinjection into the striatum. *Psychopharmacology* **78**, 336–341.

Wise, R. A. (1978). Catecholamine theories of reward: a critical review. *Brain Res.* **152**, 215–247.

Wise, R. A. and Bozarth, M. A. (1987). A psychomotor stimulant theory addiction. *Psychol. Rev.* **94**, 469–492.

Wise, R. A. and Raptis, L. (1986). Effects of naloxone and pimozide on initiation and maintenance measures of free feeding. *Brain Res.* **368**, 62–68.

Xenakis, A. and Sclafani, A. (1981). The effects of pimozide on the consumption of a palatable saccharin–glucose solution in the rat. *Pharmacol. Biochem. Behav.* **15**, 435–442.

Yoshida, M., Yokoo, H., Mizoguchi, K., Kawahara, H., Tsuda, A., Nishikawa, T. and Tanaka, M. (1992). Eating and drinking cause increased dopamine release in the nucleus accumbens and ventral tegmental area in the rat: measurement by *in vivo* microdialysis. *Neurosci. Lett.* **139**, 73–76.

11

Dopamine Receptor Subtypes and Ingestive Behaviour

PHILIP TERRY

School of Psychology, University of Birmingham, Edgbaston, Birmingham B15 2TT, UK

1 Introduction

The involvement of dopamine in the control of ingestive behaviour has been intensively studied over the past 20 years. However, it is only recently that studies have begun to examine the relative contributions of dopamine receptor subtypes to the regulation of such behaviour. In the period before the identification of dopamine receptor subtypes, the role of dopamine in feeding behaviour was investigated by studying how food intake is modified either by damage to dopaminergic pathways in the brain or by drugs that alter dopamine transmission in specifiable ways. Drugs commonly used as research tools either enhanced dopamine availability in the synapse (indirect agonists, such as amphetamine), stimulated dopamine receptors (direct agonists, such as apomorphine) or blocked dopamine receptors (antagonists, such as haloperidol). Following the classification of dopamine receptors into two subtypes (D_1 and D_2 receptors; Kebabian and Calne, 1979), it was revealed that prototypical dopamine agonists, like apomorphine, were not selective between receptor subtypes, whereas many frequently used antagonists, such as haloperidol and pimozide, had preferential affinities for the D_2 receptor class. Consequently, there are more data available for the effects of selective D_2 receptor blockade on feeding than for any other kind of drug effect at dopamine receptor subtypes.

Just as the D_1–D_2 receptor classification obliged a re-evaluation of the data concerning the effects of dopaminergic drugs on ingestive behaviour, recent developments in the categorization of dopamine receptor subtypes suggest that a further reassessment will soon be necessary. Thus the original subdivision of dopamine receptors into two subtypes has now been superseded by a six-receptor classification (for a review see Sibley and Monsma, 1992). The original identification of D_1 and D_2 receptors was based on the finding of

DRUG RECEPTOR SUBTYPES AND INGESTIVE BEHAVIOUR
ISBN 0-12-187620-9

heterogeneous signal transduction mechanisms among dopamine receptors: one subtype (D_1) was positively linked to the second-messenger cyclic AMP, whereas the other subtype (D_2) was either unlinked or negatively linked to cyclic AMP production. However, the recent isolation of novel receptor subtypes has been achieved using molecular cloning techniques (Sokoloff *et al.*, 1990, 1992; Sunahara *et al.*, 1991; Van Tol *et al.*, 1991), rather than by functional assays, and the physiology and pharmacology of the six receptors remain poorly understood. The six receptors are usually referred to as D_1, D_2, D_3, D_4 and D_5, with two isoforms of the D_2 receptor distinguished by their slightly different amino acid lengths; this difference among D_2 receptors is generally considered to have no significant functional consequences (e.g. Giros *et al.*, 1989). As regards the relationship between the resultant five dopamine receptor subtypes and the earlier two-receptor classification, it is now generally held that the previous D_1 category may be taken to incorporate the D_1 and D_5 subtypes, whereas the previous D_2 category encompasses the D_2, D_3 and D_4 subtypes. Indeed, it has been suggested that the old D_1–D_2 classification may now be used to discriminate between two receptor subtype 'families' (e.g. Sibley and Monsma, 1992; Gingrich and Caron, 1993). Such an emphasis on groupings of receptor subtypes is currently necessitated by the absence of drugs selective for individual receptor subtypes. Thus, although there are some agonists available with preferential affinity for D_3 over D_2 receptors, to date no antagonists have been presented as being selective for specific subtypes, and no drugs discriminating between D_1 and D_5 receptors are yet available. Until such tools are obtained, a dichotomous classification of dopamine receptor subtypes will remain in common use. For present purposes the terms 'D_1-type' and 'D_2-type' will be used to refer to the receptor subtype groupings, whereas individual subtypes will be referred to as D_1, D_2 etc.

As with any other neurotransmitter system, manipulations of dopaminergic activity could affect ingestive behaviour through any of several different mechanisms. Dopamine has long been considered important in the regulation of motor behaviour, and so the effects of dopaminergic drugs on feeding might be mediated by changes in motor control. Although the motor systems engaged may be separate from those required for normal ingestive behaviour, they may predispose patterns of behaviour that are incompatible with normal feeding (e.g. induction of stereotyped locomotion). Significantly, there is evidence that dopaminergic drugs can directly modulate orofacial motor control, for example by inducing chewing; thus, altered feeding patterns might reflect changes in the mechanics of eating. If it can be shown that certain dopaminergic drugs engage effector processes critical to eating, then attributing the actions of such drugs to motor effects would not necessarily undermine the presumed importance of dopamine to ingestive behaviour. However, if drug-induced changes in feeding behaviour are accompanied by the emergence of competing motor behaviours, then our understanding of dopamine involvement in ingestive behaviour would not be greatly improved; hence the importance of a comprehensive behavioural analysis to the study of neurotransmitter involvement in feeding.

The dopamine system has also been a target for the study of the neural bases of motivation and reward, and work in this field suggests that the effects of dopaminergic drugs on feeding might reflect modulation of these processes. Unfortunately an acceptable model of dopaminergic involvement in reward is yet to emerge, making it difficult to describe drug effects in terms of actions on a general (or specifically food-related) reward system. Moreover, it has proven notoriously difficult to dissociate changes in hedonic processes from changes in sensorimotor function (e.g. Salamone, 1994). These kinds of issues have scarcely been addressed from the perspective of dopamine receptor subtypes. Similarly, there are few data concerning the motivational factors underlying the effects of receptor subtype-selective drugs on feeding—for example, whether the drugs affect satiety, hunger, taste preference or macronutrient selection. Even for drugs with a long history of use as research tools in the study of ingestive behaviour (for example, amphetamine) it remains difficult to distinguish between the many processes that might underlie a drug's effects on feeding. For dopamine receptor subtype-selective drugs, the appropriate behavioural and pharmacological analyses have hardly been attempted.

This review will open with a brief overview of the effects of non-selective dopaminergic drugs on feeding, partly because such data might provide some pointers towards the normal involvement of dopamine in feeding, but also because the use of receptor-subtype antagonists in conjunction with non-selective agonists provides one means of identifying receptor subtype involvement in particular functions. Then, the roles of D_1-type and D_2-type receptors will be assessed more closely by reviewing studies that have looked at the effects of selective agonists and antagonists on feeding behaviour. Finally, a number of issues arising from the research review will be addressed. For other recent reviews of dopamine receptor subtype involvement in feeding, see Terry et al. (1995) and Cooper and Al-Naser (1993).

2 Effects of non-selective drugs

Increases in the level of synaptic dopamine by the actions of indirect dopamine agonists have long been associated with reduced feeding. Thus there are many studies of the effects of the prototypical dopamine releaser amphetamine on feeding: moderate to high doses are consistently reported to reduce food intake (e.g. Leibowitz, 1975; Blundell and Latham, 1980), whereas low doses have been variously reported either to reduce (e.g. Orthen-Gambill, 1985) or to enhance (e.g. Winn et al., 1982; Evans and Eikelboom, 1987; Evans and Vaccarino, 1987) food intake. The factors underlying these discrepant low-dose effects remain to be elucidated, although baseline level of food intake appears to be one important factor (Sills and Vaccarino, 1991; Sills et al., 1993). Microstructural analysis of the rat's anorectic response to amphetamine has suggested that reduced food intake is primarily the consequence of an extended latency to begin eating and a reduction in time spent eating; although the rate of food intake is often reported to increase, this effect is not sufficient to compensate for the changes in latency and feeding duration (e.g. Blundell and Latham, 1980; Cooper and Sweeney, 1980; Willner and Towell, 1982).

Studies of the relative contributions of D_1-type and D_2-type receptor stimulation to the anorectic effects of amphetamine have implicated both subtypes. Early studies with neuroleptic pretreatments supported a role for D_2-type receptors in amphetamine's effects: spiperone, haloperidol and pimozide (all of which show greater selectivity for D_2-type receptors) attenuated amphetamine anorexia (Heffner et al., 1977; Burridge and Blundell, 1979; Towell et al., 1988a). However, reversal by neuroleptics was most apparent at moderate-to-high doses of amphetamine, and less obvious for low-dose amphetamine anorexia (Burridge and Blundell, 1979). In fact, Gilbert and Cooper (1985) reported that the D_2-type receptor antagonist sulpiride failed to attenuate the anorexia associated with any dose of amphetamine; on the other hand, the D_1-type receptor antagonist SCH 23390 fully reversed the effects of a low dose of amphetamine. Together, these data are difficult to interpret. The possibility that D_1-type receptors underlie the low-dose amphetamine anorexia is obfuscated by the enhanced feeding sometimes reported at similar doses; also, the data from Gilbert and Cooper (1985) suggest that D_2-type receptors may not necessarily be involved in higher-dose effects of amphetamine.

Using amphetamine as a tool to examine dopamine receptor involvement is clearly complicated by its effects on other neurochemical systems. Thus, for example, its anorectic effects are also known to reflect its actions as a releaser of noradrenaline (e.g. Ahlskog, 1974; Leibowitz, 1975; Willner and Towell, 1982). Clearly there is a need to compare the effects of amphetamine with those of other indirect dopaminergic agonists. Unfortunately, most drugs studied to date also lack selectivity for dopamine. Thus the monoamine uptake inhibitors mazindol (Kruk and Zarrindast, 1976; Zambotti et al., 1976), bupropion (Zarrindast and Hosseini-Nia, 1988) and cocaine (e.g. Van Rossum and Simons, 1969; Groppetti et al., 1973) each reduce food intake, but each also has affinity for non-dopaminergic transporter sites. Only one drug selective for the inhibition of dopamine uptake has been tested, namely GBR 12909 (Van der Hoek and Cooper, 1994). Microstructural analysis of the effects of mazindol and cocaine (Cooper and Sweeney, 1980; Cooper and Van der Hoek, 1993) reveals certain commonalities with the effects of amphetamine: they extend the latency to initiate feeding, and they reduce the total time spent eating. However, of the two drugs, only mazindol appears to increase eating rate in the same manner as amphetamine. The more selective dopamine uptake inhibitor GBR 12909 also reduced food intake through a reduction in feeding duration and produced a non-significant trend towards increased eating rate (Van der Hoek and Cooper, 1994); latency to initiate eating was not reported. However, at doses that impaired feeding parameters (>15 mg/kg intraperitoneally), other aspects of behaviour were significantly changed; in particular, there was a marked increase in stereotyped sniffing. Thus it is possible that behavioural competition could account for the anorectic effect of GBR 12909. Nevertheless, feeding duration appears to be a factor that is consistently modified by drugs that increase dopaminergic transmission. Eating rate and latency to eat are less consistently affected. It might also be noted that for none of the uptake inhibitors tested to date has a low-dose hyperphagic response been reported.

It is unfortunate, given the neurochemical selectivity of GBR 12909, that there have been no attempts to antagonize the drug's anorectic effects using receptor-subtype selective antagonists. Such a study might help to determine whether the drug's effects on feeding are secondary to its effects on other behaviours. There are limited results concerning receptor subtype involvement in the effects of uptake inhibitors on feeding. For example, Zarrindast and Hosseini-Nia (1988) showed that the D_2-type antagonist pimozide blocked the hypophagia caused by bupropion. Mazindol-induced anorexia has also been reversed by pretreatment with the D_2-type antagonists pimozide (Kruk and Zarrindast, 1976; Zambotti et al., 1976) and spiperone (Cooper and Sweeney, 1980); cocaine-induced anorexia has also been blocked by spiperone (Heffner et al., 1977). The only indirect agonist (apart from amphetamine) that has been tested in combination with both D_1- and D_2-type antagonists is cocaine (Rapoza and Woolverton, 1991). In that study, results suggested that both D_1- and D_2-type antagonists were effective at attenuating cocaine-induced decreases in milk intake. Such findings are consistent with those emerging from studies of receptor subtype involvement in other behavioural effects of dopamine uptake inhibitors (e.g. Callahan et al., 1991; Melia and Spealman, 1991), but need to be examined more thoroughly with regard to feeding.

In terms of non-selective direct agonists, the anorectic effects of apomorphine have been studied over many years (e.g. Barzaghi et al., 1973; Eichler and Antelman, 1977; Heffner et al., 1977; Kruk, 1973; Willner et al., 1985; Muscat et al., 1986; Duterte-Boucher et al., 1989). Microstructural analysis of the effects of apomorphine on feeding suggests that, like the indirect agonists, it reduces the duration of eating, although, unlike the indirect agonists, it consistently reduces eating rate as well (Willner et al., 1985; Muscat et al., 1986). Furthermore, the D_2-type antagonists sulpiride and pimozide, but not antagonists of other receptors, reverse the effects of apomorphine on each feeding parameter (Muscat et al., 1986). Similar results have been reported in mice, using the D_2-type antagonists haloperidol and sulpiride (Duterte-Boucher et al., 1989). Evidence supporting a central action of apomorphine at D_2-type receptors is indicated by the failure of the peripheral D_2-type antagonist domperidone to attenuate the effects of apomorphine (Muscat et al., 1986; Duterte-Boucher et al., 1989). However, before concluding that non-selective postsynaptic agonists induce hypophagia through an action at D_2-type receptors specifically, certain qualifying factors need to be considered. First, apomorphine shows greater D_2-type selectivity in vivo than in vitro (Andersen and Jansen, 1990). Thus it may not be surprising that D_1-type selective antagonists do not appear to reverse the anorectic effects of apomorphine (e.g. Towell *et al.*, 1988b; Ladurelle *et al.*, 1991). Also, procedures expected to engender hypersensitive postsynaptic D_2-type receptors, namely chronic treatment with haloperidol or lesions by 6-hydroxydopamine, do not affect the anorectic response to apomorphine (Duterte-Boucher *et al.*, 1989). As a general point concerning antagonist studies of the effects of non-selective agonists, it needs to be borne in mind that the effects of both agonists and antagonists alone are complex. For example (as we shall see), D_2-type antagonists can produce biphasic effects on feeding dependent on dose, as can some agonists; thus dose selection for antagonist studies is difficult, and most studies to date report interactions for single doses only.

3 D_1-type receptor agonists and antagonists

Research into the role of D_1-type receptors in the regulation of feeding developed later than that into the role of D_2-type receptors, perhaps because many of the dopamine antagonists widely used before the partition of dopamine receptors were later found to be selective for the D_2-type, and perhaps also because D_2-type agonists were initially considered better able to reproduce the behavioural effects of non-selective dopamine agonists. Indeed, early studies of the prototypical D_1-type agonist SKF 38393 (Setler *et al.*, 1978) failed to reveal any marked behavioural consequences, and the drug's effects were difficult to characterize (cf. Clark and White, 1987; Waddington and O'Boyle, 1989). Nevertheless, it became apparent that the drug produced mild behavioural activation in rats habituated to a test arena, a syndrome that included modest increases in locomotor activity and time spent grooming (e.g. Molloy and Waddington, 1984, 1985, 1987). However, the observed effects were not always consistent between studies (cf. Tirelli and Terry, 1993). On the other hand, the prototypical D_1-type antagonist SCH 23390 (Hyttel, 1983; Iorio *et al.*, 1983) produced reliable effects similar to those of D_2-type antagonists: reduced locomotor activity, impaired motor control, and (at high doses) immobility or catalepsy (e.g. Christensen *et al.*, 1984; Hoffman and Beninger, 1985; Morelli and DiChiara, 1985; Loschmann *et al.*, 1991).

Gilbert and Cooper (1985) were first to report that the D_1-type agonist SKF 38393 produced a dose-dependent reduction in food intake, whereas the D_1-type antagonist SCH 23390 produced only a modest decrease in feeding. These anorectic effects were obtained in non-deprived rats given 30 min access to a palatable wet-mash diet. Using a similar procedure, Cooper *et al.* (1990) provided a microstructural analysis of the effects of SKF 38393 on feeding and other behaviours. As with the non-selective agonists, there was a significant reduction in time spent eating, but in the case of SKF 38393 this seemed directly attributable to a marked reduction in the frequency of feeding bouts. Unlike amphetamine or mazindol, but similarly to apomorphine, the local rate of eating also declined, and was accompanied by a compensatory increase in the mean duration of the feeding bouts.

Rusk and Cooper (1989a) showed that the effect of SKF 38393 on food intake was also obtainable in food-deprived rats, a result since confirmed by others (Zarrindast *et al.*, 1991; Terry and Katz, 1992, 1994), and also demonstrated in food-deprived mice (Ladurelle *et al.*, 1991). However, the relative potency of SKF 38393 on food intake is reduced in food-deprived rats in comparison with non-deprived animals (Terry and Katz, 1992). Furthermore, SKF 38393 does not only affect feeding in food-deprived animals and in those trained to eat a palatable diet: Martin-Iverson and Dourish (1988) showed that SKF 38393 reduces food intake in free-feeding rats whose intake was measured for 4 h after a single dose. In another study looking at free-feeding rats, a dose-related decrease was obtained early in the dark phase of the daily light–dark cycle, with the anorectic effect restricted to the first 6 h after drug administration (cf. Cooper and Al-Naser, 1993). Finally, with regard to the generality of the anorectic effect, SKF 38393 also inhibits sucrose sham-feeding in rats fitted with gastric fistulas (Cooper *et al.*, 1993). Thus there is considerable evidence to suggest that SKF 38393 impairs rodent food intake in a variety of different test situations.

No other D_1-type agonist has been tested across such an array of procedures. However, data are now available for a number of different D_1-type agonists in selected test procedures. SKF 38393 is a benzazepine compound with only partial agonist activity in the adenylyl cyclase assay of D_1-type agonist efficacy (e.g. O'Boyle *et al.*, 1989). However, other benzazepines with differing efficacies also reduce food intake dose-dependently, for example SKF 75670 in non-deprived rats eating palatable mash (Rusk and Cooper, 1989a), and both SKF 77434 and SKF 82958 in food-deprived rats (Terry and Katz, 1992). For none of these other benzazepines are data available concerning the parameters of feeding that underlie the anorectic effects. As regards structurally-dissimilar D_1-type agonists, three other drugs are known to reduce feeding, at least in specific test conditions: the ergoline CY 208–243 impedes sucrose sham-feeding in gastric-fistulated rats (Cooper *et al.*, 1993) and the isochroman agonists A-77636 and A-68930 reduce intake in free-feeding and non-deprived rats eating palatable mash, respectively (Al-Naser and Cooper, 1994). Comparisons with SKF 38393 in terms of drug effects on feeding parameters (other than intake alone) are available only for the latter two compounds. Thus Al-Naser and Cooper (1994) conducted a microstructural analysis of the effects of A-68930 on the consumption of palatable food by rats. They showed that, in common with SKF 38393, the drug-induced reduction in food intake was accompanied by a dose-dependent decline in the total time spent feeding, and this decline was in turn primarily the product of a reduction in the number of meals consumed. Again in common with SKF 38393, eating rate decreased with dose, whereas mean meal duration increased. Taken alone, these results might suggest a general mechanism underlying the actions of D_1-type agonists on feeding: namely, a specific effect on feeding bout frequencies. Interestingly, for this particular test procedure, a change in feeding bout frequency is also associated with reduced food intake due to pre-test satiation (Cooper and Francis, 1993); thus the microstructural analysis might be taken to suggest that the D_1-type agonists promote satiety. In this regard, it might be recalled that both SKF 38393 and CY 208-243 dose-dependently reduce sucrose sham-feeding (Cooper et al., 1993), an effect often attributed to the induction of satiety-related cues. However, there are some problems that need to be addressed before it can be claimed that D_1-type receptor stimulation is linked with satiety. One important qualification to this assumption arises from examination of the effects of A-68930 on other (non-feeding-related) behaviours. Although neither SKF 38393 nor A-68930 markedly disrupted the behavioural satiety sequence (Smith and Gibbs, 1979) associated with feeding, A-68930 significantly enhanced grooming at doses below the anorectic threshold dose. Consequently, behavioural competition from drug-induced motor effects might have contributed to the reduction in meal frequency. On the other hand, the anorectic effect of SKF 38393 was observed in the absence of drug-induced motor effects (Cooper et al., 1990). Whether these differences are due to the structural differences between the drugs and/or to possible differences between them in terms of their affinities for non-dopaminergic sites (see below) can be answered only by testing further compounds.

The only other behavioural analysis of the effects of a D_1-type agonist other than SKF 38393 in a comparable procedure is provided by Al-Naser et al. (unpublished results). They described the effects of A-77636 in free-feeding rats using a meal pattern analysis (cf. Clifton, 1987). In an earlier study, Clifton and Cooper (unpublished results, reported by Cooper and Al-Naser, 1993) found that the dopamine receptor-selective enantiomer of SKF 38393, namely $R(+)$-SKF 38393, increased the latency to start eating at the onset of the night phase of the diurnal light cycle, and reduced the average meal size without affecting the frequency of eating bouts. The hypophagic effect lasted 2–3 h. In the study using A-77636, the anorectic effect was also found to reflect a significant reduction in the average size of meals; however, there was an important difference in comparison with $R(+)$-SKF 38393: A-77636 also produced a modest increase in the frequency of meals. Thus, again, it is difficult to claim a common functional mechanism underlying the anorectic actions of D_1-type agonists. More drugs (at more than one dose) need to be tested in equivalent procedures before a reliable characterization of the effect can be advanced. Nevertheless, as we shall see, the effects of the D_1-type agonists on feeding differ markedly from those of the D_2-type agonists, which predominantly reduce food intake by a selective action on the rate of eating.

There are few studies that address the neuroanatomical basis of the effects of D_1-type agonists on ingestive behaviour. Evidence in support of a central (rather than peripheral) mechanism of D_1-type agonist effects has been provided by the failure of the peripherally-active agonist SKF 82526 (fenoldopam) to reduce feeding (Rusk and Cooper, 1989a). Despite this, recent studies looking at modulation of feeding by intracranial infusions of D_1-type agonists have not revealed *any* anorectic actions of these compounds. Thus, for example, Phillips *et al.* (1995) found no anorectic effect associated with infusions of SKF 38393 into the nucleus accumbens, and Inoue *et al.* (1995) similarly found no effect of CY 208-243 when infused into the ventrolateral striatum. Although it is difficult to generalize from such a restricted sample of findings, the implication is that the hypophagia produced by systemic administration of D_1-type agonists is not due to drug action at receptors in either the nucleus accumbens or ventrolateral striatum, regions widely considered to be important in modulating feeding and oral-motor behaviour (e.g. Dunnett and Iverson, 1982; Pisa, 1988; Salamone *et al.*, 1993; Clifton and Somerville, 1994). Hence the critical site(s) of action of D_1-type agonists remains uncertain, and might lie outside of those dopaminergic terminal areas that attract most research interest. Clarifying the issue of substrate will obviously be essential for assessing the significance of D_1-type receptor stimulation in the regulation of feeding.

Perhaps more surprising than the paucity of research into the neuroanatomical substrates underlying D_1-type agonist effects is the fact that few studies have attempted to demonstrate receptor specificity of these behavioural effects, i.e. primarily by demonstrating receptor-specific antagonism. For some time, only one experimental result was available to suggest that the anorectic effect of the prototypical agonist SKF 38393 was mediated by D_1-type receptors: testing the two enantiomers of SKF 38393 in non-deprived mice, Rusk and Cooper (1989a) showed that only the D_1-type receptor-selective enantiomer $R(+)$-SKF 38393 was effective in reducing food intake. However, studies of SKF 38393 in combination with the selective D_1-type antagonist SCH 23390 have since called into question the importance of D_1-type receptors in mediating the hypophagia induced by SKF 38393. Thus Terry and Katz (1992) found that the anorectic effect of SKF 38393 in food-deprived rats given 40 min access to powdered diet was not reliably attenuated by pretreatment with SCH 23390. On the other hand, the anorectic effects of the D_1-type agonist SKF 77434 were partially antagonized by the antagonist, and the effects of SKF 82958 were fully (and, uniquely, dose-dependently) antagonized by SCH 23390. Results from other laboratories confirm that the D_1-type antagonist SCH 23390 is at best only marginally effective at blocking the anorectic effect of SKF 38393 (e.g. Ladurelle *et al.*, 1991; Zarrindast *et al.*, 1991). These data suggest that the actions of SKF 38393 at a receptor (or receptors) other than of the D_1-type family may contribute to its anorectic effects, a significant implication given the prototypical status of SKF 38393 as a D_1-type agonist, and its use in the majority of studies examining D_1-type involvement in feeding behaviour.

As regards identifying an alternative site of action which might underlie the drug's effects on food intake, Zarrindast *et al.* (1991) reported that the non-specific 5-hydroxytryptamine (5-HT) antagonist metergoline effectively reversed the anorectic effect of SKF 38393 in rats, a finding since replicated by Terry and Katz (unpublished results; see Terry et al., 1995). Similarly, it has been reported that the drug's ability to reduce operant responding for food is also antagonized by metergoline, but not by SCH 23390 (Terry and Katz, 1993). The possibility that a serotonergic mechanism contributes to the drug's anorectic effect is supported by the finding that SKF 38393 acts as a partial agonist at the 5-HT_{2C} receptor (previously called the 5-HT_{1C} receptor) and is more efficacious than either SKF 77434 or SKF 82958 at this site (Briggs et al., 1991). It has been demonstrated that 5-HT_{2C} agonists are effective anorectic agents (Kennett and Curzon, 1988, 1991). Interestingly, the D_1-type antagonist SCH 23390 is also a partial agonist at the 5-HT_{2C} receptor (Briggs et al., 1991; Woodward et al., 1992), raising the possibility that its inability to antagonize the anorectic effect of SKF 38393 may reflect a complex additive interaction between the two drugs at a common site. Because of this, it is important to assess the effects of other D_1-type antagonists on SKF 38393-induced hypophagia. One such study (Terry and Katz, 1994) used the D_1-type antagonist SCH 39166 (Chipkin et al., 1988; McQuade et al., 1991), a drug with negligible affinity for the 5-HT_{2C} receptor (Taylor et al., 1991; Wamsley et al., 1991). Given its pharmacological profile, an enhanced antagonism of the hypophagic effect of SKF 38393 by SCH 39166 might be expected. However, like SCH 23390, SCH 39166 failed to attenuate the anorectic effect of SKF 38393; at best, both D_1-type receptor blockers produced limited antagonism when suppression of feeding by SKF 38393 was near-complete.

Thus caution is required in attributing the effects of the prototypical D_1-type agonist SKF 38393 to a specific action at D_1-type receptors. Consequently, future studies of other D_1-type compounds will be necessary in order to elucidate possible common functions underlying the effects of D_1-type agonists on feeding; comparisons with SKF 38393 might not be appropriate. As yet, behavioural analyses of other D_1-type agonists in equivalent procedures are not available.

Studies of agonist–antagonist interactions at D_1-type receptors are complicated by the fact that D_1-type antagonists themselves reduce food intake. The anorectic effects of D_1-type antagonists have not been studied as thoroughly as those of other dopaminergic agents, especially in terms of the microstructural parameters that contribute to their effects. However, it is clear that the D_1-type antagonist SCH 23390 reduces food intake both in food-deprived rats (Gilbert and Cooper, 1985; Zarrindast et al., 1991; Terry and Katz, 1992) and in free-feeding animals (Clifton et al., 1991; Naruse et al., 1991). Schneider and colleagues (1988) demonstrated that SCH 23390 inhibits sucrose sham-feeding, although its effects on corn oil sham-feeding are much weaker (Weatherford et al., 1990). There have also been several reports that SCH 23390 reduces operant responding for food reinforcement (e.g. Nakajima, 1986; Beninger et al., 1987; Sanger, 1987; Koechling et al., 1988; Rusk and Cooper, 1994). Until recently, no data were available for other D_1-type antagonists. However, Terry and Katz (1994) have now demonstrated the generality of the antagonist effect by showing that SCH 39166 inhibits deprivation-induced food intake dose-dependently. The anorectic potency of SCH 39166 was approximately half that of SCH 23390, a result that is congruent with its lower affinity at D_1-type receptors (e.g. Chipkin *et al.*, 1988; McQuade *et al.*, 1992). Given the negligible affinity of SCH 39166 for serotonergic receptors, these findings suggest that the effects of SCH 23390 are not necessarily mediated by an exclusive action at 5-HT$_2$ or 5-HT$_{2C}$ receptors, and that D_1-type receptor blockade alone can reduce food intake.

The behavioural profiles associated with the actions of D_1-type antagonists during feeding have not been well characterized. In a study of food intake across a series of discrete meal segments Koechling *et al.* (1988) demonstrated that SCH 23390 (0.025–0.10 mg/kg; route not specified) increased the latency to eat and reduced the speed of eating. A 'best scores analysis' (cf. Wise and Colle, 1984) suggested that the decrements were not due to a performance deficit, and so were taken to reflect a motivational impairment. However, other studies have questioned whether D_1-type antagonists have a specific effect on the motivation to eat. Thus, for example, using meal pattern analysis, Clifton *et al.* (1991) reported that SCH 23390 (0.01–0.10 mg/kg subcutaneously) produced a small reduction in the number of meals consumed and in the feeding rate during a meal; there was no effect on meal size, and the drug's disruptive effect on water intake was substantially greater than its effect on food intake. These findings have recently been supported by Clifton (1995), who reported no anorectic effect of the D_1-type antagonist SCH 39166 at doses that significantly disrupted drinking. Recently, in a rare study of the effects of intrastriatal infusion of SCH 23390 on food intake, Inoue *et al.* (1995) also failed to obtain any hypophagic effect, again at doses that significantly decreased water intake.

Koechling *et al.* (1988) notwithstanding the systemic dose ranges of SCH 23390 that typically reduce food intake (>0.01 mg/kg subcutaneously; >0.03 mg/kg intraperitoneally) are those that are often associated with significant disruption of motor behaviour. For example, subcutaneous doses in the range of 0.01–0.1 mg/kg are associated with potentiation of the dorsal immobility response (Meyer *et al.*, 1992), reduced locomotor activity (Meyer *et al.*, 1993) and catalepsy (Morelli and DiChiara, 1985). In a recent study questioning the behavioural specificity of the anorectic effects of D_1-type antagonists, P. Terry and colleagues (unpublished results) showed that the D_1-antagonist SCH 39166 produced no significant reduction in food intake over a range of doses (0.03–0.3 mg/kg intraperitoneally) that significantly reduced other kinds of motor behaviour: locomotion, rearing and grooming. Although total intake (grams of food consumed) did not decline significantly, there was a significant reduction in the number of meals consumed; this was apparently compensated for by a dose-dependent (but non-significant) increase in the

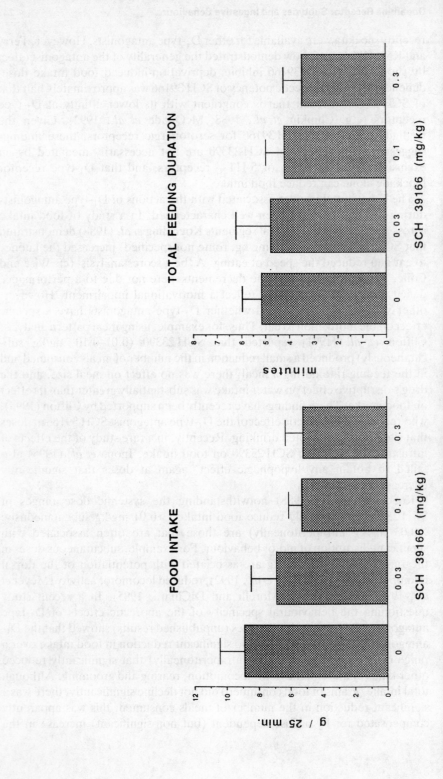

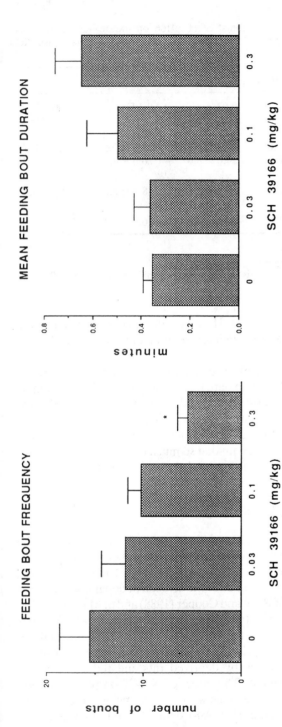

Fig. 1 Effects of the D_1-type antagonist SCH 39166 (0.03–0.3 mg/kg) on parameters of feeding behaviour. The drug was injected intraperitoneally 30 min before the rat was placed in the observation cage. Behaviours were then recorded continuously for 25 min, during which time the non-deprived rat has access to a palatable wet-mash diet. *Top left*: SCH 39166 produced a modest and non-significant reduction in food intake. *Top right*: The mean duration of feeding declined non-significantly with increasing dose. *Bottom left*: Mean bout frequency was significantly reduced, an effect primarily attributable to the 0.3 mg/kg dose. *Bottom right*: There was a non-significant trend for mean bout duration to increase with dose. See Table 1 for corresponding effects on other behaviours. All results are mean $\pm$ SE ($n = 8$). Analysis was by one-way analysis of variance *$P < 0.05$ *vs* control (Dunnett's t test).

Table 1 Effects of the D_1-type antagonist SCH 39166 on motor behaviours (not directly related to feeding) during 25-min access to a highly palatable wet-mash diet (non-deprived rats)

	SCH 39166 (mg/kg)			
	0	0.03	0.10	0.30
Locomotor activity				
Duration (min)	5.8 ± 0.6	4.4 ± 0.9	3.9 ± 0.5	2.9 ± 0.7*
Bout frequency	36.6 ± 4.1	24.0 ± 3.6*	26.6 ± 4.2	14.9 ± 3.7†
Rearing				
Bout frequency	24.9 ± 3.1	15.3 ± 2.6	18.8 ± 2.8	9.5 ± 3.0†
Grooming				
Bout frequency	9.4 ± 1.5	6.6 ± 0.9	6.9 ± 1.4	4.6 ± 0.7†

Experimental details are as in Fig. 1.
Results are expressed as mean ± SE ($n = 8$).
For each measure, overall one-way analysis of variance was significant ($P < 0.05$); *$P < 0.05$, †$P < 0.01$ vs control (Dunnett's t test).

mean duration of eating bouts (Fig. 1). However, the concomitant changes in other aspects of motor behaviour make interpretation of these effects difficult (Table 1).

Thus, with regard to the effects of D_1-type antagonists on ingestive behaviour, the limited evidence available to date fails to support a specific action on central feeding mechanisms. On the other hand, there is some indication that D_1-type agonists can produce consistent qualitative changes in feeding behaviour, albeit that more detailed behavioural studies of novel compounds still need to be undertaken. It is unfortunate that so much of the data available for D_1-type receptor ligands has been collected from a restricted number of investigators.

4 D_2-type receptor agonists and antagonists

Given the widespread interest in the D_2-type receptor as a possible site for the mediation of reward-related behaviour, it seems odd that there are few studies looking specifically at the effects of D_2-type agonists on feeding. Among the first directly relevant studies to appear after the division of dopamine receptors into two subtypes were those of Rusk and Cooper (1988) and of Martin-Iverson and Dourish (1988). In the former study the D_2-type agonists N-0437 (Van der Weide *et al.*, 1986) and RU 24213 (Euvrard *et al.*, 1979) both reduced the intake of palatable mash in non-deprived rats; N-0437 also decreased consumption of powdered laboratory chow by deprived rats and reduced operant responding for food reinforcement. The effect of N-0437 on palatable food intake was maintained over ten injections without any obvious tolerance. In contrast, Martin-Iverson and Dourish (1988) demonstrated enhanced food intake by free-feeding rats over a 4-h period following treatment with the D_2-type agonist PHNO (Martin et al., 1984) at all doses tested (7.5–120 μg/kg subcutaneously). The involvement of the D_2-type receptor in the mediation of this effect was supported by its reversal following pretreatment with the D_2-type antagonist haloperidol. However, this hyperphagia was specific to a particular kind of diet: standard laboratory food pellets. Over the same dose range, PHNO significantly reduced the intake of both sweetened milk and liquid chow diets. The authors concluded that the increased feeding observed when solid pellets were available was most likely due to the stimulation of chewing behaviour. The specificity of the hyperphagic effect is supported by the fact that PHNO has since been found only to decrease consumption of powdered chow by free-feeding rats (cf. Cooper and Al-Naser, 1993) and of palatable mash by non-deprived rats (cf. Terry et al., 1995). Given that the hyperphagic effect of PHNO was specific to one diet, and occurred over a wide dose range, it seems unlikely that it could be attributable to the drug preferentially stimulating autoreceptors. Nevertheless, there is some evidence that, at low doses, D_2-type agonists might interact with autoreceptors to enhance food intake. For example, intraventricular bromocriptine can stimulate feeding at low doses (Morley et al., 1982), although the preferential D_2-type agonist lisuride, at systemic doses presumed to act at autoreceptors, has the opposite effect (Carruba et al., 1980). However, in accordance with the possibility that dopamine D_2-type agonists might stimulate feeding at low doses (by autoreceptor activation) and inhibit feeding at higher doses (by postsynaptic receptor activation), Clifton et al. (1989) showed that N-0437 produced just such a biphasic dose–effect function in free-feeding rats. Ferrari et al. (1992a) also reported that, at doses considered autoreceptor selective (0.01–0.5 mg/kg intraperitoneally), the D_2-type agonist B-HT 920 (Anden et al., 1982) decreased the latency to initiate feeding and increased food intake over a 6-h period in food-deprived rats. However, studying the effects of the D_2-type agonists lisuride and CQ 32-084 on feeding in two different test situations (a modified X-maze and the home cage), Ferrari et al. (1992b) suggested that the hyperphagic effect was apparent only in a stressful test situation (in this case, the X-maze) and might reflect an anxiolytic action of D_2-type autoreceptor activation, rather than a specific interaction with mechanisms regulating food intake.

Interestingly, infusion of quinpirole into the ventrolateral striatum has been shown to produce hyperphagia (Inoue et al., 1995), whereas infusion into the nucleus accumbens is without effect (Phillips et al., 1995), suggesting a possible neuroanatomical site for the hyperphagic response to D_2-type agonists. However, there are two caveats. First, sucrose ingestion is significantly *reduced* by intra-accumbens infusions of the D_3 subtype-selective agonist 7-OH-DPAT (Gilbert and Cooper, 1995), a drug that actually has a similar D_2–D_3 selectivity to quinpirole (e.g. Levesque et al., 1992). Second, systemic injection of quinpirole routinely *inhibits* food intake (e.g. Zarrindast et al., 1991; Cooper and Al-Naser, 1993), and in fact D_2-type agonist-induced hyperphagia has not been reported elsewhere (albeit that there are few studies that adopt closely comparable procedures in terms of prototypical drug, dose range, deprivation status or diet). With regard to the possibility that hyperphagia occurs as a result of the stimulation of chewing-related behaviour, it is notable that Zarrindast *et al.* (1991) showed only dose-dependent inhibition of feeding by the D_2-type agonists bromocriptine and quinpirole, despite (presumably) using standard laboratory pellets as the diet (the nature of the diet was not specified). In mice tested for consumption of solid pellets, the D_2-type agonist RU 24926 produced dose-dependent anorexia (Ladurelle *et al.*, 1991). Similarly, most other reports, using different diets, demonstrate dose-dependent reductions in food intake following D_2-type agonist treatment (cf. Cooper and Al-Naser, 1993; Terry *et al.*, 1995).

In the only published study of the microstructure of feeding in response to a D_2-type agonist (Rusk and Cooper, 1989b), only dose-dependent decreases in food intake were reported, even though the drug used, N-0437, produced a behavioural profile congruent with autoreceptor stimulation at the lowest dose. The predominant effect of the drug was to reduce the local rate of eating, with no effect on total feeding duration, and no consistent effect on the frequency of feeding bouts; the time course of feeding was also unaffected. The drug modified a number of non-feeding behaviours over the full dose range (0.3–3.0 mg/kg intraperitoneally), although it is not easy to relate these changes to the effects on food intake. For example, at the anorectic doses (1.0 and 3.0 mg/kg), the frequency of grooming was significantly reduced and the total duration of sniffing behaviour increased; locomotor activity was unaffected. It is not clear how such a pattern of effects might indirectly influence the rate of eating specifically. However, the same doses also increased the frequency, and thereby the total duration, of oral behaviours. This effect was dose dependent, although being a composite category of various behaviours (e.g. yawning, licking, vacuous chewing), it is difficult to determine how the various aspects might have modulated the action of feeding. Unfortunately, there are no other studies in the literature that provide a microstructural analysis of the effects of a different D_2-type agonist, although Al-Naser (1993) reported that quinpirole also produces dose-dependent anorexia through a reduction in local rate of eating, suggesting a common mechanism of action. However, using a meal-pattern analysis, Clifton *et al.* (1989) obtained a biphasic dose–response profile for the effects of N-0437 on feeding, with enhanced food intake at an intraperitoneal dose of 0.3 mg/kg and decreased consumption at 1.0 and 3.0 mg/kg. The primary effect throughout was on meal size, although duration also increased at the lowest dose. In contrast with the microstructural analysis of D_2-type agonist effects, rate of feeding was only slightly reduced.

It is interesting to note that the conflicting reports of enhanced *vs* reduced food intake at low doses of D_2-type agonists find a parallel in studies using low doses of the non-selective indirect agonist, D-amphetamine (as described above). However, the similarities extend no further: at higher doses, D-amphetamine produces its anorectic effect by reducing feeding duration and tends to increase the local rate of eating, exactly the opposite effect of N-0437. Indeed, none of the indirect agonists tested to date has produced a selective reduction in eating rates. However, this particular effect, namely a slowed rate of feeding, is characteristic of the action of the (purportedly) non-selective direct agonist, apomorphine. Again, this might support the notion that apomorphine's effects on feeding are mediated through D_2-type receptors and/ or that the drug is more reliably categorized as a D_2-type agonist *in vivo*. On the other hand, it should be noted that apomorphine also reduces total feeding duration, whereas N-0437 does not, and there are no reports of apomorphine stimulating food intake at low doses. This latter point raises important questions concerning the proposed autoreceptor mediation of hyperphagia, since apomorphine at low doses is widely regarded as a selective D_2-type autoreceptor agonist, and its non-feeding behavioural effects are consistent with this view. The issue of presynaptic *vs* postsynaptic effects needs to be addressed in the light of these inconsistencies. A reconceptualization of these effects might emerge from recent developments in dopamine receptor classification and the suggestion that certain behavioural effects previously attributed to autoreceptor binding might instead be due to drug action at a postsynaptic receptor subtype (e.g. Stahle, 1992), perhaps the D_3 receptor subtype (Waters *et al.*, 1994).

Given that D_2-type agonists effectively inhibit feeding across a range of test situations, it is perhaps surprising that N-0437 has been shown to be without effect in terminating sucrose sham-feeding, even though it reduces sucrose intake by non-fistulated rats (Cooper *et al.*, 1989). The absence of an effect on sham-feeding is in marked contrast with the actions of D_1-type agonists, which produce strong dose-dependent suppressions of intake (Cooper *et al.*, 1993; see above). Rusk and Cooper (1989b) suggested that this profile of effects implies that D_2-type agonists act to reduce feeding only in the presence of normal satiety cues. However, other D_2-type agonists need to be tested on sham-feeding before broad conclusions can be drawn.

Receptor specificity of the anorectic effects of D_2-type agonists has been demonstrated, even though, as is the case for D_1-type agonists, agonist–antagonist interaction experiments have concentrated only on measures of total food intake. Thus Rusk and Cooper (1988) showed that the effect of N-0437 (1.0 mg/kg intraperitoneally) on palatable mash consumption was blocked by pretreatment with 0.01 mg/kg (route not specified) of the selective D_2-type antagonist YM 09151-2 (Terai *et al.*, 1983). This accords with results from earlier studies which found antagonism of the anorectic effects of the D_2-type agonists pergolide, lisuride and lergotrile by drugs such as haloperidol, spiperone and pimozide (e.g. Greene *et al.*, 1985; Hawkins *et al.*, 1986). Ladurelle and colleagues (1991) also showed reversal of the anorectic effects of

RU 24926 by sulpiride in food-deprived mice. However, there are some anomalous results. For example, Zarrindast *et al*. (1991) found that, whereas the anorectic effects of quinpirole were reversed by pretreatment with either of the D_2-type antagonists sulpiride or pimozide, only the former antagonist was able to reverse the effects of a different agonist, bromocriptine. Perhaps these results might be explained when a clearer characterization of the relative affinities of the various drugs for D_2, D_3 and D_4 receptors emerges.

As mentioned in the introduction, antagonists at D_2-type receptors have been studied more thoroughly than most other kinds of drugs interacting with dopamine receptors, especially with regard to various motivated behaviours, including eating. This is largely due to continuing interest in the hypothesis that dopamine transmission represents a crucial substrate for reward (e.g. Wise, 1982). Consequently, the impaired transmission associated with postsynaptic receptor blockade has been linked with anhedonia, an insensitivity to the reward value of biologically salient stimuli (Wise, 1982). Most of the relevant studies were conducted before the general acceptance of subtypes of dopamine receptors, and they typically used neuroleptic drugs which were later found to have preferential affinity for D_2-type receptors. The issue as to whether these drugs affect the motivational properties of reward or disrupt sensorimotor functions crucial to consummatory responses remains highly contentious (for a recent review see Salamone, 1994). There is even some debate as to whether D_2-type antagonists consistently modify food intake (cf. Blackburn *et al*., 1992). Many of the earlier studies on dopamine antagonists and feeding used the D_2-type antagonist pimozide, and showed that it reduced lever-pressing for food (Wise *et al*., 1978), free-feeding in rats given access to serial meal segments (Wise and Colle, 1984), deprivation-induced feeding (Wise and Raptis, 1986), feeding provoked by electrical stimulation of the lateral hypothalamus (Streather and Bozarth, 1987), and both sham-feeding and normal intake of saccharin or saccharin–sucrose solutions (Xenakis and Sclafani, 1981; Geary and Smith, 1985). Schneider and co-workers (1986) demonstrated that the inhibitory potencies of a series of four D_2-type antagonists tested on sham-feeding corresponded with their binding potencies at D_2-type receptors. Furthermore, these effects on sham and real feeding appear to be centrally mediated, since domperidone, a D_2-type antagonist that is excluded from the central nervous system, is unable to reproduce the effects of pimozide in these tasks (Duong and Weingarten, 1993).

Nevertheless, there are many reported failures to inhibit food intake with D_2-type antagonists. For example, although in an early study Heffner *et al*. (1977) showed an effect of spiperone on food intake, another D_2-type antagonist, haloperidol, had no effect. Others who have reported no effects include Kruk (1973), Zis and Fibiger (1975), Tombaugh *et al*. (1979), Willis *et al*. (1983), Hoffman and Beninger (1986) and Blackburn *et al*. (1987). Drug dose and test procedure appear to be important variables, but it seems clear that the motivational salience of attractive cues, rather than feeding behaviour specifically, is particularly sensitive to the effects of these drugs (cf. Blackburn *et al.*, 1992). However, it might be noted that the various kinds of theoretical formulation that have emerged to address the actions of neuroleptics have not yet effectively integrated the findings associated with the other categories of dopamine receptor ligand: D_1-type agonists and antagonists, and D_2-type agonists.

In line with the proposal that operant responding for food is more easily disrupted than the consummatory response of eating, Rusk and Cooper (1994) recently demonstrated that the D_2-type antagonist YM 09151-2 significantly reduced lever-pressing for food at a dose (0.03 mg/kg intraperitoneally) lower than that which reduced deprivation-induced feeding or the consumption of palatable wet mash (0.1 mg/kg in both cases). Interestingly, the 0.01 mg/kg dose actually enhanced food intake in the food-deprived rats, although no such low-dose effect was obtained with pimozide. Similar increases in feeding following low doses of D_2-type antagonists have previously been reported: for spiperone (Rowland and Engle, 1977; Cooper and Sweeney, 1980), pimozide (Lawson *et al.*, 1984), haloperidol (Hobbs *et al.*, 1994) and sulpiride injected into the lateral hypothalamus (Parada *et al.*, 1988). The less selective dopamine receptor antagonists chlorpromazine and clozapine have also been reported to stimulate food intake (Reynolds and Carlisle, 1961; Stolerman, 1970; Antelman *et al.*, 1977). In a microstructural analysis of the effects of the D_2-type antagonist haloperidol injected directly into various striatal regions (Bakshi and Kelley, 1991), a dose-dependent enhancement of feeding duration was obtained following injection into the nucleus accumbens (although total intake was not significantly increased), whereas injection into the ventrolateral striatum reduced feeding duration. The anorectic effect of injections into the ventrolateral striatum has been confirmed by Inoue *et al.* (1995) using sulpiride as a D_2-type antagonist.

In the study by Bakshi and Kelley (1991), the increased duration of feeding associated with accumbens infusions was a consequence of extended mean bout duration, rather than of increased bout frequency. Meal-pattern analysis has highlighted similar parameters as being important to the effects of D_2-type antagonists on feeding. Clifton *et al.* (1991) showed that mean meal duration, in addition to average meal size, was significantly enhanced by both YM 09151-2 and remoxipride, although a trend was evident for raclopride only. Remoxipride and raclopride produced short-term increases in food intake. Despite this, all three D_2-type antagonists significantly reduced eating rate, a parameter not affected by striatal infusion of haloperidol. However, systemic injection of haloperidol has been shown to reduce feeding through the same mechanism, with feeding duration also declining (Salamone, 1988; Salamone *et al.*, 1990). Thus D_2-type antagonists have one feature in common with D_2-type agonists: a decrease in the local rate of eating, regardless of whether intake is stimulated or inhibited. However, the primacy of eating rate as the parameter affected by D_2-type antagonists has been questioned in a recent study of palatable food

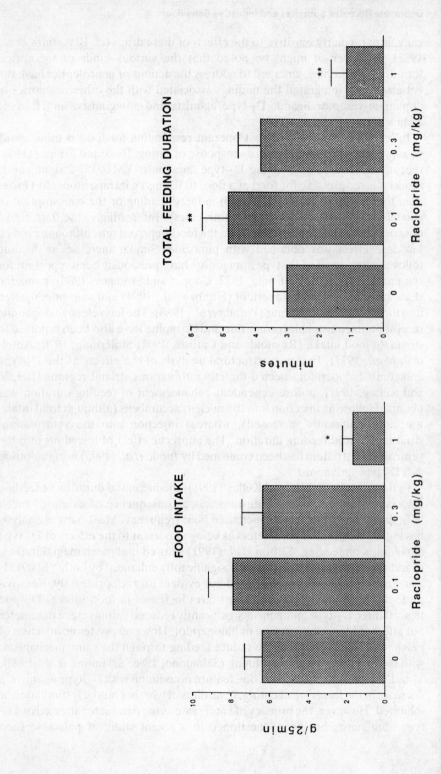

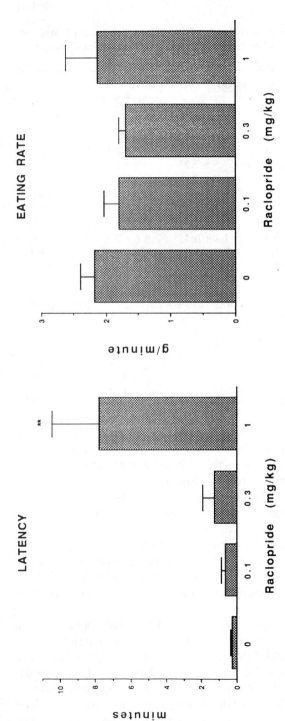

Fig. 2 Effects of the D₂-type antagonist raclopride (0.1–1.0 mg/kg) on parameters of feeding behaviour. The drug was injected intraperitoneally 30 min before the rat was placed in the observation cage. Behaviours were then recorded continuously for 25 min, during which time the non-deprived rat had access to a palatable wet-mash diet. *Top left*: Biphasic effect of raclopride on food intake. The overall effect was significant ($P < 0.0001$), but individual comparisons revealed a significant difference only between the 1.0 mg/kg dose and control conditions. *Top right*: There was a significant biphasic effect of raclopride on mean duration of feeding; duration increased significantly at 0.1 mg/kg and decreased significantly at 1.0 mg/kg. *Bottom left*: Eating latency was significantly increased by raclopride ($P < 0.01$)), with a considerable increase at 1.0 mg/kg. *Botttom right*: Raclopride did not affect the rate of eating at any dose. See Table 2 for corresponding effects on other behaviours. All results are mean ± SE ($n = 8$). Analysis was by one-way analysis of variance; $^*P < 0.05$, $^{**}P < 0.01$ *vs* control (Dunnett's t test).

Table 2 Effects of the D_2-type antagonist raclopride on motor behaviours (not directly related to feeding) during 25-min access to a highly palatable wet-mash diet (non-deprived rats)

	Raclopride (mg/kg)			
	0	0.1	0.3	1.0
Locomotor activity				
Duration (min)	5.5 ± 1.1	5.6 ± 0.6	3.9 ± 0.6	0.4 ± 0.1†
Bout frequency	60.8 ± 9.6	57.5 ± 7.2	43.8 ± 8.5	6.0 ± 1.5†
Rearing				
Duration (min)	5.3 ± 0.7	5.5 ± 0.5	3.0 ± 0.9*	0.3 ± 0.1†
Bout frequency	50.8 ± 7.1	47.4 ± 6.7	26.6 ± 8.9†	3.6 ± 1.3†
Grooming				
Duration (min)	3.6 ± 0.3	2.4 ± 0.5	2.6 ± 0.5	1.1 ± 0.4†
Bout frequency	12.3 ± 1.2	9.9 ± 1.2	8.6 ± 1.7	3.1 ± 3.0†

Experimental details are as in Fig. 2.
Results are expressed as mean ± SE ($n = 8$).
For each measure, overall one-way analysis of variance was significant ($P < 0.05$); *$P < 0.05$, †$P < 0.01$ vs control (Dunnett's t test).

consumption by non-deprived rats (P. Terry *et al.* unpublished results). This study demonstrated a biphasic dose–effect of raclopride on feeding, and the only parameters significantly affected were feeding duration and latency to start eating; eating rate did not change over doses (Fig. 2). The low-dose hyperphagic effect reflected modest increases in the number of feeding bouts and mean bout duration, whereas the high-dose hypophagia was a product of increased latency to eat and reduced number of feeding bouts. Thus it is not necessary for eating rate to be the only factor underlying D_2-type antagonist effects on feeding. It is also important to note that the hypophagic effect occurred at and above those doses of raclopride that significantly disrupted other aspects of motor behaviour: only the low-dose hyperphagia was unaccompanied by changes in other behavioural parameters (Table 2). Hence it is difficult to assume behavioural specificity of the D_2-type antagonist anorectic effect.

Clearly, the effects of D_2-type antagonists on ingestive behaviour are difficult to assimilate within a single model. The functional heterogeneity of different striatal subfields, and differential effects across hypothalamic and ventral forebrain structures (e.g. Parada *et al.*, 1988; Bakshi and Kelley, 1991), might help explain some of the different effects of the antagonists, and also perhaps of the agonists, although comparisons of systemic and intrastriatal infusions of several drugs by microstructural analysis will be necessary. The factors contributing to the observation of biphasic effects of D_2-type antagonists are also likely related to baseline intake levels, as suggested by Rusk and Cooper (1994), and as has been suggested for the biphasic effects of amphetamine (Sills and Vaccarino, 1991). Baseline levels of food intake were low when hyperphagia was observed by Rusk and Cooper (1994) and by P. Terry and co-workers (unpublished results, see above). However, more generally, the presence of biphasic effects in both agonist and antagonist studies presents special difficulties of interpretation which do not arise with regard to drugs interacting at D_1-type receptors. They also create problems in the design and interpretation of agonist–antagonist studies. In addition, the increased eating that sometimes follows injection of D_2-type antagonists at low doses has not been effectively accommodated within models of dopaminergic involvement in reward-related behaviour. If the effect is mediated by autoreceptor blockade (thereby perhaps enhancing dopamine release), it is hard to explain why D_2-type agonists at low doses produce the same outcome. Thus, whereas an assessment of the roles of D_1-type receptors in feeding is impeded by dependence on particular drugs and the limited number of studies, an interpretation of the roles of D_2-type receptors is hindered by the weight of ostensibly conflicting findings.

5   Interactions between D_1- and D_2-type receptors

There has been considerable interest in the possibility that D_1- and D_2-type receptors interact to modulate each other's effects. Thus D_1-type antagonists have been shown to attenuate the motor effects of D_2-type agonists in rats, leading to the proposal that D_1-type receptor stimulation might serve an 'enabling' role in modulating the effects of D_2-type receptor stimulation (e.g. Molloy et al., 1986). Studies of D_1- and D_2-type agonists in combination have also indicated that D_1-type agonists can interact synergistically with D_2-type agonists to enhance the behavioural effects associated with D_2-type receptor agonists (e.g. Braun and Chase, 1986). However, a model of receptor subtype interactions based on a simple cooperative relationship has been challenged by findings which demonstrate a functional opposition in the regulation of certain behaviours (cf. Waddington and Daly, 1993). It has also been shown that, in some circumstances, D_2-type receptor agonists can potentiate the effects of D_1-type receptor agonists, although findings in this regard have been less consistent than those describing how D_2-type effects are modified by D_1-type ligands (e.g. Chandler et al., 1990; cf. Waddington and Daly, 1993).

The data regarding receptor subtype interactions in the control of feeding are limited, since the issue has not been addressed systematically. To some extent this is understandable, given that the effects of individual categories of drug remain only partially characterized. However, in an early study, Martin-Iverson and Dourish (1988) showed that the D_1-type antagonist SCH 23390 reversed the hyperphagia induced by the D_2-type agonist PHNO, suggesting an enabling role of the D_1-type receptor in the production of this unusual response. The only study looking at the effects of D_1-type antagonists on D_2-type agonist-induced anorexia was that of Zarrindast et al. (1991). They found that SCH 23390 was unable to reverse the anorectic effects of either bromocriptine or quinpirole, suggesting that the hypophagic effect (as distinct from the hyperphagic effect) of D_2-type agonists is not modulated by D_1-type receptors. In this respect the inhibition of feeding behaviour is unusual, since few other behavioural effects of D_2-type agonists show such receptor specificity. The converse experiment, looking at the effects of D_2-type antagonists on D_1-type agonist-induced anorexia, is equally rare. Zarrindast et al. (1991) reported that sulpiride failed to reverse the effects of SKF 38393, although only a single dose of sulpiride was tested. Terry and Katz (1992), on the other hand, showed a clear antagonism of the effects of the D_1-type agonist SKF 82958 by the D_2-type antagonist spiperone: the relative potency of the agonist was decreased by a factor of 3.6. Thus, from antagonism studies, there is clearer evidence of D_2-type receptor modulation of D_1-type receptor effects on feeding than there is of D_1-type receptor modulation of D_2-type receptor effects.

The other basis for claiming synergistic interactions between D_1- and D_2-type receptors arises from studies that involved co-administration of agonists at the two sites. Martin-Iverson and Dourish (1988), looking at the hyperphagia induced by the D_2-type agonist PHNO, found that the D_1-type agonist SKF 38393 reduced the size of the hyperphagic effect to an extent commensurate with its own hypophagic effect. In more typical circumstances, where D_2-type agonists reduce feeding, Zarrindast et al., (1991) showed negligible potentiation when SKF 38393 and quinpirole were administered in combination. Lack of potentiation was also reported by Ladurelle et al. (1991), although the two drugs tested (RU 24926 and SKF 38393) produced an additive inhibition of food intake. The only examples of potentiated anorexia have been reported by Cooper and colleagues (Cooper and Al-Naser, 1993; Terry et al., 1995), using SKF 38393 in combination with PHNO or quinpirole, and testing either palatable mash consumption in partially-satiated rats or free-feeding intake. Combined administration of the D_1-type agonist A-68930 with the D_2-type agonist quinpirole, at doses that have no effect on their own, also suppresses sucrose drinking, suggesting a potentiation (H. A. Al-Naser and S. J. Cooper, unpublished results; see Cooper and Al-Naser, 1993). Although these studies typically use only single doses of the various agonists, they suggest a combination effect in excess of being simply additive. It is not clear why others have not reported similar effects.

Thus antagonist studies tend to support a modulatory role of D_2-type receptors in the anorectic actions of D_1-type agonists, rather than vice versa. The agonist studies support this view, since potentiation has been found only when behaviourally inactive doses of D_2-type agonists are combined with active or inactive doses of D_1-type agonists.

6 Interactions of subtype-selective drugs with other systems

There are few studies of the ways in which drug actions at particular dopamine receptor subtypes might interact with other neurochemical systems to modulate feeding. Indeed, such studies might seem premature in light of the many questions that remain concerning the drugs' individual profiles of effects. However, a number of results have raised the possibility that relevant interactions might occur: for example, both D_1- and D_2-type antagonists can attenuate the hyperphagia produced by injection of the benzodiazepine diazepam in non-deprived rats (Naruse *et al.*, 1991), and the opioid antagonist naltrexone interacts with both D_1- and D_2-type antagonists to potentiate a reduction in food intake by deprived rats (Hobbs *et al.*, 1994). As regards direct modulation of the effects of dopamine receptor subtype-selective drugs, it has been shown that the cholecystokinin receptor antagonist devazepide can block the anorectic effects of the D_1-type antagonist SCH 23390 (Cooper and Barber, 1990). The extent to which this effect is specific to this drug (or receptor subtype) remains to be determined. Thus it is too early even to begin describing the nature of dopamine receptor subtype interactions with other neurochemical systems; however, there is clearly an enormous potential for further study.

7 Conclusions

After reviewing the available evidence it should be apparent that the effects of dopamine receptor-selective drugs on feeding remain incompletely characterized. D_1-type agonists consistently produce anorexia, but the role of competing behavioural responses and the receptor-specificity of the hypophagic effect need to be further investigated. There is some suggestion that D_1-type agonists specifically affect eating duration through an effect on meal frequency, but more drugs need to be studied. Similarly, D_1-type antagonists can reduce food intake, perhaps also through an action on meal frequency, but disruptions of feeding occur in conjunction with decrements in motor behaviour, and water intake is more potently inhibited. D_2-type agonists and antagonists present even greater interpretative difficulties: both classes of drug produce biphasic effects on intake, with low doses enhancing food intake and high doses suppressing it. Both classes tend to reduce eating rate, and the enhanced feeding sometimes reported following low doses of a D_2-type antagonist most often reflects an increase in average meal duration. Stimulation of chewing might explain some instances of increased feeding at low doses of D_2-type agonists, but otherwise the cause is not well understood. One scheme that has been presented to organize these findings (Terry *et al.*, 1995) proposes that D_1-type agonists might actually contribute a satiety signal which promotes meal termination, whereas D_2-type agonists simply modify the manner of eating. However, it remains difficult to incorporate the antagonist data into this kind of formulation. Nevertheless, we suggest an increased emphasis on elaborating the role of D_1-type receptors in the mediation of motivated behaviours, an area that has recently begun to attract more attention in the field of drug abuse research (e.g. Cabib *et al.*, 1991; Self and Stein, 1992; Terry *et al.*, 1994).

A number of important issues, as yet unanswered, have been highlighted. Whether these might be clarified with the availability of new compounds selective for individual receptor subtypes, or with the publication of more thorough receptor binding characterizations of currently used drugs, remains to be seen. Further study of the critical sites of action of these drugs is also clearly warranted; until recently, most work looking at the neural substrates underlying the anorectic effects of dopaminergic drugs focused on non-selective (primarily indirect) agonists. Finally, making comparisons between the limited numbers of relevant studies to date is hindered by the need to compare across different kinds of procedure; there are wide variations between studies in terms of food deprivation status, scheduling of food, type of diet, drug and test history. For dopamine receptor subtype agents, it is not yet possible to determine how these factors interact with drug class to determine outcome. It has already been pointed out that much of the work reviewed here has emerged from a small number of laboratories; clearly, only with more widespread study will the role of dopamine receptor subtypes in the regulation of ingestive behaviour be understood.

Acknowledgements

The author would like to thank Steve Cooper and Pete Clifton for comments on an earlier draft of the manuscript, and Alison Cooper for assistance during its preparation.

References

Ahlskog, J. E. (1974). Food intake and amphetamine anorexia after selective forebrain norepinephrine loss. *Brain Res.* **82**, 211–240.

Al-Naser, H. A. (1993). Cholecystokinin and dopamine in relation to ingestional behaviour of rats. PhD thesis, University of Birmingham, UK.

Al-Naser, H. A. and Cooper, S. J. (1994). A-68930, a novel, potent dopamine D_1 receptor agonist: a microstructural analysis of its effects on feeding and other behaviour in the rat. *Behav. Pharmacol.* **5**, 210–218.

Anden, N. E., Golembioska-Nikitin, K. and Thormstrom, V. (1982). Selective stimulation of dopamine and noradrenaline autoreceptors by B-HT 920 and B-HT 933, respectively. *Naunyn Schmiedebergs Arch. Pharmacol.* **321**, 100–104.

Andersen, P. H. and Jansen, J. A. (1990). Dopamine receptor agonists: selectivity and dopamine D_1 receptor efficacy. *Eur. J. Pharmacol.* **188**, 335–347.

Antelman, S. M., Black, C. A. and Rowland, N. E. (1977). Clozapine induces hyperphagia in undeprived rats. *Life Sci.* **21**, 1747–1750.

Bakshi, V. P. and Kelley, A. E. (1991). Dopaminergic regulation of feeding behavior: I. Differential effects of haloperidol microinfusion into three striatal subregions. *Psychobiology* **19**, 223–232.

Barzaghi, R., Groppetti, A., Mantegazza, P. and Muller, E. E. (1973). Reduction of food intake by apomorphine: a pimozide-sensitive effect. *J. Pharm. Pharmacol.* **25**, 909–911.

Beninger, R. J., Cheng, M., Hahn, B. L., Hoffman, D. C., Mazurski, E. J., Morency, M. A., Ramm, P. and Stewart, R. J. (1987). Effects of extinction, pimozide, SCH 2330, and metoclopramide on food-rewarded operant responding of rats. *Psychopharmacology* **92**, 343–349.

Blackburn, J. R., Phillips, A. G. and Fibiger, H. C. (1987). Dopamine and preparatory behavior. I. Effects of pimozide. *Behav. Neurosci.* **101**, 352–360.

Blackburn, J. R., Pfaus, J. G. and Phillips, A. G. (1992). Dopamine functions in appetitive and defensive behaviours. *Prog. Neurobiol.* **39**, 247–279.

Blundell, J. E. and Latham, C. J. (1980). Characterisation of adjustments to the structure of feeding behaviour following pharmacological treatment: effects of amphetamine and fenfluramine and the antagonism produced by pimozide and methergoline. *Pharmacol. Biochem. Behav.* **12**, 717–722.

Braun, A. R. and Chase, T. N. (1986). Obligatory D-1/D-2 receptor interactions in the generation of dopamine agonist related behaviors. *Eur. J. Pharmacol.* **131**, 301–306.

Briggs, C. A., Pollock, N. J., Frail, D. E., Paxson, C. L., Rakowski, R. F., Kang, C. H. and Kebabian, J. W. (1991). Activation of the 5-HT$_{1C}$ receptor expressed in *Xenopus* oocytes by the benzazepines SCH 23390 and SKF 38393. *Br. J. Pharmacol.* **104**, 1038–1044.

Burridge, S. L. and Blundell, J. E. (1979). Amphetamine anorexia: antagonism by typical but not atypical neuroleptics. *Neuropharmacology* **18**, 453–457.

Cabib, S., Castellano, C., Cestari, V., Filibeck, U. and Puglisi-Allegra, S. (1991). D$_1$ and D$_2$ receptor antagonists differently affect cocaine-induced locomotor hyperactivity in the mouse. *Psychopharmacology* **105**, 335–339.

Callahan, P. M., Appel, J. B. and Cunningham, K. A. (1991). Dopamine D$_1$ and D$_2$ mediation of the discriminative stimulus properties of *d*-amphetamine and cocaine. *Psychopharmacology* **103**, 50–55.

Carruba, M. O., Ricciardi, S., Miller, E. E. and Mantegazza, P. (1980). Anorectic effect of lisuride and other ergot derivatives in the rat. *Eur. J. Pharmacol.* **64**, 133–141.

Chandler, C. J., Wohab, W., Starr, B. S. and Starr, M. S. (1990). Motor depression: a new role for D$_1$ receptors? *Neuroscience* **38**, 437–445.

Chipkin, R. E., Iorio, L. C., Coffin, V. L., McQuade, R. D., Berger, J. G. and Barnett, A. (1988). Pharmacological profile of SCH 39166: a dopamine D$_1$ selective benzonaphthazepine with potential antipsychotic activity. *J. Pharmacol. Exp. Ther.* **247**, 1093–1102.

Christensen, A. V., Arnt, J., Hyttel, J., Lars, J.-J. and Svendsen, O. (1984). Pharmacological effects of a specific dopamine D$_1$ antagonist SCH 23390 in comparison with neuroleptics. *Life Sci.* **34**, 1529–1540.

Clark, D. and White, F. J. (1987). Review: D$_1$ dopamine receptor—the search for a function: a critical evaluation of the D$_1$/D$_2$ dopamine receptor classification and its functional implications. *Synapse* **1**, 347–388.

Clifton, P. G. (1987). Analysis of feeding and drinking patterns. In *Methods for the Study of Feeding and Drinking* (F. M. Toates and N. Rowland, eds), pp. 19–35. Elsevier, Amsterdam.

Clifton, P. G. (1995) Effects of SCH 39166 and domperidone on the meal patterning of male rats. *Pharmacol. Biochem. Behav.* **52**, 265–270.

Clifton, P. G. and Somerville, E. M. (1994). Disturbance of meal patterning following nucleus accumbens lesions in the rat. *Brain Res.* **667**, 123–128.

Clifton, P. G., Rusk, I. N. and Cooper, S. J. (1989). Stimulation and inhibition of food intake by the selective dopamine D_2 agonist, N-0437: a meal pattern analysis. *Pharmacol. Biochem. Behav.* **33**, 21–26.

Clifton, P. G., Rusk, I. N. and Cooper, S. J. (1991). Effects of dopamine D_1 and dopamine D_2 antagonists on the free feeding and drinking patterns of rats. *Behav. Neurosci.* **105**, 272–281.

Cooper, S. J. and Al-Naser, H. A. (1993). D_1:D_2 receptor interactions in relation to feeding responses and food intake. In *D_1:D_2 Dopamine Receptor Interactions* (J. Waddington, ed.). pp. 203–233. Academic Press, London.

Cooper, S. J. and Barber, D. J. (1990). SCH 23390-induced hypophagia is blocked by the selective CCK-A receptor antagonist devazepide, but not by the CCK-B/gastrin receptor antagonist L-365 260. *Brain Res. Bull,* **24**, 631–633.

Cooper, S. J. and Francis, J. A. (1993). A microstructural analysis of the effects of presatiation on feeding behavior in the rat. *Physiol. Behav.* **53**, 413–416.

Cooper, S. J. and Sweeney, K. F. (1980). Effects of spiperone alone and in combination with anorectic agents on feeding parameters in the rat. *Neuropharmacology* **19**, 997–1003.

Cooper, S. J. and Van der Hoek, G. A. (1993). Cocaine: a microstructural analysis of its effects on feeding and associated behaviour in the rat. *Brain Res.* **608**, 45–51.

Cooper, S. J., Rusk, I. N. and Barber, D. J. (1989). Sucrose sham-feeding in the rat after administration of the selective D_2 receptor agonist N-0437, *d*-amphetamine and cocaine. *Pharmacol. Biochem. Behav.* **32**, 447–452.

Cooper, S. J., Francis, J. and Rusk, I. N. (1990). The anorectic effect of SK&F 38393, a selective dopamine D_1 receptor agonist: a microstructural analysis of feeding and related behavior. *Psychopharmacology* **100**, 182–187.

Cooper, S. J., Francis, J. and Barber, D. J. (1993). Selective dopamine D-1 receptor agonist, SK and F 38393 and CY 208-243 reduce sucrose sham-feeding in the rat. *Neuropharmacology* **32**, 101–102.

Dunnett, S. B. and Iverson, S. D. (1982). Regulatory impairments following selective 6-OHDA lesions of the neostriatum. *Behav. Brain Res.* **4**, 195–202.

Duong, A. and Weingarten, H. P. (1993). Dopamine antagonists act on central, but not peripheral, receptors to inhibit sham and real feeding. *Physiol. Behav.* **54**, 449–454.

Duterte-Boucher, D., Naudin, B. and Costentin, J. (1989). Characteristics of the dopamine receptors involved in the anorectic effects of apomorphine in mice. *Fundam. Clin. Pharmacol.* **3**, 337–346.

Eichler, A. J. and Antelman, S. M. (1977). Apomorphine: feeding or anorexia depending on internal state. *Commun. Psychopharm.* **1**, 533–540.

Euvrard. C., Ferland, L., Dipaolo, T., Beaulieu, M., Labrie, F., Oberlander, C., Raynaud, J. P. and Boissier, J. R. (1979). Activity of two new potent dopaminergic agonists at the striatal and anterior pituitary levels. *Naunyn Schmiedebergs Arch. Pharmacol.* **309**, 241–245.

Evans, K. R. and Eikelboom, R. (1987). Feeding induced by ventricular bromocriptine and amphetamine: a possible excitatory role for dopamine in eating behavior. *Behav. Neurosci.* **101**, 591–593.

Evans, K. R. and Vaccarino, F. J. (1987). Intra-nucleus accumbens amphetamine: dose-dependent effects on food intake. *Pharmacol. Biochem. Behav.* **27**, 649–652.

Ferrari, F., Pelloni, F. and Giuliani, D. (1992a). B-HT 920-induced effects on rat feeding behaviour. *Pharmacol. Res.* **26**, 285–292.

Ferrari, F., Pelloni, F. and Giuliani, D. (1992b). Effects of the dopamine D_2 agonists lisuride and CQ 32-084 on rat feeding behaviour. *Pharmacol. Biochem. Behav.* **41**, 683–688.

Geary, N. and Smith, G. P. (1985). Pimozide decreases the positive reinforcing effect on sham fed sucrose in the rat. *Pharmacol. Biochem. Behav.* **22**, 787–790.

Gilbert, D. B. and Cooper, S. J. (1985). Analysis of dopamine D_1 and D_2 receptor involvement in d- and l-amphetamine-induced anorexia in rats. *Brain Res. Bull.* **15**, 385–389.

Gilbert, D. B. and Cooper, S. J. (1995). 7-OH-DPAT injected into the accumbens reduces locomotion and sucrose ingestion: D_3 autoreceptor-mediated effects? *Pharmacol. Biochem. Behav.* **52**, 275–280.

Gingrich, J. A. and Caron, M. G. (1993). Recent advances in the molecular biology of dopamine receptors. *Annu. Rev. Neurosci.* **16**, 299–321.

Giros, B., Sokoloff, P., Martres, M. P., Riou, J. F., Emorine, L. J. and Schwartz, J. C. (1989). Alternative splicing directs the expression of two D_2 dopamine isoforms. *Nature* **342**, 923–926.

Greene, S. B., Mathews, D., Hollingsworth, E. M. and Garbin, C. P. (1985). Behavioral effects of pergolide mesylate on food intake and body weight. *Pharmacol. Biochem. Behav.* **23**, 161–167.

Groppetti, A., Zambotti, F., Biazzi, A. and Mantegazza, P. (1973). Amphetamine and cocaine on amine turnover. In *Frontiers in Catecholamine Research* (E. Usdin and S. H. Snyder, eds). pp. 917–925. Pergamon Press, New York.

Hawkins, M. F., Barkemeyer, C. A. and Tulley, R. T. (1986). Synergistic effects of dopamine agonists and centrally-administered neurotensin on feeding. *Pharmacol. Biochem. Behav.* **24**, 1195–1201.

Heffner, T. G., Zigmond, M. J. and Stricker, E. M. (1977). Effects of dopaminergic agonists and antagonists on feeding in intact and 6-hydroxydopamine-treated rats. *J. Pharmacol. Exp. Ther.* **201**, 386–399.

Hobbs, D. J., Koch, J. E. and Bodnar, R. J. (1994). Naltrexone, dopamine receptor agonists and antagonists, and food intake in rats: 1. Food deprivation. *Pharmacol. Biochem. Behav.* **49**, 197–204.

Hoffman, D. C. and Beninger, R. J. (1985). The D_1 dopamine receptor antagonist SCH 23390 reduces locomotor activity and rearing in rats. *Pharmacol. Biochem. Behav.* **22**, 341–342.

Hoffman, D. C. and Beninger, R. J. (1986). Feeding behaviour in rats is differentially affected by pimozide treatment depending on prior experience. *Pharmacol. Biochem. Behav.* **24**, 259–262.

Hyttel, J. (1983). SCH 23390: the first selective dopamine D_1 antagonist. *Eur. J. Pharmacol.* **91**, 153–154.

Inoue, K., Kirike, N., Fujisaki, Y., Okuno, M., Ito, H. and Yamagami, S. (1995). D_2 receptors in the ventrolateral striatum are involved in feeding behaviour in rats. *Pharmacol. Biochem. Behav.* **50**, 153–161.

Iorio, L. C., Barnett, A., Leitz, F. H., Houser, V. P. and Korduba, C. A. (1983). SCH 23390, a potential benzazepine antipsychotic with unique interactions on dopaminergic systems. *J. Parmacol. Exp. Ther.* **226**, 462–468.

Kebabian, J. W. and Calne, D. B. (1979). Multiple receptors for dopamine. *Nature* **277**, 93–96.

Kennett, G. A. and Curzon, G. (1988). Evidence that hypophagia induced by mCPP and TFMPP require $5\text{-}HT_{1C}$ and $5\text{-}HT_{1B}$ receptors; hypophagia induced by RU 24969 only requires $5\text{-}HT_{1B}$ receptors. *Psychopharmacology* **96**, 93–100.

Kennett, G. A. and Curzon, G. (1991). Potencies of antagonists indicate that $5\text{-}HT_{1C}$ receptors mediate 1–3(chlorophenyl)piperazine-induced hypophagia. *Br. J. Pharmacol.* **103**, 2016–2020.

Koechling, U., Colle, L. M. and Wise, R. A. (1988). Effects of SCH 23390 on motivational aspects of deprivation-induced feeding. *Psychobiology* **16**, 207–212.

Kruk, Z. L. (1973). Dopamine and 5-hydroxytryptamine inhibit feeding in rats. *Nature New Biol.* **246**, 52–53.

Kruk, Z. L. and Zarrindast, M. R. (1976). Mazindol anorexia is mediated by activation of dopaminergic mechanisms. *Br. J. Pharmacol.* **58**, 367–372.

Ladurelle, N., Duterte-Boucher, D. and Costentin, J. (1991). Stimulation of D_1 and D_2 dopamine receptors produces additive anorectic effects. *Fundam. Clin. Pharmacol.* **5**, 481–490.

Lawson, W. B., Byrd, J. and Reed, D. (1984). Effects of neuroleptics on food intake. *Soc. Neurosci. Abstr.* **10**, 303.

Leibowitz, S. F. (1975). Amphetamine: possible site and mode of action for producing anorexia in the rat. *Brain Res.* **84**, 160–167.

Levesque, D., Diaz, J., Pilon, C., Martres, M.-P., Giros, B., Souil, E., Schott, D., Morgat, J. L., Schwartz, J.-C. and Sokoloff, P. (1992). Identification, characterization and localization of the dopamine D_3 receptor in rat brain using 7-[^{3}H]hydroxy-N,N-di-n-propyl-2-aminotetralin. *Proc. Natl. Acad. Sci. USA* **89**, 8155–8159.

Loschmann, P.-A., Smith, L. A., Lange, K. W., Jaehnig, P., Jenner, P. and Marsden, C. D. (1991). Motor activity following the administration of selective D-1 and D-2 dopaminergic drugs to normal common marmosets. *Psychopharmacology* **105**, 303–309.

McQuade, R. D., Duffy, R. A., Anderson, C. C., Crosby, G., Coffin, V. L., Chipkin, R. E. and Barnett, A. (1991). SCH 39166: a new D_1-selective radioligand: *in vitro* and *in vivo* binding analyses. *J. Neurochem.* **57**, 2001.

McQuade, R. D., Duffy, R. A., Coffin, V. L. and Barnett, A. (1992). *In vivo* binding to dopamine receptors: a correlate of potential antipsychotic activity. *Eur. J. Pharmacol.* **215**, 29–34.

Martin, G. E., Williams, M., Pettibone, D. J., Yarbrough, G. G., Clineschmidt, B. V. and Jones, J. H. (1984). Pharmacologic profile of a novel potent direct-acting dopamine agonist (+)-4-propyl-9-hydroxynaphthoxazine ([+]-PHNO). *J. Pharmacol. Exp. Ther.* **230**, 569–576.

Martin-Iverson, M. T. and Dourish, C. T. (1988). Role of dopamine D-1 and D-2 receptor subtypes in mediating dopamine agonist effects on food consumption in rats. *Psychopharmacology* **96**, 370–374.

Melia, K. F. and Spealman, R. D. (1991). Pharmacological characterization of the discriminative-stimulus effects of GBR 12909. *J. Pharmacol. Exp. Ther.* **258**, 626–632.

Meyer, M. E., Cottrell, G. A. and Van Hartesveldt, C. (1992). Dopamine D_1 antagonist potentiate the durations of bar and cling catalepsy and the dorsal immobility response in rats. *Pharmacol. Biochem. Behav.* **41**, 507–510.

Meyer, M. E., Cottrell, G. A., Van Hartesveldt, C. and Potter, T. J. (1993). Effects of dopamine D_1 antagonists SCH 23390 and SK & F 83566 on locomotor activities in rats. *Pharmacol. Biochem. Behav.* **44**, 429–432.

Molloy, A. G. and Waddington, J. L. (1984). Dopaminergic behavior stereospecifically promoted by the D-1 agonist R-SK & F 38393 and selectively blocked by the D-1 antagonist SCH 23390. *Psychopharmacology* **82**, 409–410.

Molloy, A. G. and Waddington, J. L. (1985). Sniffing, rearing and locomotor responses to the D-1 dopamine agonist R-SK & F 38393 and to apomorphine: differential interactions with the selective D-1 and D-2 antagonists SCH 23390 and metoclopramide. *Eur. J. Pharmacol.* **108**, 305–308.

Molloy, A. G. and Waddington, J. L. (1987). Assessment of grooming and other behavioural responses to the D-1 receptor agonist SK & F 38393 and its R- and S-enantiomers in intact adult rats. *Psychopharmacology* **92**, 164–168.

Molloy, A. G., O'Boyle, K. M., Pugh, M. T. and Waddington, J. L. (1986). Locomotor behaviors in response to new selective D-1 and D-2 dopamine receptor agonists, and the influence of selective antagonists. *Pharmacol. Biochem. Behav.* **25**, 249–253.

Morelli, M. and DiChiara, G. (1985). Catalepsy induced by SCH 23390 in rats. *Eur. J. Pharmacol.* **117**, 179–185.

Morley, J. E., Levine, A. S., Grace, M. and Kneip, J. (1982). Dynorphin-(1–13), dopamine and feeding in rats. *Pharmacol. Biochem. Behav.* **16**, 701–705.

Muscat, R., Willner, P. and Towell. (1986). Apomorphine anorexia: a further pharmacological characterization. *Eur. J. Pharmacol.* **123**, 123–131.

Nakajima, S. (1986). Suppression of operant responding in the rat by dopamine D_1 receptor blockage with SCH 23390. *Physiol. Psychol.* **14**, 111–114.

Naruse, T., Amano, H. and Koizumi, Y. (1991). Possible involvement of dopamine D-1 and D-2 receptors in diazepam-induced hyperphagia in rats. *Fundam. Clin. Pharmacol.* **5**, 677–693.

O'Boyle, K. M., Gaitanopoulos, D. E., Brenner, M. and Waddington, J. L. (1989). Agonist and antagonist properties of benzazepine and thienopyridine derivatives at the D_1 dopamine receptor. *Neuropharmacology* **28**, 401–405.

Orthen-Gambill, N. (1985). Sucrose intake unaffected by fenfluramine but suppressed by amphetamine administration. *Psychopharmacology* **87**, 25–29.

Parada, M. A., Hernandez, L. and Hoebel, B. G. (1988). Sulpiride injections in the lateral hypothalamus induce feeding and drinking in rats. *Pharmacol. Biochem. Behav.* **30**, 917–923.

Phillips, G. D., Howes, S. R., Whitelaw, R. B., Robbins, T. W. and Everitt, B. J. (1995). Analysis of the effects of intra-accumbens SKF 38393 and LY 171555 upon the behavioral satiety sequence. *Psychopharmacology* **117**, 82–90.

Pisa, M. (1988). Motor functions of the striatum in the rat: critical role of the lateral region in tongue and forelimb reaching. *Neuroscience* **24**, 453–463.

Rapoza, D. and Woolverton, W. L. (1991). Attenuation of the effects of cocaine on milk consumption in rats by dopamine antagonists. *Pharmacol. Biochem. Behav.* **40**, 133–137.

Reynolds, R. W. and Carlisle, H. J. (1961). The effect of chlorpromazine on food intake in the normal rat. *J. Comp. Physiol. Psychol.* **54**, 354–356.

Rowland, N. and Engle, D. J. (1977). Feeding and drinking interactions after acute butyrophenone administration. *Pharmacol. Biochem. Behav.* **7**, 295–301.

Rusk, I. N. and Cooper, S. J. (1988). Profile of the selective dopamine D-2 receptor agonist N-0437: its effect on palatability and deprivation-induced feeding, and operant responding for food. *Physiol. Behav.* **44**, 545–553.

Rusk, I. N. and Cooper, S. J. (1989a). The selective dopamine D_1 agonist SK & F 38393: its effects on palatability and deprivation-induced feeding, and operant responding for food. *Pharmacol. Biochem. Behav.* **34**, 17–22.

Rusk, I. N. and Cooper, S. J. (1989b). Microstructural analysis of the anorectic effect of N-0437, a highly selective dopamine D_2 agonist. *Brain Res.* **494**, 350–358.

Rusk, I. N. and Cooper, S. J. (1994). Parametric studies of selective D_1 or D_2 antagonists: effects on appetitive and feeding behaviour. *Behav. Pharmacol.* **5**, 615–622.

Salamone, J. D. (1988). Dopaminergic involvement in activational aspects of motivation: effects of haloperidol on schedule-induced activity, feeding and foraging in rats. *Psychobiology* **16**, 196–206.

Salamone, J. D. (1994). The involvement of nucleus accumbens dopamine in appetitive and aversive motivation. *Behav. Brain Res.* **61**, 117–133.

Salamone, J. D., Zigmond, M. J. and Stricker, E. M. (1990). Characterization of the impaired feeding behaviour in rats given haloperidol or dopamine-depleting brain lesions. *Neuroscience* **39**, 17–24.

Salamone, J. D., Mahan, K. and Rogers, S. (1993). Ventrolateral striatal dopamine depletions impair feeding and food handling in rats. *Pharmacol. Biochem. Behav.* **44**, 605–610.

Sanger, D. J. (1987). The actions of SCH 23390, a D_1 receptor antagonist, on operant and avoidance behaviour in rats. *Pharmacol. Biochem. Behav.* **26**, 509–513.

Schneider, L. H., Gibbs, J. and Smith, G. P. (1986). D-2 selective antagonists suppress sucrose sham feeding in the rat. *Brain Res. Bull.* **17**, 605–611.

Schneider, L. H., Greenberg, D. and Smith, G. P. (1988). Comparison of the effects of selective D-1 and D-2 receptor antagonists on sucrose sham feeding and water sham drinking. In *The Mesocorticolimbic Dopamine System* (P. W. Kalivas and C. B. Nemeroff, eds). *Ann. N.Y. Acad. Sci.* **537**, 534–537.

Self, D. W. and Stein, L. (1992). The D_1 agonists SKF 82958 and SKF 77434 are self-administered by rats. *Brain Res.* **582**, 349–352.

Setler, P. E., Sarau, H. M., Zirckle, C. I. and Saunders, H. J. (1978). The central effects of a novel dopamine agonist. *Eur. J. Pharmacol.* **50**, 419–430.

Sibley, D. R. and Monsma, F. J., Jr. (1992). Molecular biology of dopamine receptors. *Trends Pharm. Sci.* **13**, 61–69.

Sills, T. L. and Vaccarino, F. J. (1991). Facilitation and inhibition of feeding by a single dose of amphetamine: relationship to baseline intake and accumbens cholecysto-kinin. *Psychopharmacology* **105**, 329–334.

Sills, T. L., Baird, J. P. and Vaccarino, F. J. (1993). Individual differences in the feeding effects of amphetamine: role of nucleus accumbens dopamine and circadian factors. *Psychopharmacology* **112**, 211–218.

Smith, P. G. and Gibbs, J. (1979). Postprandial satiety. In *Progress in Psychobiology and Physiological Psychology,* Vol. 8, pp. 179–242. Academic Press, New York.

Sokoloff, P. B., Giros, B., Martres, M.-P., Bouthenet, M.-L. and Schwartz, J. C. (1990). Molecular K cloning and characterization of a novel dopamine receptor (D_3) as a target for neuroleptics. *Nature* **347**, 146–151.

Sokoloff, P. B., Andrieux, M., Besancon, R., Pilon, C., Martres, M.-P., Giros, B. and Schwartz, J. C. (1992). Pharmacology of human dopamine D_3 receptor expressed in a mammalian cell line: comparison with D_2 receptor. *Eur. J. Pharmacol.* **225**, 331–337.

Stahle, L. (1992). Do autoreceptors mediate dopamine agonist-induced yawning and suppression of exploration? A critical review. *Psychopharmacology* **106**, 1–13.

Stolerman, I. P. (1970). Eating, drinking and spontaneous activity in rats after the administration of chlorpromazine. *Neuropharmacology* **9**, 405–411.

Streather, A. and Bozarth, M. A. (1987). Effect of dopamine-receptor blockage on stimulation-induced feeding. *Pharmacol. Biochem. Behav.* **27**, 521–524.

Sunahara, R. K., Guan, H.-C., O'Dowd, B. F., Seeman, P., Laurier, L. G., Ng. G., George, S. R., Torchia, J., Van Tol, H. H. M. and Niznik, H. B. (1991). Cloning of the gene for a human dopamine D_5 deceptor with higher affinity for dopamine than D_1. *Nature* **350**, 614–619.

Taylor, L. A., Tedford, C. E. and McQuade, R. D. (1991). The binding of SCH 39166 and SCH 23390 to 5-HT_{1C} receptors in porcine choroid plexus. *Life Sci.* **49**, 1505–1511.

Terai, M., Usuda, S., Kuroiwa, I., Noshiro, O. and Maeno, H. (1983). Selective binding of YM-09151-2, new potent neuroleptic, to D_2-dopaminergic receptors. *Jpn. J. Pharmacol.* **33**, 749–755.

Terry, P. and Katz, J. L. (1992). Differential antagonism of the effects of dopamine D_1 receptor agonists on feeding behaviour in the rat. *Psychopharmacology* **109**, 403–409.

Terry, P. and Katz, J. L. (1993). Differential effects of dopaminergic and serotonergic antagonists on the behavioral actions of dopamine D-1 agonists. *Soc. Neurosci. Abstr.* **19**, 760.

Terry, P. and Katz, J. L. (1994). A comparison of the effects of the D-1 receptor antagonists SCH 23390 and SCH 39166 on suppression of feeding behaviour by the D-1 agonist SKF 38393. *Psychopharmacology* **113**, 328–333.

Terry, P., Witkin, J. M. and Katz, J. L. (1994). Pharmacological characterization of the novel discriminative stimulus effects of a low dose of cocaine. *J. Pharmacol. Exp. Ther.* **270**, 1041–1048.

Terry, P., Gilbert, D. B. and Cooper, S. J. (1995). Dopamine receptor subtype agonists and feeding behaviour. *Obesity Res.* (in press).

Timmerman, W., Rusk, I. N., Tepper, P. G., Horn, A. S. and Cooper, S. J. (1989). The effects of the enantiomers of the dopamine agonist N-0437 on food consumption and yawning behaviour in rats. *Eur. J. Pharmacol.* **174**, 107–114.

Tirelli, E. and Terry, P. (1993). Biphasic locomotor effects of the dopamine D-1 agonist SKF 38393 and their attenuation in non-habituated mice. *Psychopharmacology* **110**, 69–75.

Tombaugh, T. N., Tombaugh, J. and Anisman, H. (1979). Effects of dopamine receptor blockade on alimentary behaviors: home cage food consumption, magazine training, operant acquisition and performance. *Psychopharmacology* **66**, 219–225.

Towell, A., Muscat, R. and Willner, P. (1988a). Behavioural microanalysis of the role of dopamine in amphetamine anorexia. *Pharmacol. Biochem. Behav.* **30**, 641–648.

Towell, A., Willner, P. and Muscat, R. (1988b). Apomorphine anorexia: the role of dopamine receptors in the ventral forebrain. *Psychopharmacology* **96**, 135–141.

Van der Hoek, G. A. and Cooper, S. J. (1994). The selective dopamine uptake inhibitor GBR 12909: its effects on the microstructure of feeding in rats. *Pharmacol. Biochem. Behav.* **48**, 135–140.

Van der Weide, J., de Vries, J. B., Tepper, P. G. and Horn, A. S. (1986). Pharmacological profiles of three new, potent and selective dopamine receptor agonists: N-0434, N-0437 and N-0734. *Eur. J. Pharmacol.* **125**, 273–282.

Van Rossum, J. M. and Simons, F. (1969). Locomotor activity and anorexigenic action. *Psychopharmacology* **14**, 248–254.

Van Tol, H. H. M., Bunzow, J. R., Guan, H. C., Sunahara, R. K., Seeman, P., Niznik, H. B. and Civelli, O. (1991). Cloning of the gene for a human dopamine D_4 receptor with high affinity for the antipsychotic clozapine. *Nature* **350**, 610–614.

Waddington, J. L. and Daly, S. A. (1993). Regulation of unconditioned motor behaviour by D_1:D_2 interaction. In *D_1:D_2 Dopamine Receptor Interactions* (J. Waddington, ed.). pp. 203–233. Academic Press, London.

Waddington, J. L. and O'Boyle, K. M. (1989). Drugs acting on brain dopamine receptors: a conceptual re-evaluation five years after the first selective D-1 antagonist. *Pharmacol. Ther.* **43**, 1–52.

Wamsley, J. K., Hunt, M. E., McQuade, R. D. and Alburges, M. E. (1991). [^{3}H]SCH39166, a D_1 dopamine receptor antagonist: binding characteristics and localization. *Exp. Neurol.* **111**, 145–151.

Waters, N., Lofberg, L., Haadsma-Svensson, S., Svennson, K., Sonesson, C. and Carlsson, A. (1994). Differential effects of dopamine D_2 and D_3 receptor antagonists in regard to dopamine release, *in vivo* receptor displacement and behaviour. *J. Neural Transm. [Gen. Sect.]* **98**, 39–55.

Weatherford, S. C., Greenberg, D., Gibbs, J. and Smith, G. B. (1990). The potency of dopamine D-1 and D-2 receptor antagonists is inversley related to the reward value of sham-fed corn oil and sucrose in rats. *Pharmacol. Biochem. Behav.* **37**, 317–323.

Willis, G. L., Smith, G. P. and Kinchington, P. C. (1983). Neuroleptic-like anorexia produced by an extra-cerebral DA antagonist. *Brain Res. Bull.* **11**, 21–24.

Willner, P. and Towell, A. (1982). Microstructural analysis of the involvement of beta-receptors in amphetamine anorexia. *Pharmacol. Biochem. Behav.* **17**, 255–262.

Willner, P., Towell, A. and Muscat, R. (1985). Apomorphine anorexia: a behavioural and neuropharmacological analysis. *Psychopharmacology* **87**, 351–356.

Winn, P., Williams, S. F. and Herberg, L. J. (1982). Feeding stimulated by very low doses of *d*-amphetamine administered systemically or by microinjection into the striatum. *Psychopharmacology* **78**, 336–341.

Wise, R. A. (1982). Neuroleptics and operant behavior: the anhedonia hypothesis. *Behav. Brain Sci.* **5**, 39–87.

Wise, R. A. and Colle, L. M. (1984). Pimozide attenuates free-feeding: best scores analysis reveals a motivational deficit. *Psychopharmacology* **84**, 446–451.

Wise, R. A. and Raptis, L. (1986). Effects of naloxone and pimozide on initiation and maintenance measures of free feeding. *Brain Res.* **368**, 62–68.

Wise, R. A., Spindler, J., de Wit, H. and Gerber, G. J. (1978). Neuroleptic induced 'anhedonia' in rats: pimozide blocks reward quality of food. *Science* **201**, 262–264.

Woodward, R. M., Panicker, M. M. and Miledi, R. (1992). Actions of dopamine and dopaminergic drugs on cloned serotonin receptors expressed in *Xenopus* oocytes. *Proc. Natl. Acad. Sci.* **89**, 4708–4712.

Xenakis, S. and Sclafani, A. (1981). The effects of pimozide on the consumption of a palatable saccharin–glucose solution in the rat. *Pharmacol. Biochem. Behav.* **15**, 435–442.

Zambotti, F., Carruba, M. O., Barzaghi, F., Vicentini, L., Gropetti, A. and Mantegazza, P. (1976). Behavioural effects of a new non-phenylethylamine anorexigenic agent: mazindol. *Eur. J. Pharmacol.* **36**, 405–512.

Zarrindast, M. R. and Hosseini-Nia, T. (1988). Anorectic and behavioural effects of bupropion. *Gen. Pharmacol.* **19**, 201–204.

Zarrindast, M. R., Owji, A. A. and Hosseini-Nia, T. (1991). Evaluation of dopamine receptor invovement in rat feeding behaviour. *Gen. Pharmacol.* **22**, 1011–1016.

Zis, A. P. and Fibiger, H. C. (1975). Neuroleptic-induced deficits in food and water regulation: similarities to the lateral hypothalamic syndrome. *Psychopharmacology* **43**, 63–68.

12

Imidazoline Receptors and Ingestion

HELEN C. JACKSON* and DAVID J. NUTT

Psychopharmacology Unit, University of Bristol, School of Medical Sciences, University Walk, Bristol BS8 1TD, UK
*Current address: Knoll Pharmaceuticals Research Department, 1 Thane Road West, Nottingham NG2 3AA, UK

1 Introduction

The α_2-adrenoceptor antagonist idazoxan (Fig. 1) was synthesized in 1978 by Reckitt and Colman as part of a project investigating the pharmacological effects of imidazoline analogues (Doxey *et al.*, 1983, 1985). For several years it was used extensively to investigate α_2-adrenoceptor function in animals and humans. However, in the late 1980s, receptor binding studies showed that tritiated idazoxan was only partially displaced from its binding sites by catecholamines (see Michel and Insel, 1989). These findings suggested that [³H]idazoxan bound with high affinity, not only to α_2-adrenoceptors, but also to non-α_2-adrenoceptor binding sites. These sites are distinct from α_2-adrenoceptors in both their pharmacology and anatomical distribution, and have recently been termed I_2 (imidazoline-$_2$) receptor sites (Ernsberger, 1992). I_2 sites have been shown to exist in a variety of different species including rabbits (Convents *et al.*, 1989; Hudson *et al.*, 1992a; Renouard *et al.*, 1993), guinea-pigs (Wikberg and Uhlen, 1990), rats (Brown *et al.*, 1990; Mallard *et al.*, 1992) and humans (Michel *et al.*, 1989; Langin *et al.*, 1990; De Vos *et al.*, 1991, 1994). They are present in the central nervous system (e.g. Convents *et al.*, 1989; Brown *et al.*, 1990; Wikberg and Uhlen, 1990; Mallard *et al.*, 1992) and also in a number of peripheral tissues including urethral smooth muscle (Yablonsky and Dausse, 1991), adipocytes (Langin and Lafontan, 1989; MacKinnon *et al.*, 1989; Langin *et al.*, 1990), kidney (Michel *et al.*, 1989; Hamilton *et al.*, 1991) and liver (Tesson *et al.*, 1991).

The α_2-adrenoceptor agonist clonidine has low affinity for I_2 receptors labelled by [³H]idazoxan (Brown *et al.*, 1990) but high affinity for non-adrenoceptor imidazoline sites designated I_1 receptors (Ernsberger, 1992). These sites were first described in the cow (Ernsberger *et al.*, 1987) but are also present in rats, rabbits and humans (Bricca *et al.*, 1989; Ernsberger *et al.*, 1990,

DRUG RECEPTOR SUBTYPES AND INGESTIVE BEHAVIOUR
ISBN 0-12-187620-9

IDAZOXAN

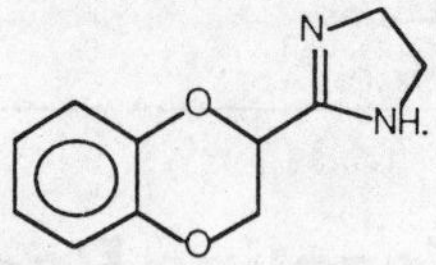

RX821029

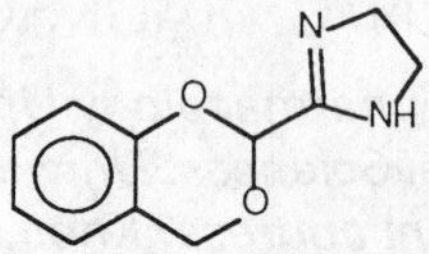

RX801077

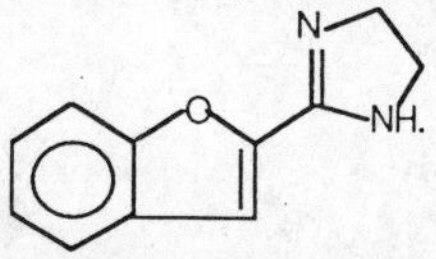

LSL 60101

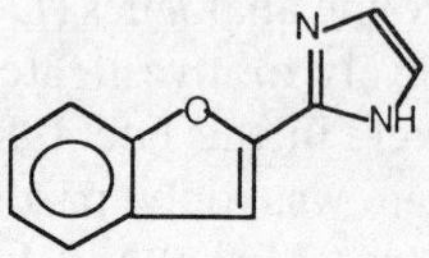

Fig. 1 Structures of I_2 receptor ligands.

1993). It has been proposed by some workers that the vasodepressor effects of clonidine within the brainstem may be primarily due to activation of I_1 receptors (Bousquet et al., 1984; Ernsberger et al., 1990; Gomez et al., 1991). Receptor binding studies with [^{3}H]clonidine have shown that idazoxan has some affinity for I_1 receptors (Bricca et al., 1989). In this chapter compounds have been characterized as I_2 receptor ligands because they act at non-adrenoceptor sites labelled by [^{3}H]idazoxan, but it should be noted that these compounds may also have affinity for I_1 receptors. The physiological functions of either I_1 or I_2 receptors are still not fully understood; however, in this chapter we have reviewed preliminary findings which suggest that I_2 receptor sites may play a role in the control of food intake.

2   Idazoxan and food intake

One of the first indications that imidazolines may affect appetite was a report by Sleight et al. (1988) at a meeting of the British Pharmacological Society. These authors used idazoxan (2 mg/kg intraperitoneally) to investigate the

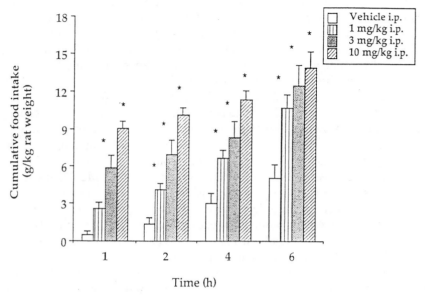

Fig. 2   Effect of idazoxan on food intake in freely feeding rats. Individually housed male Wistar rats (250–350 g) were injected with saline or idazoxan, and intake of powdered standard rat diet was measured during the following 6 h. Procedures began at 09.00 hours so that measurements were carried out during the light period. Values represent mean ± SEM intakes for groups of six rats. *$P < 0.05$ vs vehicle-treated control (one-way analysis of variance and Dunnett's test). From Jackson et al. (1991), with kind permission of Macmillan Press.

possible involvement of α_2-adrenoceptors in the hyperphagic effects of the 5-hydroxytryptamine$_{1A}$ (5-HT$_{1A}$) agonist 8-OH-DPAT (8-hydroxy-(2-di-*n*-propylamino)tetralin) and observed that it significantly increased food intake in freely-feeding rats when given alone. This finding was unexpected. A number of different workers had shown that α_2-adrenoceptor agonists such as clonidine stimulated eating behaviour (Sanger, 1983; McCabe et al., 1984; Goldman et al., 1985); therefore α_2-adrenoceptor antagonists would have been expected to exert the opposite effect, i.e. to decrease food intake.

Following this report, we decided to investigate the effects of idazoxan on appetite more thoroughly and observed that in male Wistar rats it produced a dose-related (1, 3, 10 mg/kg intraperitoneally) increase in food intake in the 6 h following injection (Jackson et al., 1991; Fig. 2). Idazoxan (10 and 30 mg/kg) has since been shown to increase food intake by two other groups (Hartley et al., 1994; Menargues et al., 1994). In all these experiments the effect of idazoxan on food intake was measured in freely feeding Wistar or Sprague–Dawley rats and feeding studies were performed in the light phase, i.e. under conditions when the food intake of control animals was minimal. Similar doses of idazoxan did not increase (or decrease) food intake during the dark period or in food-deprived animals (Menargues *et al.*, 1994). In these situations the food intake of control animals is much higher than during the light period and it may simply be difficult to produce any further stimulation of eating behaviour. Another possibility is that endogeneous I_2 ligands may exist (as discussed below) and that changes in their levels may influence the effects of idazoxan on food intake. For example, I_2 sites may be maximally occupied by endogenous ligand at night and hence idazoxan would have no further effect on food intake.

The stimulatory effects of idazoxan on food intake in rats appear to be relatively short lived. Food intake was not significantly affected by this drug when measured over a 24 h period (Jackson *et al.*, 1991; Menargues *et al.*, 1994). This may reflect the pharmacokinetics of the drug and/or be due to compensatory mechanisms, since animals treated with the highest dose of idazoxan (10 mg/kg) were observed to eat significantly less than controls in the 4–24 h period after injection (Jackson *et al.*, 1991).

As mentioned above, the stimulatory effects of idazoxan on food intake seem unlikely to be related to its α_2-antagonist properties since it has been well established that α_2-adrenoceptor agonists increase food intake in rats. In rat brain homogenates, [^{3}H]idazoxan exhibits roughly equal affinity for both α_2-adrenoceptors and I_2 receptor sites (it has a K_i of 8.5 nmol/l at I_2 sites, compared with 11.2 at α_2-adrenoceptors; Hudson *et al.*, 1992b). In this tissue 70–80% of specific [^{3}H]idazoxan binding is to α_2-adrenoceptors and 20–30% is to I_2 receptor sites (Mallard *et al.*, 1992). Quantitative autoradiography has demonstrated that several brain nuclei in the rat contain higher densities of I_2 receptors than α_2-adrenoceptors (Mallard *et al.*, 1992). These brain areas include the hypothalamus and the area postrema, i.e. brain regions that have traditionally been associated with control of food intake (see Bernstein *et al.*, 1985; Sugrue, 1987).

One possibility, therefore, is that the effects of idazoxan on food intake may be due to its high affinity at I_2 sites. Initial studies into the function of I_2 receptors compared the pharmacological effects of idazoxan with those of other α_2-adrenoceptor antagonists since selective I_2 receptor ligands were not available. In this context, a range of doses of the 2-ethoxy and 2-methoxy analogues of idazoxan, RX 811059 (Doxey *et al.*, 1985) and RX 821002 (Langin *et al.*, 1989) failed to increase food consumption in the freely feeding rat model (Jackson *et al.*, 1991). These are highly selective α_2-adrenoceptor antagonists with only negligible affinity for I_2 binding sites (Langin *et al.*, 1990; Mallard *et al.*, 1992). An increase in food intake following administration of RX 821002 was reported by Menargues *et al.* (1994); however, this was relatively small compared with the increase produced by idazoxan. These results support the notion that the effects of idazoxan on food intake may be dissociated from its α_2-antagonist properties.

3 I₂ receptor ligands and food intake

Recently a number of imidazolines have been described which act selectively at
I_2 receptor sites compared with α_2-adrenoceptors. For example, in rat brain the
1,3-benzodioxan isomer of idazoxan, RX 821029 (2-(1,3-benzodioxanyl)-2-
imidazoline) has a K_i of 1.8 nmol/l at I_2 receptors and of 244 nmol/l at α_2-
adrenoceptors, i.e. it has 130-fold selectivity for I_2 sites over α_2 receptors
(Hudson *et al.*, 1992b). Furthermore, RX 801077 (2-(2-benzofuranyl)-2-
imidazoline) has a K_i of 1.2 nmol/l at I_2 receptors in rat brain and of 1860 nmol/l
at α_2-adrenoceptors, i.e. it has 1550-fold selectivity for I_2 receptors (Hudson *et
al.*, 1995). By comparison, idazoxan has only 1.3-fold selectivity for I_2 sites
(Hudson *et al.*, 1992b). In our studies, both RX 821029 and RX 801077
produced a marked increase in food intake in the hour following intraperitoneal administration of a 10 mg/kg dose (Figs 3 and 4). This dose of RX 821029
and RX 801077 did not significantly alter food intake when measured over a 24-
h period, i.e. the results were consistent with those obtained with idazoxan.

In accordance with these findings, Garcia-Sevilla *et al.* (1993) have recently
patented a series of benzofuranylimidazole derivatives as appetite stimulants/

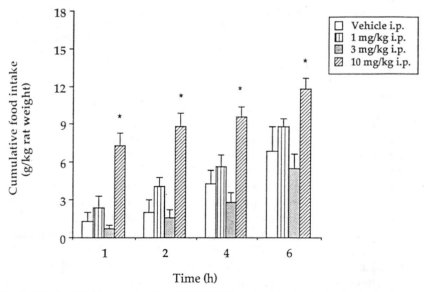

Time (h)

Fig. 3   Effect of the I_2 receptor ligand RX 821029 on food intake in the freely feeding rat.
Individually housed male Wistar rats (250–350 g) were injected with saline or RX 821029, and
intake of powdered standard rat diet was measured during the following 6 h. Procedures began at
09.00 hours so that measurements were carried out during the light period. Values represent
mean ± SEM intakes for groups of six rats. $^*P < 0.05$ *vs* vehicle-treated control (one-way analysis of
variance and Dunnett's test).

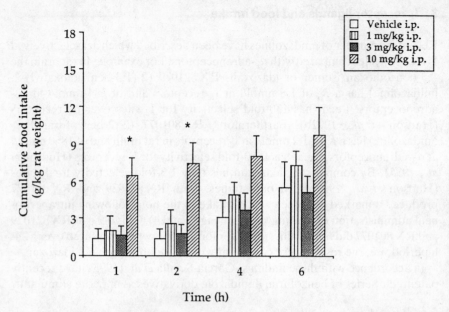

Fig. 4 Effect of the I_2 receptor ligand RX 801077 on food intake in the freely feeding rat. Individually housed male Wistar rats (250–350 g) were injected with saline or RX 801077, and intake of powered standard rat diet was measured during the following 6 h. Procedures began at 09.00 hours so that measurements were carried out during the light period. Values represent mean ± SEM intakes for groups of six rats. *$P < 0.05$ vs vehicle-treated control (one-way analysis of variance and Dunnett's test). From Nutt et al. (1995), with kind permission of the New York Academy of Sciences.

antianorexic agents. Intraperitoneal administration of a high dose (25 mg/kg) of three of the compounds increased food intake (7–10 times that of controls) in freely feeding rats. These compounds (2-(benzofuran-2-yl)imidazole hydrochloride; 1-methyl-2-(benzofuran-2-yl)imidazole hydrochloride and 2-(6-methoxybenzofuran-2-yl)imidazole hydrochloride) were shown to have selectivity for I_2 receptors over α_2-adrenoceptors in rat cerebral cortex. The effects of 2-(benzofuran-2-yl)imidazole hydrochloride (LSL 60101) on appetite were also reported in an abstract by Menargues et al. (1994). This compound is similar in structure to RX 801077. In rat cortex it has a K_i at I_2 receptors of 350 nmol/l and an I_2 vs α_2 selectivity of 280 (Menargues et al., 1994). LSL 60101 (30 mg/kg intraperitoneally) significantly increased food intake in rats in the 4 h following injection. However, it did not alter 24 h food intake. Furthermore LSL 60101 did not modify food intake if injected during the dark phase and failed to affect food intake in food-deprived rats, i.e. it acted in a similar manner to idazoxan.

As mentioned in the introduction, idazoxan and its analogues may also act at I_1 receptors. Selective I_1 ligands are available, for example moxonidine

(Ernsberger *et al.*, 1993), but their effects on feeding behaviour have not been reported; therefore it is unclear whether I_1 receptors play a role in control of food intake, although this would not be predicted from current knowledge of their anatomical distribution in the central nervous system (Ernsberger *et al.*, 1987; Kamisaki *et al.*, 1990).

4 Pharmacological mechanisms underlying the effects of idazoxan and I_2 ligands on food intake

Idazoxan and other α_2-adrenoceptor antagonists increase noradrenaline levels in the central nervous system by inhibition of presynaptic autoreceptors (Dennis *et al.*, 1987; Thomas and Holman, 1991). Noradrenaline has been demonstrated to increase food intake in rats. However, this is believed to be due to activation of postsynaptic α_2-adrenoceptors located in the paraventricular nucleus of the hypothalamus (Goldman *et al.*, 1985), which would be blocked by idazoxan. It is unlikely that idazoxan-induced hyperphagia is mediated by other types of adrenoceptor. There have been no reports of stimulatory effects of α_1 agonists on food intake. On the contrary, α_1-adrenoceptor agonists decrease food intake (Wellman *et al.*, 1993) and the α_1-adrenoceptor antagonist prazosin has recently been shown to increase food intake in rats (Routledge *et al.*, 1994). Furthermore, the β-adrenoceptor agonist isoprenaline has no effect on food intake in freely feeding rats (Jackson and Nutt, 1992) and selective β-adrenoceptor antagonists do not attenuate idazoxan-induced feedings, as discussed below. In addition, the selective α_2-adrenoceptor antagonists, RX 811059 and RX 821002, which also increase synaptic levels of noradrenaline and indirectly activate α_1- and β-adrenoceptors, have little or no effect on food intake (Jackson *et al.*, 1991; Menargues *et al.*, 1994). Thus it seems unlikely that noradrenaline, acting via α_1 or β-adrenoceptors, plays a role in idazoxan-induced hyperphagia.

By contrast, the possibility that activation of α_2-adrenoceptors by noradrenaline may contribute to the effects of I_2 ligands on food intake cannot be precluded. RX 801077 has been shown to increase potassium-evoked release of [^{3}H]noradrenaline from slices of rat hippocampus, and microdialysis studies have shown that both RX 821029 and RX 801077 increase extracellular levels of noradrenaline in the frontal cortex and hippocampus (Nutt *et al.*, 1995). This is presumably through a different mechanism to the α_2-adrenoceptor antagonists, possibly by inhibition of monoamine oxidase activity (Nutt *et al.*, 1995). α_2-adrenoceptors will not be blocked in the presence of I_2-selective ligands, and it would be interesting to investigate the effects of RX 811059 or RX 821002 on the hyperphagic response to RX 801077. These observations suggest that the neurochemical pathways underlying the food intake induced by idazoxan and I_2 receptor ligands may not be identical.

Another neurotransmitter implicated in the control of appetite is 5-HT, as reviewed elsewhere in this book. The effect of I_2 ligands on the 5-HT system have not yet been fully explored. However, 5-HT$_{1A}$ agonists such as 8-OH-DPAT increase food intake in rats (Dourish et al., 1985); hence it is possible that the 5-HT system may be involved to some extent in the effects of idazoxan and other I$_2$ ligands on feeding behaviour.

Our studies with propranolol were consistent with this hypothesis since idazoxan-induced feeding was blocked by the (−)-isomer but not by similar doses of (+)-propranolol (Jackson and Nutt, 1992). The (−)-enantiomer of propranolol antagonizes both 5-HT$_1$ receptors and β-adrenoceptors; however, it seems unlikely that β-adrenoceptors are involved in idazoxan-induced hyperphagia since it is not attenuated by the selective β_1-adrenoceptor antagonist betaxolol or by the selective β_2-adrenoceptor antagonist ICI 118551 (Jackson and Nutt, 1992). The inhibitory effects of (−)-propranolol on idazoxan induced feeding have been confirmed by Hartley et al. (1994). However, these authors also showed that the feeding response to idazoxan was not attenuated by the selective 5-HT$_{1A}$ receptor antagonist WAY-100135 or by 24 h pretreatment with 8-OH-DPAT, which desensitizes 5-HT$_{1A}$ somatodendritic autoreceptors. These findings argue against the involvement of 5-HT$_{1A}$ receptors in idazoxan-induced food intake.

It has recently been shown that blockade of 5-HT$_{2C}$ receptors, for example by metergoline, can increase daytime food intake in rats (Dourish et al., 1989). This is presumably due to inhibition of the effects of endogenous 5-HT at 5-HT$_{2C}$ receptors. Interestingly, metergoline potentiated idazoxan-induced food intake in our studies (Jackson and Nutt, 1992) and the 5-HT reuptake inhibitor WY-27587, which would increase 5-HT levels in the synaptic cleft, reduced the hyperphagic effects of idazoxan (Hartley et al., 1994).

Further studies are clearly required to clarify the possible interactions between I$_2$ receptor ligands and the 5-HT system which may contribute to their effects on food intake. One approach would be to use the microdialysis technique in conscious rats to try to correlate the effects of I$_2$ ligands on food intake with their effects on extracellular levels of 5-HT in different brain regions.

Opioid receptors have also been implicated in the increase in food intake induced by I$_2$ receptor ligands. The increase in food consumption induced by idazoxan was antagonized in a stereoselective fashion by low doses of the opioid antagonist naloxone and by low doses of naltrexone, suggesting that it may be mediated through the release of endogenous opioids and subsequent activation of opioid receptors (Jackson et al., 1992). Preliminary experiments with selective opioid antagonists suggest that κ, as opposed to μ or δ opioid receptors, maybe involved in this response. Thus, the increase in food intake induced by idazoxan was not blocked by the selective δ opioid antagonist naltrindole nor by the μ/δ opioid antagonist 16-methyl cyprenorphine, which clearly discriminates between μ/δ and κ opioid receptor function in vivo (Jackson et al., 1992). We have also shown that the increase in food intake induced by RX 801077 in freely feeding rats may be completely abolished by

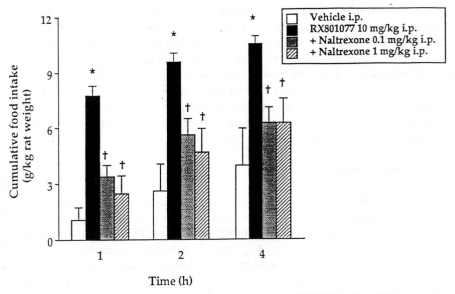

Time (h)

Fig. 5 Inhibition of the increase in food intake induced by RX 801077 by the opioid antagonist naltrexone. Individually housed male Wistar rats (250–350 g) were injected concurrently with RX 801077 and naltrexone, and intake of powdered standard rat diet was measured during the following 4 h. Procedures began at 09.00 hours so that measurements were carried out during the light period. Values represent mean ± SEM intakes for groups of six rats. $*P < 0.05$ vs vehicle-treated control; $\dagger P < 0.05$ vs RX 801077-treated group (one-way analysis of variance and Dunnett's test).

pretreatment with low doses of naltrexone (Fig. 5), which had no effect on food intake by itself. The involvement of different types of opioid receptors in RX 801077-induced feeding should be investigated more closely since it could be argued that the potency of naltrexone (0.1 mg/kg) against this response is not consistent with κ opioid mediation.

Finally, it should be noted that there is no evidence as yet that idazoxan and the I_2 receptor ligands may act directly at other receptors involved in the control of food intake. Idazoxan has high selectivity for α_2 over α_1-adrenoceptors (Doxey et al., 1983, 1985). Hence blockade of α_1-adrenoceptors cannot account for idazoxan-induced feeding. Furthermore, idazoxan does not displace [^{3}H]5-HT from its binding sites in the cerebral cortex of the rat (A. Lane, personal communication) and is inactive at opioid receptors (Doxey et al., 1983). The receptor profiles of the benzofuranylimidazole derivatives patented by Garcia-Sevilla and co-workers as appetite stimulants (see above) have not been fully defined; however, they do not have any appreciable affinity for α_1-adrenoceptors, as reported in the patent application. In addition, receptor binding studies carried out by a contract research organization (NOVASCREEN®, Oceanix Biosciences Corporation, Maryland, USA) demonstrated that RX 801077 was inactive (less than 20% displacement at 10 μmol/l) at a wide range of different receptors including those implicated in control of feeding behaviour such as α-adrenoceptors and 5-HT, benzodiazepine and peptide receptors (unpublished results).

To summarize, preliminary studies suggest that the 5-HT and opioid systems may contribute to the effects of idazoxan and I_2 ligands on food intake. However, further interaction studies with antagonists of monoamine and peptide receptors are required to determine fully the neurochemical substrates underlying the effects of these compounds on appetite.

5   Water intake studies

Idazoxan also increases water intake in rats (Jackson et al., 1991). However, this effect appears to be related to blockade of α_2-adrenoceptors since the selective α_2-adrenoceptor antagonists RX 811059 and RX 821002 also produce drinking in freely feeding rats. An increase in water consumption was also observed following treatment with the α_2 adrenoceptor antagonist L-659 066, which does not readily cross the blood–brain barrier. This finding suggests that the α_2-adrenoceptor antagonists increase water intake via action in the periphery or via α_2-adrenoceptors located in the circumventricular organs (see Jackson et al., 1991). In our studies the imidazoline I_2 receptor ligand RX 821029 increased both food and water intake at a dose of 10 mg/kg. However, RX 801077, which acts more selectively at I_2 receptors than at α_2-adrenoceptors, did not significantly increase drinking at a dose that stimulated feeding behaviour (Fig. 6).

6   Effect of idazoxan and RX 801077 on locomotor activity

The effects of drugs on food intake may be secondary to drug-induced changes in activity levels. Thus, food intake may be induced as a consequence of increased activity during the light period when animals are normally quiescent. Idazoxan has been shown to increase locomotor activity in rats (Dickinson et al., 1990); however, it is unlikely that its effects on food intake are due to this because selective α_2-adrenoceptor antagonists such as RX 811059 increase locomotor activity in rats (Dickinson et al., 1990) but do not alter food intake as mentioned above. Furthermore, the dose of RX 801077 that increases food intake does not alter locomotor activity in rats (Fig. 7). These results suggest that idazoxan and RX 801077 may exert specific effects on food intake.

7   General considerations and future directions

In this chapter we have described the stimulatory effects of idazoxan and other I_2 receptor ligands on food intake in rats. A number of questions still need to be answered. For instance, do I_2 receptor ligands increase food consumption via

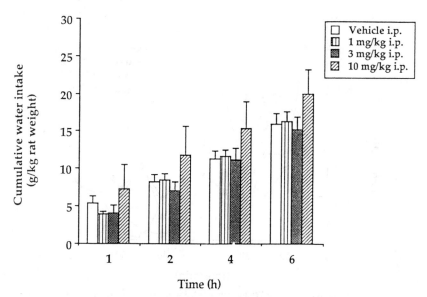

Time (h)

Fig. 6   Effect of RX 801077 on water intake in the rat. Individually housed male Wistar rats (250–350 g) were injected with saline or RX 801077, and water intake was measured during the following 6 h. Procedures began at 09.00 hours so that measurements were carried out during the light period. Values represent mean ± SEM intakes for groups of six rats. RX 801077 had no significant effect on water intake (one-way analysis of variance and Dunnett's test).

central or peripheral mechanisms? The bioavailability and pharmacokinetics of I_2 ligands has not been explored, but we would predict from their structure that the imidazolines would readily enter the brain following systemic administration. In this context, intravenous injections of RX 801077 in doses of 1, 3 and 10 mg/kg have been shown to increase the rate of metabolic activity in discrete brain areas (French, 1994), including the arcuate nucleus of the hypothalamus which contains a high density of I_2 receptors, as mentioned above. It would be particularly interesting, therefore, to measure food intake following site-specific injections of idazoxan and the I_2-selective ligands into different brain regions.

Another approach has been used by Miralles and colleagues (1993), who compared the density and affinity states of central I_2 receptors in lean and obese Zucker rats. No differences were found in I_2 receptor binding in the cerebral cortex or hypothalamus of the lean and obese rats. These authors also reported that the density of I_2 receptors in the cerebral cortex of the Zucker rats was not modified by chronic administration of the anorexic agent mazindol. However, the possibility that changes in I_2 receptors occurred in discrete brain areas cannot be precluded without further study. It should also be noted that, although mazindol is an imidazoline derivative, it has only low affinity for I_2 sites (K_i 900 nmol/l; Miralles et al., 1993).

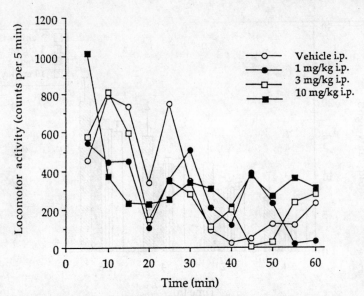

Fig. 7 Locomotor activity of male Wistar rats (250–350 g) following administration of saline or RX 801077. Animals were tested individually in automated activity boxes (60 × 60 × 30 cm high) to which they were accustomed for 40 min before the experiment began. Fifteen sets of infrared emitters and detectors were located at floor level of the activity boxes and activity counts were measured as the number of beam breaks per unit time. Results are expressed as mean values for groups of eight animals. RX 801077 had no significant effect on locomotor activity in habituated rats (Kruskal–Wallis test).

At present it is unclear whether idazoxan, RX 821029, RX 801077 and LSL 60101 are agonists or antagonists at I_2 receptors. They may stimulate food intake during the day by direct agonist action or by blocking the inhibitory effects of endogenous agonists at I_2 receptors. It is possible that changes in central levels of endogenous I_2 ligands may contribute towards the increase in food intake observed in rats during the dark period or in food-deprived animals. A number of workers have been searching for endogenous ligands for imidazoline receptors. One recent proposal is agmatine (decarboxylated arginine), which has affinity for both I_1 and I_2 receptors (Li *et al.*, 1994). It will be interesting to investigate the effects of putative endogenous I_2 ligands on food intake and to examine whether their levels are altered throughout the day or in food-deprived animals.

Further information about the effects of idazoxan and I_2 ligands on food intake could be obtained by more detailed analysis of feeding behaviour following their administration, particularly in comparison with other appetite stimulants. For instance, do these compounds selectively increase intake of fat, carbohydrate or protein, and would they be able to stimulate food intake in rats fed on more or less palatable diets? It would also be relevant to study the effects of I_2 receptor ligands on satiation using, for example, the paradigm developed by Jackson and Cooper (1986). In this model, non-deprived rats are adapted to eat a sweetened palatable mash. The animals are given access to this food for a short period before drug administration, i.e. they are partially satiated at the start of the feeding experiment. The effects of drugs on parameters such as latency to eat, duration of feeding and rate of eating can then be monitored. If the effects of I_2 ligands on food intake are mediated by κ opioid receptors, they would be expected to produce similar effects to the κ opioid agonist U-50 488H in this paradigm, i.e. to increase duration of feeding by increasing the frequency of feeding bouts and also to increase the latency to the final feeding bout (see Jackson and Cooper, 1986). It would also be pertinent to investigate the effects of I_2 ligands in the taste reactivity test (Grill and Norgren, 1978), which can be used to explore whether compounds affect taste perception. For instance, do they increase food intake by increasing the reward value of food? In this context, benzodiazepines have been shown to selectively enhance positive taste reactions in the rat (Treit and Berridge, 1990), although not all compounds that increase food intake act in this way. It would therefore be interesting to compare the effects of I_2 ligands in this procedure with those of other appetite stimulants, including opioid agonists and drugs acting on the 5-HT system.

A further important question that needs to be addressed is whether idazoxan and selective I_2 receptor ligands increase food intake in species other than the rat. Imidazoline receptors in different species may not necessarily be the same or have the same anatomical distribution. Furthermore, the ratio of I_2 receptors to α_2-adrenoceptors appears to vary from species to species (Hudson et al., 1992a). For example, in rabbit brain about 70% of [^{3}H]idazoxan binding is to I_2 sites. The food intake of rabbits was found to be unaltered during chronic administration of idazoxan (2 mg/kg subcutaneously twice daily; Portillo et al., 1991). However, food intake was measured as the cumulative daily value over the 7-day experimental period, and increases in food consumption immediately after drug administration would not have been detected. It would also be interesting to study the effects of idazoxan and I_2 receptor ligands on food intake in guinea-pigs. In these animals about 60% of [^{3}H]idazoxan binding is to I_2 receptors, which appear to be concentrated in several brain nuclei including the hypothalamus (Hudson et al., 1992a). As mentioned in the introduction, I_2 receptors have been detected in human tissues. Human brain has about an equal density of I_2 receptors and α_2-adrenoceptors (De Vos et al., 1991). Idazoxan has been administered to healthy volunteers and to patients suffering from a number of different psychiatric disorders; however, its effects on food intake in humans have not been monitored.

In conclusion, the results presented in this chapter show that I_2 receptor ligands increase food intake in rats. Further studies are required to assess the physiological role of these sites in the regulation of feeding behaviour. However, it is interesting to speculate that drugs designed either to stimulate or to antagonize I_2 sites may provide a novel therapeutic approach for the control of eating disorders such as obesity and anorexia nervosa.

References

Bernstein, I. L., Treneer, C. M. and Kott, J. N. (1985). Area postrema mediates tumor effects on food intake, body weight, and learned aversions. *Am. J. Physiol.* **249**, R296–R300.

Bousquet, P., Feldman, J., Bloch, R. and Schwartz, J. (1984). Central cardiovascular effects of α adrenergic drugs: differences between catecholamines and imidazolines. *J. Pharmacol. Exp. Ther.* **230**, 232–236.

Bricca, G., Dontenwill, M., Molines, A., Feldman, J., Belcourt, A. and Bousquet, P. (1989). The imidazoline preferring receptor: binding studies in bovine, rat and human brainstem. *Eur. J. Pharmacol.* **162**, 1–9.

Brown, C. M., MacKinnon, A. C., McGrath, J. C., Spedding, M. and Kilpatrick, A. T. (1990). α_2-Adrenoceptor subtypes and imidazoline-like binding sites in the rat brain. *Br. J. Pharmacol.* **99**, 803–809.

Convents, A., Convents, D., De Backer, J.-P., De Keyser, J. and Vauquelin, G. (1989). High affinity binding of [^{3}H]rauwolscine and [^{3}H]RX 781094 to α_2-adrenergic receptors and non-stereoselective sites in human and rabbit brain cortex membranes. *Biochem. Pharmacol.* **38**, 455–463.

De Vos, H., Convents, A., De Keyser, J., De Backer, J.-P., Van Meggen, I. J. B., Ebinger, G. and Vauquelin, G. (1991). Autoradiographic distribution of α_2 adrenoceptors, NAIBS, and 5-HT$_{1A}$ receptors in human brain using [^{3}H]idazoxan and [^{3}H]rauwolscine. *Brain Res.* **566**, 13–20.

De Vos, H., Bricca, G., De Keyser, J., De Backer, J.-P., Bousquet, P. and Vauquelin, G. (1994). Imidazoline receptors, non-adrenergic idazoxan binding sites and α_2-adrenoceptors in the human central nervous system. *Neuroscience* **59**, 589–598.

Dennis, T., L'Heureux, R., Carter, C. and Scatton, B. (1987). Pre-synaptic alpha-2 adrenoceptors play a major role in the effects of idazoxan on cortical noradrenaline release (as measured by *in vivo* dialysis) in the rat. *J. Pharmacol. Exp. Ther.* **241**, 642–649.

Dickinson, S. L., Gadie, B. and Tulloch, I. F. (1990). Specific α_2-adrenoceptor antagonists induce behavioural activation in the rat. *J. Psychopharmacol.* **4**, 90–99.

Dourish, C. T., Hutson, P. H. and Curzon, G. (1985). Low doses of the putative serotonin agonist 8-hydroxy-2-(di-*n*-propyl amino)tetralin (8-OH-DPAT) elicit feeding in the rat. *Psychopharmacology* **86**, 197–204.

Dourish, C. T., Clark, M. L., Fletcher, A. and Iversen, S. D. (1989). Evidence that blockade of post-synaptic 5-HT$_1$ receptors elicits feeding in satiated rats. *Psychopharmacology* **97**, 54–58.

Doxey, J. C., Roach, A. G. and Smith, C. F. C. (1983). Studies on RX 781094: a selective, potent and specific antagonist of α_2-adrenoceptors. *Br. J. Pharmacol.* **78**, 489–505.

Doxey, J. C., Lane, A. C., Roach, A. G., Smith, C. F. C. and Walter, D. S. (1985). Selective α_2-adrenoceptor agonists and antagonists. In *Pharmacology of Adrenoceptors* (E. Szabadi, C. M. Bradshaw and S. R. Nahorski, eds), pp. 13–22. Macmillan, New York.

Ernsberger, P. (1992). Heterogeneity of imidazoline binding sites: proposed I_1 and I_2 subtypes. *Fundam. Clin. Pharmacol.* **6 (supplement 1)**, 55S.

Ernsberger, P., Meeley, M. P., Mann, J. J. and Reis, D. J. (1987). Clonidine binds to imidazole binding sites as well as α_2-adrenoceptors in the ventrolateral medulla. *Eur. J. Pharmacol.* **134**, 1–13.

Ernsberger, P., Giuliano, R., Willette, R. N. and Reis, D. J. (1990). Role of imidazole receptors in the vasodepressor response to clonidine analogs in the rostral ventrolateral medulla. *J. Pharmacol. Exp. Ther.* **253**, 408–418.

Ernsberger, P., Damon, T. H., Graff, L. M., Christen, M. O. and Schafer, S. G. (1993). Moxonidine, a centrally acting antihypertensive agent, is a selective ligand for I_1-imidazoline sites. *J. Pharmacol. Exp. Ther.* **264**, 172–182.

French, N. (1994). *Functional evaluation of α_2-adrenoceptors and imidazoline-preferring I_2 sites in the central nervous system.* PhD thesis, University of Strathclyde, Glasgow.

Garcia-Sevilla, J. A., Meana Martinez, J. J., Barturen Fernandez, F., Geijo Caballero, F. A., Menargues Banos, A., Obach Vidal, R. and Pla Rodas, F. (1993). Benzofuranylimidazole derivatives. *UK Patent Application GB 2 262 739 A.*

Goldman, C. K., Marino, L. and Leibowitz, S. F. (1985). Postsynaptic α_2-noradrenergic receptors mediate feeding induced by paraventricular nucleus injection of norepinephrine and clonidine. *Eur. J. Pharmacol.* **115**, 11–19.

Gomez, R., Ernsberger, P., Feinland, G. and Reis, D. J. (1991). Rilmenidine lowers arterial pressure via imidazole receptors in brainstem C1 area. *Eur. J. Pharmacol.* **195**, 181–191.

Grill, H. J. and Norgren, R. (1978). The taste-reactivity test: I. Mimetic response to gustatory stimuli in neurologically normal rats. *Brain Res.* **143**, 263–279.

Hamilton, C. A., Yakubu, M. A., Jardine, E. and Reid, J. L. (1991). Imidazole binding sites in rabbit kidney and forebrain membranes. *J. Auton. Pharmacol.* **11**, 277–283.

Hartley, J. E., Brown, G., Dourish, C. T. and Fletcher, A. (1994). Evidence indicating that 5-HT$_{1A}$ receptor mechanisms are not involved in idazoxan-induced hyperphagia. *Br. J. Pharmacol.* **111**, 145P.

Hudson, A., Mallard, N. and Nutt, D. (1992a). Autoradiographic localisation of non-Adrenoceptor idazoxan binding sites in the mammalian central nervous system. *Fundam. Clin. Pharmacol.* **6 (supplement 1)**, 52S.

Hudson, A., Mallard, N., Nutt, D. and Chapleo, C. (1992b). RX 821029: a selective ligand for non-adrenoceptor idazoxan binding sites in mammalian brain. *Fundam. Clin. Pharmacol.* **6 (supplement 1)**, 45S.

Hudson, A., Mallard, N. J., Nutt, D. J. and Chapleo, C. B. (1995). Affinity and selectivity of 2-(2-benzofuranyl)-2-imidazoline for mammalian brain non-adrenoceptor idazoxan binding sites (I_2-sites). *Br. J. Pharmacol.* **114**, 411.

Jackson, A. and Cooper, S. J. (1986). An observational analysis of the effect of the selective κ opioid agonist, U-50 488H, on feeding and related behaviours in the rat. *Psychopharmacology* **90**, 217–221.

Jackson, H. C. and Nutt, D. J. (1992). Are 5-HT receptors or β-adrenoceptors involved in idazoxan-induced food and water intake? *Neuropharmacology* **31**, 1081–1087.

Jackson, H. C., Griffin, I. J. and Nutt, D. J. (1991). The effects of idazoxan and other α_2-adrenoceptor antagonists on food and water intake in the rat. *Br. J. Pharmacol.* **104**, 258–262.

Jackson, H. C., Griffin, I. J. and Nutt, D. J. (1992). Endogenous opioids may be involved in idazoxan-induced food intake. *Neuropharmacology* **31**, 771–776.

Kamisaki, Y., Ishikawa, T., Takao, Y., Omodani, H., Kuno, N. and Itoh, T. (1990). Binding of [^{3}H]p-aminoclonidine to two sites, alpha 2-adrenoceptors and imidazoline binding sites: distribution of imidazoline binding sites in rat brain. *Brain Res.* **514**, 15–21.

Langin, D. and Lafontan, M. (1989). [^{3}H]Idazoxan binding at non-α_2-adrenoceptors in rabbit adipocyte membranes. *Eur. J. Pharmacol.* **159**, 199–203.

Langin, D., Lafontan, M., Stillings, M. R. and Paris, H. (1989). [^{3}H]RX 821002: a new tool for the identification of α_2-adrenoceptors. *Eur. J. Pharmacol.* **167**, 95–104.

Langin, D., Paris, H. and Lafontan, M. (1990). Binding of [^{3}H]idazoxan and of its methoxy derivative [^{3}H]RX 821002 in human fat cells: [^{3}H]idazoxan but not [^{3}H]RX 821002 labels additional non-α_2-adrenergic binding sites. *Mol. Pharmacol.* **37**, 876–885.

Li, G., Regunathan, S., Barrow, C. J., Eshraghi, J., Cooper, R. and Reis, D. J. (1994). Agmatine: an endogenous clonidine-displacing substance in the brain. *Science* **263**, 966–969.

McCabe, J. T., De Bellis, M. and Leibowitz, S. F. (1984). Clonidine-induced feeding: analysis of central sites of action and fibre projections mediating this response. *Brain Res.* **309**, 85–104.

MacKinnon, A. C., Brown, C. M., Spedding, M. and Kilpatrick, A. T. (1989). [^{3}H]Idazoxan binds with high affinity to two sites on hamster adipocytes: an α_2-adrenoceptor and a non-adrenoceptor site. *Br. J. Pharmacol.* **98**, 1143–1150.

Mallard, N. J., Hudson, A. L. and Nutt, D. J. (1992). Characterization and autoradiographical localization of non-adrenoceptor idazoxan binding sites in the rat brain. *Br. J. Pharmacol.* **106**, 1019–1027.

Menargues, A., Cedo, M., Artiga, O., Obach, R. and Garcia-Sevilla, J. A. (1994). Modulation of food intake by α_2-adrenoceptor antagonists and I_2-imidazoline drugs in rats: LSL 60101 as a novel and selective ligand for I_2-imidazoline sites. *Br. J. Pharmacol.* **111**, 298P.

Michel, M. C. and Insel, P. A. (1989). Are there multiple imidazoline binding sites? *Trends Pharmacol. Sci.* **10**, 342–344.

Michel, M. C., Brodde, O.-E., Schnepel, B., Behrendt, J., Tschada, R., Motulsky, H. J. and Insel, P. A. (1989). [^{3}H]Idazoxan and some other α_2-adrenergic drugs also bind with high affinity to a nonadrenergic site. *Mol. Pharmacol.* **35**, 324–330.

Miralles, A., Ribas, C., Olmos, G. and Garcia-Sevilla, J. A. (1993). No effect of genetic obesity and mazindol on imidazoline I_2 binding sites in the brain of Zucker rats. *Eur. J. Pharmacol.* **243**, 305–308.

Nutt, D. J., French, N., Handley, S., Hudson, A., Husbands, S., Jackson, H., Jordan, S., Lalies, M. D., Lewis, J., Lione, L., Mallard, N. and Pratt, J. (1995). Functional studies of specific imidazoline-2 receptor ligands. In *The Imidazoline Receptor, Pharmacology, Functions, Ligands and Relevance to Biology & Medicine* (D. J. Reis, P. Bousquet and A. Panini, eds), pp. 125–129. New York Academy of Science, New York.

Portillo, M., Reverte, M., Langin, D., Senard, J. M., Tran, M. A., Berlan, M. and Montastruc, J. L. (1991). Effect of a 7-day treatment with idazoxan and its 2-methyoxy derivative RX 821002 on alpha$_2$-adrenoceptors and non-adrenoceptor idazoxan binding sites in rabbits. *Br. J. Pharmacol.* **104**, 190–194.

Renouard, A., Widdowson, P. S. and Cordi, A. (1993). [^{3}H]idazoxan binding to rabbit cerebral cortex recognises multiple imidazoline. I_2-type receptors: pharmacological characterization and relationship to monoamine oxidase. *Br. J. Pharmacol.* **109**, 625–631.

Routledge, C., Hartley, J., Gurling, J., Ashworth-Preece, M., Brown, G. and Dourish, C. T. (1994). *In vivo* characterization of the putative 5-HT$_{1A}$ receptor antagonist SDZ 216525 using two models of somatodendritic 5-HT$_{1A}$ receptor function. *Neuropharmacology* **33**, 359–366.

Sanger, D. J. (1983). An analysis of the effects of systemically administered clonidine on the food and water intake of rats. *Br. J. Pharmacol.* **78**, 159–164.

Sleight, A. J., Smith, R. J., Marsden, C. A. and Palfreyman, M. G. (1988). Is the hyperphagic response to 8-OH-DPAT a model for 5HT$_{1A}$ receptor responsiveness? *Br. J. Pharmacol.* **95**, 875P.

Sugrue, M. F. (1987). Neuropharmacology of drugs affecting food intake. *Pharmacol. Ther.* **32**, 145–182.

Tesson, F., Prip-Buus, C., Lemoine, A., Pegorier, J. P. and Parini, A. (1991). Subcellular distribution of imidazoline–guanidinium-receptive sites in human and rabbit liver. *J. Biol. Chem.* **266**, 155–160.

Thomas, D. N. and Holman, R. B. (1991). A microdialysis study of the regulation of endogenous noradrenaline release in the rat hippocampus. *J. Neurochem.* **56**, 1741–1746.

Treit, D. and Berridge, K. C. (1990). A comparison of benzodiazepine, serotonin, and dopamine agents in the taste-reactivity paradigm. *Pharmacol. Biochem. Behav.* **37**, 451–456.

Wellman, P. J., Davies, B. T., Morien, A. and McMahon, L. (1993). Modulation of feeding by hypothalamic paraventricular nucleus α_1- and α_2-adrenoreceptors. *Life Sci.* **53**, 669–679.

Wikberg, J. E. S. and Uhlen, S. (1990). Further characterization of the guinea pig cerebral cortex idazoxan receptor: solubilization, distinction from the imidazole site, and demonstration of cirazoline as an idazoxan receptor-selective drug. *J. Neurochem.* **55**, 192–203.

Yablonsky, F. and Dausse, J. P. (1991). Nonadrenergic binding sites for the α_2-antagonist [^{3}H]idazoxan in the rabbit urethral smooth muscle. *Biochem. Pharmacol.* **41**, 701–707.

13

Medial Hypothalamic α2-Adrenergic and Serotonergic Effects on Ingestive Behaviour

PAUL J. CURRIE

Department of Psychology, Wayne State University, 71 W. Warren
Avenue, Detroit, MI 48202, USA

1 Introduction

Brain monoamines are believed to play a critical role in the control of ingestive behaviour. Considerable evidence suggests that the hypothalamus, a forebrain structure which receives and integrates multiple metabolic, hormonal and thermogenic inputs (Leibowitz, 1988, 1992), is uniquely sensitive to the feeding-modulatory effects of these neurochemicals. For example, it has been demonstrated that injection of noradrenaline (norepinephrine) into the hypothalamic paraventricular nucleus (PVN) potentiates food intake, whereas serotonergic stimulation of this nucleus reliably inhibits feeding and, in particular, eating induced by exogenous noradrenaline (Weiss et al., 1986; Leibowitz, 1988, 1990; Fletcher and Paterson, 1989a; Currie and Coscina, 1994).

Recent neuropharmacological and biochemical data have further shown that noradrenaline and 5-hydroxytryptamine (5-HT, serotonin) are most effective in modifying food intake when administered at the onset of the nocturnal cycle (Leibowitz et al., 1990b; Tempel and Leibowitz, 1990; Currie, 1993) and that, within the PVN, there is an increase in the release or metabolism of these neurotransmitters in association with eating during the early dark period (Stanley et al., 1989a,b; Paez et al., 1993). These findings in turn suggest that a diurnal rhythm of adrenergic and serotonergic activity exists within the PVN, specifically in relation to feeding behaviour. Based on this evidence it is proposed that noradrenaline and 5-HT systems function in a circadian-related manner whereby 5-HT interacts antagonistically with PVN adrenergic receptor mechanisms to modulate episodes of spontaneous eating at the start of the rat's active feeding cycle.

DRUG RECEPTOR SUBTYPES AND INGESTIVE BEHAVIOUR
ISBN 0-12-187620-9

2 Adrenergic stimulation of feeding

Central injection of noradrenaline has been shown to enhance food intake in several animal species (Leibowitz, 1986; Sugrue, 1987; Currie and Wilson, 1993) and cannula-mapping studies have demonstrated that the PVN is highly sensitive to the feeding-stimulant action of this neurochemical (Leibowitz, 1978, 1988). When administered into the PVN, noradrenaline produces eating in satiated rats and potentiates eating in hungry rats (Leibowitz, 1978; Leibowitz *et al.*, 1985a,b). The feeding response induced by noradrenaline, which has been observed at doses as low as 0.025–0.1 nmol (Leibowitz, 1978), is believed to result from the selective activation of postsynaptic α_2-adrenoceptors. Thus, adrenergically stimulated food intake is prevented by pretreatment with the general α-adrenergic receptor antagonist phentolamine and the selective α_2-adrenergic antagonists idazoxan and yohimbine, but is unaffected by the α_1-adrenoceptor antagonist prazosin (Goldman *et al.*, 1985; Fletcher and Paterson, 1989b; Currie and Coscina, 1993b). Moreover, the destruction of adrenergic presynaptic nerve terminals has little impact on eating induced by exogenous noradrenaline, consistent with a postsynaptic site of action (Leibowitz and Brown, 1980; Goldman *et al.*, 1985).

The α_2-adrenergic agonist clonidine has also been reported to stimulate food intake when injected systemically, intraventricularly or directly into the PVN (Sanger, 1983; Leibowitz *et al.*, 1985a; Shor-Posner *et al.*, 1988; Koulu *et al.*, 1990; Currie, 1993). The hyperphagic effects of both noradrenaline and clonidine are blocked in a dose-dependent fashion by α_2-receptor antagonism (Goldman *et al.*, 1985; Currie and Wilson 1992b, 1993; Currie and Coscina, 1993b) and attenuated by PVN lesion (Leibowitz *et al.*, 1983; Shor-Posner *et al.*, 1988; Fletcher *et al.*, 1993). Other selective α_2 agonists reportedly increase feeding when injected systemically (Majeed *et al.*, 1991). However, the impact of peripherally and centrally administered clonidine on food intake appears to be biphasic, such that low doses of drug stimulate appetite whereas higher doses tend to suppress feeding behaviour (Currie and Wilson, 1991; Wellman and Davies, 1991). While the inhibition of food intake could result from the induction of sedation or other non-specific behavioural effects, alternatively an effect of clonidine on α_1-adrenoceptors may explain, in part, why high doses of this compound decrease ingestion. Specifically, at high doses clonidine may show affinity for α_1-adrenoceptors (U'Prichard, 1981) and it has recently been suggested that the α_1 receptor subtype may mediate feeding suppression (Wellman, 1992). Microinjection into the PVN of the various α_1 agonists including cirazoline, methoxamine, phenylephrine and phenylpropanolamine attenuate feeding, an effect that is reversed by pretreatment with α_1-adrenergic receptor antagonists (Wellman and Davies, 1990, 1991; Wellman *et al.*, 1993).

Multiple injection of either noradrenaline or clonidine, giving rise to chronic activation of PVN α_2-adrenoceptors, elicits a continuing, robust hyperphagia and enhanced gains in body weight (Leibowitz et al., 1984; Lichtenstein et al., 1984). Paradoxically, radiofrequency or electrolytic lesions of the PVN also produce overeating and increases in body weight (Leibowitz et al., 1981; Fletcher et al., 1993). The apparently conflicting data can be reconciled if it is assumed that noradrenaline has an inhibitory effect at a cellular level in the PVN, and that this serves to inhibit a satiety mechanism, thus leading to the disinhibition of feeding (Hoebel, 1985). Damage to local PVN satiety neurons would therefore be predicted to elicit hyperphagia and obesity under such a model. Noradrenaline is known to inhibit the firing rate of hypothalamic neurons, particularly in the parvocellular PVN, and it is this subregion that is believed to mediate adrenergic feeding (Inenaga et al., 1986; Leibowitz, 1988). This is consistent with the finding that PVN infusion of the selective catecholamine neurotoxin, 6-hydroxydopamine (6-OHDA), which depletes presynaptic noradrenaline stores resulting in impaired postsynaptic adrenoceptor stimulation, produces a suppression of food intake and a decrease in body weight (Shor-Posner et al., 1986a).

While the effects of 6-OHDA on feeding and body weight appear to be in direct contrast to the impact of radiofrequency or electrolytic lesions of the PVN, it is somewhat surprising that axon-sparing excitotoxic lesions of this nucleus have not consistently been reported to produce excessive weight gain or sustained disturbances in food intake. Whereas a number of studies have found little or no change in feeding and body weight following PVN lesions with N-methyl-D-aspartic acid (NMDA) or kainic acid (Zhang and Ciriello, 1985; Rockhold et al., 1990), others have demonstrated accelerated body weight gain following ibotenate lesion of the PVN (Touzani and Velley, 1992). In another report, unilateral ibotenic acid lesions of the PVN induced changes in body weight, although food intake was not affected (Hajnal et al., 1993). These findings suggest that such disturbances in energy intake and body mass homoeostasis may result from more widespread tissue damage, including fibres of passage, rather than the exclusive destruction cell bodies within the PVN itself.

The PVN is extensively innervated by ascending noradrenaline fibres that arise from the brainstem. The specific adrenergic innervation to the PVN that controls feeding appears to derive, in part, from noradrenaline-containing neurons in the dorsal pons, possibly the locus ceruleus and subceruleus (Leibowitz and Brown, 1980). The efferent projection follows a periventricular course and returns to hindbrain structures such as the dorsal vagal complex, en route to the peripheral autonomic nervous system (McCabe et al., 1984; Weiss and Leibowitz, 1985). It has been demonstrated that the adrenergic control of eating is dependent on an intact vagus nerve, including its pancreatic branch (Sawchenko et al., 1981), and that feeding elicited by PVN noradrenaline is abolished by hypophysectomy or adrenalectomy and restored by corticosterone replacement (Roland et al., 1985, 1986; Leibowitz, 1988). Consequently, the integrity of the noradrenaline feeding response requires not only the activation of postsynaptic α_2 receptors, but is additionally dependent on other neural and hormonal inputs.

3 Serotonergic inhibition of feeding

In marked contrast to the feeding-stimulant action of noradrenaline, converging pharmacological evidence supports a selective inhibitory role for 5-HT in the control of ingestive behaviour. Peripheral administration of drugs that increase 5-HT neurotransmission reduce food intake in laboratory animals and humans (Sugrue, 1987; Samanin and Garattini, 1989; Garattini et al., 1990; Blundell, 1992). These drugs include D-fenfluramine, which releases 5-HT and inhibits its reuptake (Rowland and Carlton, 1986; Neill and Cooper, 1989; Dourish, 1992), the 5-HT uptake inhibitor fluoxetine (Wong et al., 1988; Clifton et al., 1989; Fuller, 1994; Fuller et al., 1994) and the direct 5-HT receptor agonists 1-(m-chlorophenyl)piperazine (m-CPP), 1-(m-trifluoro-methylphenyl)piperazine (TFMPP) and RU 24969 (Kennett and Curzon, 1988; Dourish, 1992; Luo and Li, 1992). Interestingly, certain compounds that reduce 5-HT function, including the $5\text{-HT}_{1/2}$ antagonists metergoline and methysergide (Fletcher, 1988; Dourish et al., 1989; Currie and Coscina, 1994; Coscina et al., 1994), as well as the selective 5-HT_{1A} agonist 8-hydroxy-2-(di-n-propylamino)tetralin (8-OH-DPAT) (Dourish et al., 1985; Bendotti and Samanin, 1986; Fletcher and Davies, 1990; Currie and Coscina, 1993a), have been shown to potentiate food intake under certain experimental conditions.

With respect to a central mechanism of action, autoradiographic and immunofluorescence studies have identified 5-HT-containing terminals in the medial region of the hypothalamus (Sawchenko et al., 1983) as well as dense patterns of serotonergic receptors, including 5-HT_1 receptors (Pazos and Palacios, 1985; Leibowitz and Jhanwar-Uniyal, 1989) which are reported to mediate the satiety-inducing effect of 5-HT (Curzon, 1990). The serotonergic innervation of the medial hypothalamus arises from 5-HT projections of the midbrain raphe nuclei (Steinbusch, 1981). Several studies have indicated that the PVN is particularly sensitive to the feeding-inhibitory effect of 5-HT. Thus, local injections of 5-HT have been found to suppress food intake in a dose-dependent manner (Shor-Posner et al., 1986b; Leibowitz et al., 1988, 1989). This effect has been reproduced by PVN treatment with indirect and direct 5-HT agonists (Shor-Posner et al., 1986b; Hutson et al., 1988; Weiss et al., 1990, 1991) and blocked by metergoline (Currie and Coscina, 1994).

Despite the above evidence, it is generally acknowledged that the impact of various serotonergic compounds on feeding is not mediated exclusively by the PVN. Lesions to this nucleus fail to modify the anorectic effects of peripherally administered D-fenfluramine, fluoxetine and TFMPP (Fletcher et al., 1993). Further, PVN injections of the 5-HT_{1B} agonists TFMPP and RU 24969, although effective in suppressing food intake when injected systemically

(Bendotti and Samanin, 1987; Kennett and Curzon, 1988; Fletcher et al., 1993), fail to reduce food intake consistently when injected directly into the PVN (Fletcher et al., 1992). More recent evidence indicates that other medial hypothalamic sites, specifically the ventromedial nucleus (VMN) and the suprachiasmatic nucleus (SCN), are also highly responsive to the anorectic action of exogenous 5-HT (Leibowitz et al., 1990a,b), suggesting that the 5-HT axis implicated in feeding suppression may involve the coordinated impact of several medial hypothalamic nuclei. Clearly, however, the PVN would appear to play an integral role in mediating this neurotransmitter's anorectic action.

4 Diurnal rhythm of PVN noradrenaline and 5-HT

Natural feeding behaviour in the rat has been shown to exhibit a strong circadian rhythm, with larger episodes of eating characteristic of the beginning and end of the dark phase (Armstrong, 1980). Recent studies indicate that a rhythm of adrenergic and serotonergic activity in relation to feeding may also occur across the light–dark cycle. This rhythm is expressed in temporal shifts in the responsiveness of medial hypothalamic noradrenaline and 5-HT receptors to neurochemical stimulation, and in the release and utilization of both neurotransmitters (Table 1). Specifically, exogenous noradrenaline is most effective in disinhibiting feeding at onset of the dark period, compared with

Table 1 Antagonistic effects of medial hypothalamic α₂-adrenergic and serotonergic systems in the control of feeding

	Noradrenaline	5-HT	References
Extracellular PVN levels during the early dark period	↑	↑	Stanley et al. (1989a,b), Paez et al. (1993)
Effects on dark-onset feeding	↑	↓	Currie and Wilson (1992a, 1993) Currie and Coscina (1994)
Carbohydrate intake	↑	↓	Leibowitz et al. (1989, 1990b), Tempel and Leibowitz (1990), Currie (1993)
Meal size, duration and eating rate	↑	↓	Shor-Posner et al. (1986b, 1988) Leibowitz et al. (1993b)
Body weight gain	↑	↓	Lichtenstein et al. (1984), Leibowitz (1990, 1992)

↑, increased; ↓, decreased.

other points in the diurnal cycle (Tempel and Leibowitz, 1990; Currie, 1993; Currie and Wilson, 1993). The feeding-stimulatory effect of noradrenaline is associated with a selective increase in the intake of carbohydrate (Leibowitz, 1988; Tempel and Leibowitz, 1990; Currie, 1993), a macronutrient that is generally preferred over protein and fat at this point in the dark period (Leibowitz, 1988; Tempel et al., 1989; Currie, 1993). In addition, at this time, a peak in PVN extracellular noradrenaline levels is evident (Stanley et al., 1989a), associated with an increase in α_2-adrenergic receptor density (Jhanwar-Uniyal et al., 1986) and an increase in circulating corticosterone, a hormone that is critical for the expression of adrenergic feeding (Leibowitz, 1986; Rowland et al., 1986).

Other work has shown that extracellular noradrenaline concentrations within the PVN may increase in response to food deprivation (Stanley et al., 1989a), although this increase is associated with a downregulation of α_2-receptors, particularly at the onset of the dark period (Jhanwar-Uniyal et al., 1988). The downregulation of α_2-adrenoceptors may be in response to enhanced noradrenaline turnover in the PVN or to a decline in circulating glucose levels (Chafetz et al., 1986; Jhanwar-Uniyal et al., 1987). Taken together, and in light of the recent finding demonstrating a strong positive correlation between the extracellular PVN concentration of noradrenaline and the amount of food (carbohydrate) ingested (Paez et al., 1993), these findings strongly suggest that enhanced release of noradrenaline in the PVN may participate in the initiation or maintenance of the spontaneous eating behaviour that naturally occurs in the rat at the start of the nocturnal period as well as after food deprivation.

Similarly, the impact of 5-HT on ingestive behaviour appears to be most pronounced at the start of the active feeding period, as demonstrated by medial hypothalamic administration of 5-HT or indirectly acting serotonergic agonists (Leibowitz et al., 1989, 1990a; Rogacki et al., 1989; Currie and Wilson, 1992a; Currie, 1993). At this time, serotonergic stimulation of the PVN is found to be most effective in suppressing food intake, particularly carbohydrate ingestion (Leibowitz et al., 1989, 1990a; Rogacki et al., 1989; Weiss et al., 1990, 1991). This temporally dependent anorectic effect of 5-HT has also been reported in the VMN and the SCN (Leibowitz et al., 1990b; Weiss et al., 1990, 1991).

The proposal that medial hypothalamic serotonergic control of feeding is expressed phasically, primarily at the start of the natural feeding cycle, is also supported by earlier studies examining 5-HT synthesis, metabolism and re-uptake (Hery et al., 1982; Faradji et al., 1983; Martin and Marsden, 1985; Mason, 1986). More recently, extracellular levels of the 5-HT metabolite 5-hydroxyindoleacetic acid (5-HIAA) have been shown to exhibit a marked transient peak immediately following dark onset in free-feeding rats (Stanley et al., 1989b). Since the peak in 5-HIAA is abolished under conditions of food deprivation (Stanley et al., 1989b), this has been taken as evidence to suggest that 5-HT may play a critical role in controlling food intake during the early portion of the nocturnal eating period. Specifically, 5-HT may act to terminate the initial eating bouts that occur during the early dark phase, possibly by stimulating PVN and VMN satiety neurons (Leibowitz, 1990; Leibowitz et al., 1990b), as well as SCN neurons which are critically involved in the circadian rhythms of physiological systems (Martin and Marsden, 1985; Mason, 1986; Hermes and Renaud, 1993).

In partial support of this hypothesis, several studies have shown that administration of 5-HT or its agonists, including DL-norfenfluramine, directly into the PVN produces a significant decrease in the size and duration of individual meals, associated with a reduced rate of eating (Shor-Posner et al., 1986b; Leibowitz et al., 1988; Leibowitz, 1990). Because the latency to meal onset and the frequency of meals consumed remain unaltered, it is argued that endogenous 5-HT may primarily influence the termination of feeding rather than its initiation. Similar effects on meal patterns have been observed in animals receiving systemic injections of serotonergic agonists (Blundell, 1986; Fletcher and Burton, 1986; Leibowitz et al., 1988), suggesting that centrally and peripherally administered 5-HT compounds share, at some level, a common mechanism of action. Moreover, these effects are generally opposite to those produced by PVN injection of noradrenaline or clonidine (Shor-Posner et al., 1988; Leibowitz et al., 1993b).

5 Antagonistic function of PVN noradrenaline and 5-HT

In addition to the above evidence demonstrating that PVN noradrenaline and 5-HT evoke essentially the opposite effects on natural feeding patterns, further microinjection studies in brain-cannulated rats have provided more direct evidence to indicate that endogenous 5-HT interacts antagonistically with noradrenaline to control ingestive behaviour. Specifically, medial hypothalamic 5-HT is believed to act to suppress ingestion at the onset of the nocturnal period, in part through its inhibitory interaction with noradrenaline. PVN injections of low doses (2.5–10 nmol) of 5-HT have recently been reported to block the feeding-stimulant action of noradrenaline in a dose-dependent manner at the start of the dark period, and this effect is reversed by metergoline pretreatment (Fig. 1) (Currie and Coscina, 1994). This work is in agreement with earlier findings showing that 5-HT injected into the PVN during the mid-light cycle also inhibits noradrenaline-induced eating, and that serotonergic receptor antagonists as opposed to dopaminergic, cholinergic or histaminergic antagonists effectively and dose-dependently block the inhibitory influence of 5-HT on adrenergic feeding (Weiss et al., 1986; Leibowitz et al., 1988; Fletcher and Paterson, 1989a). Moreover, the 5-HT agonists DL-fenfluramine, DL-norfenfluramine, fluoxetine and quipazine, when injected systemically or directly into the PVN, appear to be similarly effective in suppressing the adrenergic eating response (Weiss et al., 1986; Leibowitz et al., 1988; Fletcher et al., 1992).

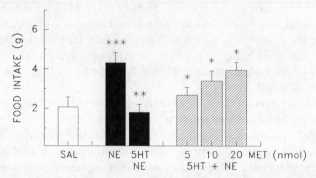

Fig. 1 Blockade of the serotonergic inhibition of noradrenaline (norepinephrine, NE)-stimulated eating at the beginning of the dark period following PVN infusion of metergoline. Values represent mean ± SEM food intake 90 min after treatment. *$P < 0.05$ vs intake after co-injection of 5-hydroxytryptamine (5-HT) (10 nmol) and NE (20 nmol); **$P < 0.05$ vs NE; ***$P < 0.05$ vs saline (SAL).

These findings are consistent with biochemical data indicating a direct inhibitory effect of 5-HT on hypothalamic noradrenaline release *in vitro* (Blandina *et al.*, 1991), and with other evidence showing that 5-HT projections to the hypothalamus tonically inhibit the *in vivo* activity of adrenergic neurons terminating in this region (Tian *et al.*, 1993). It should be noted, however, that while peripheral injections of the 5-HT agonists TFMPP and RU 24969 have been found reliably to suppress food intake elicited by PVN noradrenaline infusion, this effect was not reproduced when either compound was administered into the PVN (Fletcher *et al.*, 1992). Furthermore, although it has been proposed that PVN noradrenaline and 5-HT interact specifically to control the ingestion of carbohydrate at the beginning of the dark cycle, the ability of 5-HT to inhibit an adrenergically stimulated carbohydrate preference at this time has yet to be demonstrated.

In an attempt to characterize more fully the functional boundaries within which brain 5-HT systems may interact with noradrenaline to modulate feeding behaviour, several recent studies have examined whether treatments which impede 5-HT neurotransmission might enhance feeding, specifically noradrenaline-induced eating. Indeed, there is evidence that acute depletion of brain 5-HT is associated with a reliable increase in food intake. One such example is the increase in feeding that results from administration of the 5-HT$_{1A}$ agonist 8-OH-DPAT, injected either systemically or into the midbrain raphe nuclei (Dourish *et al.*, 1985; Fletcher and Davies, 1990; Currie and Coscina, 1993a). 8-OH-DPAT has been shown to inhibit forebrain 5-HT neurotransmission (for a review see Hjorth, 1992), including extracellular levels of medial hypothalamic 5-HT (Schwartz *et al.*, 1990), through the preferential activation of somatodendritic 5-HT$_{1A}$ receptors in the raphe nuclei. It has been proposed that the feeding effects of this compound may

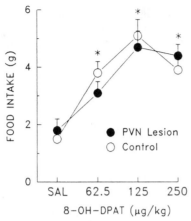

Fig. 2 The dose–response effects of 8-OH-DPAT on food intake in PVN-lesioned rats and sham-operated controls. Values represent mean ± SEM intake over 2 h. *$P < 0.05$ vs saline (SAL). From Fletcher et al. (1993), with kind permission of Elsevier Science.

result from the diminished release of 5-HT specifically within the medial hypothalamus. However, extensive work has shown that neither systemic nor raphe injection of 8-OH-DPAT modifies feeding induced by PVN noradrenaline or peripherally administered clonidine (de Rooy and Coscina, 1990; Coscina and de Rooy, 1993; Currie et al., 1994). Moreover, localized damage to PVN 5-HT terminals following infusion of the 5-HT neurotoxin 5,7-dihydroxytryptamine (5,7-DHT) also fails to alter the magnitude of eating elicited by microinjection of noradrenaline into the PVN (Coscina and de Rooy, 1992). Taken together, these findings suggest that decrements in 5-HT function within the PVN do not potentiate adrenergic feeding and further imply that the interactive effect of PVN 5-HT and noradrenaline on ingestive behaviour is not bidirectional.

In fact, even the feeding effects of 5-HT$_{1A}$ agonists such as 8-OH-DPAT are unlikely to be mediated by reduced serotonergic release within the PVN. This is consistent with the finding that systemic, but not PVN, injection of metergoline is effective in potentiating feeding (Leibowitz et al., 1993a; Currie and Coscina, 1994). Injection of 5-HT into the PVN does not reverse the feeding-stimulant action of 8-OH-DPAT (Fletcher and Coscina, 1993), nor does the blockade of PVN α₂-adrenoceptors alter the ability of this compound to potentiate food intake when administered into either the dorsal or median raphe (Currie and Coscina, 1993b). Furthermore, discrete PVN lesions leave intact the 8-OH-DPAT eating response (Fig. 2) (Fletcher et al., 1993), which is perhaps the most convincing evidence that feeding elicited by 5-HT$_{1A}$ agonists is independent of PVN mechanisms. However, widespread depletion of brain 5-HT has been shown to impair the short-term feeding response of 8-OH-DPAT (Coscina and de Rooy, 1992), indicating the underlying importance of central 5-HT systems in mediating this effect. In addition, dopamine receptor blockade in the nucleus accumbens attenuates eating elicited by 8-OH-DPAT (Fletcher and Davies, 1990; Fletcher, 1991), suggesting that dopaminergic neurons are also involved in mediating the effect of 8-OH-DPAT on food intake.

6 Conclusions

Diurnal variations in brain neurotransmitter release and activity are believed to be closely related to the expression of natural eating behaviour and to variations in the feeding response to exogenous neurotransmitter administration (Tempel and Leibowitz, 1990; Currie and Coscina, 1993a, 1994). The findings summarized above suggest that, with respect to medial hypothalamic noradrenaline and 5-HT, the impact of these two monoamine systems, mediated respectively by the inhibition or activation of satiety neurons, may occur specifically in the PVN, where 5-HT interacts antagonistically with noradrenaline to control food intake. The competitive antagonism between PVN adrenergic and serotonergic receptor mechanisms appears to be unidirectional and is hypothesized to occur at the beginning of the dark period. At this time, an increase in the release of endogenous 5-HT may act directly to inhibit the increase in feeding resulting from enhanced PVN postsynaptic α_2-adrenoceptor stimulation. It is likely that activation of these systems, in association with other neuroactive hormones and peptides, also enables an animal to modulate various temporal aspects of ingestive behaviour as well as appetite for specific macronutrients.

However, while microinjection of 5-HT into the PVN reliably suppresses feeding, and in particular eating induced by noradrenaline, acute depletion of 5-HT within this nucleus does not appear to be associated with a reliable increase in food intake or potentiation of adrenergic feeding. Consequently the PVN is unlikely to be a critical brain site mediating the feeding-stimulant action of the 5-HT$_{1A}$ agonist 8-OH-DPAT. This is consistent with additional evidence indicating that peripherally administered compounds which alter 5-HT function, such as metergoline, fenfluramine and fluoxetine, do not appear to modify feeding behaviour by an action limited to the PVN. Collectively these data should draw to our attention the underlying importance of multiple hypothalamic, possibly extrahypothalamic, 5-HT systems, which may be critically involved in the expression of such 5-HT-related changes in food intake.

References

Armstrong, S. (1980). A chronometric approach to the study of feeding behavior. *Neurosci. Biobehav. Rev.* **4**, 27–53.
Bendotti, C. and Samanin, R. (1986). 8-Hydroxy-2-(di-*n*-propylamino)tetralin (8-OH-

DPAT) elicits feeding in free feeding rats by acting on central serotonin neurons. *Eur. J. Pharmacol.* **121**, 147–150.

Bendotti, C. and Samanin, R. (1987). The role of putative 5-HT$_{1A}$ and 5-HT$_{1B}$ receptors in the control of feeding in rats. *Life Sci.* **41**, 635–642.

Blandina, P., Goldfarb, J., Walcott, J. and Green, J. P. (1991). Serotonergic modulation of the release of endogenous norepinephrine from rat hypothalamic slices. *J. Pharmacol. Exp. Ther.* **256**, 341–347.

Blundell, J. E. (1986). Serotonin manipulations and the structure of feeding. *Appetite* **7** (supplement), 39–56.

Blundell, J. E. (1992). Serotonin and the biology of feeding. *Am. J. Clin. Nutr.* **55**, 155S–159S.

Chafetz, M. D., Parko, K., Diaz, S. and Leibowitz, S. F. (1986). Relationships between medial hypothalamic α_2 receptor binding, norepinephrine and circulating glucose. *Brain Res.* **384**, 404–408.

Clifton, P. G., Barnfield, A. M. and Philcox, L. (1989). A behavioural profile of fluoxetine-induced anorexia. *Psychopharmacology* **97**, 89–95.

Coscina, D. V. and de Rooy, E. C. H. (1992). Effects of intracisternal *vs.* intrahypothalamic 5,7-DHT on feeding elicited by hypothalamic infusion of noradrenaline. *Brain Res.* **597**, 310–320.

Coscina, D. V. and de Rooy, E. C. H. (1993). Lack of synergistic feeding enhancement by systemic clonidine and 8-OH-DPAT. *Pharmacol. Biochem. Behav.* **44**, 777–781.

Coscina, D. V., Feifel, D., Nobrega, J. N. and Currie, P. J. (1994). Intraventricular but not intraparaventricular nucleus metergoline elicits feeding in satiated rats. *Am. J. Physiol.* **266**, R1562–R1567.

Currie, P. J. (1993). Differential effects of NE, CLON and 5-HT on feeding and macronutrient selection in genetically obese (*ob/ob*) and lean mice. *Brain Res. Bull.* **32**, 133–142.

Currie, P. J. and Coscina, D. V. (1993a). Diurnal variations in the feeding response to 8-OH-DPAT injected into the dorsal or median raphe. *NeuroReport* **4**, 1105–1107.

Currie, P. J. and Coscina, D. V. (1993b). Paraventricular nucleus injections of idazoxan block feeding induced by paraventricular nucleus norepinephrine but not intraraphe 8-hydroxy-2-(di-*n*-propylamino)tetralin. *Brain Res.* **627**, 153–158.

Currie, P. J. and Coscina, D. V. (1994). Effects of metergoline on feeding, 5-HT anorexia and 5-HT inhibition of NE-induced eating. *Int. J. Obes.* **18** (supplement 2), 71.

Currie, P. J. and Wilson, L. M. (1991). Bidirectional effects of clonidine on carbohydrate intake in genetically obese (*ob/ob*) mice. *Pharmacol. Biochem. Behav.* **38**, 177–184.

Currie, P. J. and Wilson, L. M. (1992a). Central injection of 5-hydroxytryptamine reduces food intake in obese and lean mice. *NeuroReport* **3**, 59–61.

Currie, P. J. and Wilson, L. M. (1992b). Yohimbine attenuates clonidine-induced feeding and macronutrient selection in genetically obese (*ob/ob*) mice. *Pharmacol. Biochem. Behav.* **43**, 1039–1046.

Currie, P. J. and Wilson, L. M. (1993). Potentiation of dark onset feeding in genetically obese (genotype *ob/ob*) mice following central injection of norepinephrine and clonidine. *Eur. J. Pharmacol.* **232**, 227–234.

Currie, P. J., Fletcher, P. J. and Coscina, D. V. (1994). Administration of 8-OH-DPAT into the midbrain raphe nuclei: effects on medial hypothalamic NE-induced feeding. *Am. J. Physiol.* **266**, R1645–R1651.

Curzon, G. (1990). Serotonin and appetite. *Ann. N.Y. Acad. Sci.* **600**, 521–531.

de Rooy, E. C. H. and Coscina, D. V. (1990). Effects of 8-OH-DPAT on the feeding induced by hypothalamic NE infusion. *Pharmacol. Biochem. Behav.* **36**, 937–943.

Dourish, C. T. (1992). 5-HT receptor subtypes and feeding behaviour. *Advances in the Biosciences* **85**, 179–202.

Dourish, C. T., Hutson, P. H. and Curzon, G. (1985). Low doses of the putative serotonin agonist 8-hydroxy-2-(di-*n*-propylamino)tetralin (8-OH-DPAT) elicit feeding in the rat. *Psychopharmacology* **86**, 197–204.

Dourish, C. T., Clark, M. L., Fletcher, A. and Iversen, S. D. (1989). Evidence that blockade of post-synaptic 5-HT$_1$ receptors elicits feeding in satiated rats. *Psychopharmacology* **97**, 54–58.

Faradji, H., Despuglio, R. and Jouvet, M. (1983). Voltametric measurements of 5-hydroxyindole compounds in the suprachiasmatic nuclei: circadian fluctuations. *Brain Res.* **279**, 111–119.

Fletcher, P. J. (1988). Increased food intake in satiated rats induced by the 5-HT antagonists methysergide, metergoline and ritanserin. *Psychopharmacology* **96**, 237–242.

Fletcher, P. J. (1991). Dopamine receptor blockade in the nucleus accumbens or caudate nucleus differentially affects feeding induced by 8-OH-DPAT injected into dorsal or median raphe. *Brain Res.* **552**, 181–189.

Fletcher, P. J. and Burton, M. J. (1986). Microstructural analysis of the anorectic action of peripherally administered 5-HT. *Pharmacol. Biochem. Behav.* **24**, 1133–1136.

Fletcher, P. J. and Coscina, D. V. (1993). Injecting 5-HT into the PVN does not prevent feeding induced by injecting 8-OH-DPAT into the raphe. *Pharmacol. Biochem. Behav.* **46**, 487–491.

Fletcher, P. J. and Davies, M. (1990). A pharmacological analysis of the eating response induced by 8-OH-DPAT injected into the dorsal raphe nucleus reveals the involvement of dopaminergic mechanisms. *Psychopharmacology* **100**, 188–194.

Fletcher, P. J. and Paterson, I. A. (1989a). A comparison of the effects of tryptamine and 5-hydroxytryptamine on feeding following injection into the paraventricular nucleus of the hypothalamus. *Pharmacol. Biochem. Behav.* **32**, 907–911.

Fletcher, P. J. and Paterson, I. A. (1989b). *m*-Octopamine injected into the paraventricular nucleus induces eating in rats: a comparison with noradrenaline-induced eating. *Br. J. Pharmacol.* **97**, 483–489.

Fletcher, P. J., Ming, Z.-H., Zack, M. H. and Coscina, D. V. (1992). A comparison of the effects of the 5-HT$_1$ agonists TFMPP and RU 24969 on feeding following peripheral or medial hypothalamic injection. *Brain Res.* **580**, 265–272.

Fletcher, P. J., Currie, P. J., Chambers, J. W. and Coscina, D. V. (1993). Radio-frequency lesions of the PVN fail to modify the effects of serotonergic drugs on food intake. *Brain Res.* **630**, 1–9.

Fuller, R. W. (1994). Uptake inhibitors increase extracellular serotonin concentration measured by brain microdialysis. *Life Sci.* **55**, 163–167.

Fuller, R. W., Hemrick-Luecke, S. K. and Snoddy, H. D. (1994). Fluoxetine at anorectic doses does not have properties of a dopamine uptake inhibitor. *J. Neural Transm.* **92**, 165–177.

Garattini, S., Caccia, S., Mennini, T. and Samanin, R. (1990). Serotonin transmission and food intake. In *Serotonin: From Cell Biology to Pharmacology and Therapeutics* (R. Paoletti, ed.), pp. 193–202. Kluwer Academic Publishers, Dordrecht.

Goldman, C., Marino, L. and Leibowitz, S. F. (1985). Postsynaptic α_2-noradrenergic receptors in the paraventricular nucleus mediate feeding induced by paraventricular nucleus injection of norepinephrine and clonidine. *Eur. J. Pharmacol.* **115**, 11–19.

Hajnal, A. Czurko, A., Thornton, S. N., Karadi, Z., Sandor, P., Nicolaidis, S. and Lenard, L. (1993). Feeding deficits after unilateral ibotenate lesion of the rat paraventricular nucleus of the hypothalamus. *Appetite* **21**, 181.

Hermes, M. L. J. and Renaud, L. P. (1993). Differential responses of identified rat hypothalamic paraventricular neurons to suprachiasmatic nucleus stimulation. *Neuroscience* **56**, 823–832.

Hery, M., Faudon, M., Dusticier, G. and Hery, F. (1982). Daily variations in serotonin metabolism in the suprachiasmatic nucleus of the rat: influence of oestradiol impregnation. *J. Endocrinol.* **94**, 157–166.

Hjorth, S. (1992). Functional differences between ascending 5-HT systems. *Advances in the Biosciences* **85**, 203–218.

Hoebel, B. G. (1985). Brain neurotransmitters in food and drug reward. *Am. J. Clin. Nutr.* **42**, 1133–1150.

Hutson, P. H., Donohoe, T. P. and Curzon, G. (1988). Infusion of the 5-hydroxytryptamine agonists RU 24969 and TFMPP into the paraventricular nucleus of the hypothalamus causes hypophagia. *Psychopharmacology* **97**, 550–552.

Inenaga, K., Dyball, R. E. J., Okuya, S. and Yamashita, H. (1986). Characterization of hypothalamic noradrenaline receptors in the supraoptic nucleus and periventricular region of the paraventricular nucleus of mice *in vivo*. *Brain Res.* **369**, 37–47.

Jhanwar-Uniyal, M., Roland, C. R. and Leibowitz, S. F. (1986). Diurnal rhythm of α_2-noradrenergic receptors in the paraventricular nucleus and other brain areas: relation to circulating corticosterone and feeding behavior. *Life Sci.* **38**, 473–482.

Jhanwar-Uniyal, M., Darwish, M., Levin, B. E. and Leibowitz, S. F. (1987). Alterations in catecholamine levels and turnover in discrete brain areas after food deprivation. *Pharmacol. Biochem. Behav.* **26**, 271–275.

Jhanwar-Uniyal, M., Papamichael, M. J. and Leibowitz, S. F. (1988). Glucose-dependent changes in α_2-noradrenergic receptors in hypothalamic nuclei. *Physiol. Behav.* **44**, 611–617.

Kennett, G. A. and Curzon, G. (1988). Evidence that hypophagia induced by mCPP and TFMPP requires 5-HT$_{1C}$ and 5-HT$_{1B}$ receptors; hypophagia induced by RU 24969 only requires 5-HT$_{1B}$ receptors. *Psychopharmacology* **96**, 93–100.

Koulu, M., Huupponen, R., Hanninen, H., Pesonen, U., Rouru, J. and Seppala, T. (1990). Hypothalamic neurochemistry and feeding behavioral responses to clonidine, an alpha-2-agonist, and to trifluoromethylphenylpiperazine, a putative 5-hydroxytryptamine-1B agonist, in genetically obese Zucker rats. *Neuroendocrinology* **52**, 503–510.

Leibowitz, S. F. (1978). Adrenergic stimulation of the paraventricular nucleus and its effects on ingestive behavior as a function of drug dose and time of injection in the light–dark cycle. *Brain Res. Bull.* **3**, 357–363.

Leibowitz, S. F. (1986). Brain monoamines and peptides: role in the control of eating behavior. *Fed. Proc.* **45**, 1396–1403.

Leibowitz, S. F. (1988). Hypothalamic paraventricular nucleus: interaction between α_2-noradrenergic system and circulating hormones and nutrients in relation to energy balance. *Neurosci. Biobehav. Rev.* **12**, 101–109.

Leibowitz, S. F. (1990). The role of serotonin in eating disorders. *Drugs* **39 (supplement 3)**, 33–48.

Leibowitz, S. F. (1992). Neurochemical–neuroendocrine systems in the brain controlling macronutrient intake and metabolism. *Trends Neurosci.* **15**, 491–497.

Leibowitz, S. F. and Brown, L. L. (1980). Histochemical and pharmacological analysis of noradrenergic projections to the paraventricular hypothalamus in relation to feeding stimulation. *Brain Res.* **201**, 289–314.

Leibowitz, S. F. and Jhanwar-Uniyal, M. (1989). 5-HT$_{1A}$ and 5-HT$_{1B}$ receptor binding sites in discrete hypothalamic nuclei: relation to feeding. *Soc. Neurosci. Abstr.* **15**, 655.

Leibowitz, S. F., Hammer, N. J. and Chang, K. (1981). Hypothalamic paraventricular nucleus lesions produce overeating and obesity in the rat. *Physiol. Behav.* **27**, 1031–1040.

Leibowitz, S. F., Hammer, N. J. and Chang, K. (1983). Feeding behavior induced by central norepinephrine injection is attenuated by discrete hypothalamic paraventricular nucleus lesions. *Pharmacol. Biochem. Behav.* **19**, 945–950.

Leibowitz, S. F., Roosin, P. and Rosenn, M. (1984). Chronic norepinephrine injection into the paraventricular nucleus produces hyperphagia and increases body weight gain in the rat. *Pharmacol. Biochem. Behav.* **21**, 801–808.

Leibowitz, S. F., Brown, O., Tretter, J. R. and Kirschgessner, A. (1985a). Norepinephrine, clonidine and tricyclic antidepressants selectively stimulate carbohydrate ingestion through noradrenergic system of the paraventricular nucleus. *Pharmacol. Biochem. Behav.* **23**, 541–550.

Leibowitz, S. F., Weiss, G. F., Yee, F. and Tretter, J. R. (1985b). Noradrenergic innervation of the paraventricular nucleus: specific role in control of carbohydrate ingestion. *Brain Res. Bull.* **14**, 561–567.

Leibowitz, S. F., Weiss, G. F. and Shor-Posner, G. (1988). Hypothalamic serotonin: pharmacological, biochemical and behavioral analyses of its feeding-suppressive action. *Clin. Neuropharmacol.* **11**, S51–S71.

Leibowitz, S. F., Weiss, G. F., Walsh, U. A. and Viswanath, D. (1989). Medial hypothalamic serotonin: role in circadian patterns of feeding and macronutrient selection. *Brain Res.* **503**, 132–140.

Leibowitz, S. F. Shor-Posner, G. and Weiss, G. F. (1990a). Serotonin in medial hypothalamic nuclei controls circadian patterns of macronutrient intake. In *Serotonin: From Cell Biology to Pharmacology and Therapeutics* (R. Paoletti, ed.), pp. 203–211. Kluwer Academic Publishers, Dordrecht.

Leibowitz, S. F., Weiss, G. F. and Suh, J. S. (1990b). Medial hypothalamic nuclei mediate serotonin's inhibitory effect on feeding behavior. *Pharmacol. Biochem. Behav.* **37**, 735–742.

Leibowitz, S. F., Alexander, J. T., Cheung, W. K. and Weiss, G. F. (1993a). Effects of serotonin and the serotonin blocker metergoline on meal patterns and macronutrient selection. *Pharmacol. Biochem. Behav.* **45**, 185–194.

Leibowitz, S. F., Shor-Posner, G., Brennan, G. and Alexander, J. T. (1993b). Meal pattern analysis of macronutrient intake after PVN norepinephrine and peripheral clonidine administration. *Obes. Res.* **1**, 29–39.

Lichtenstein, S. S., Marinescu, C. M. and Leibowitz, S. F. (1984). Chronic infusion of norepinephrine and clonidine into the hypothalamic paraventricular nucleus. *Brain Res. Bull.* **13**, 591–595.

Lou, S. and Li, E. T. S. (1992). Effect of 5-HT agonists on rats fed single diets with varying proportions of carbohydrate and protein. *Psychopharmacology* **109**, 212–216.

McCabe, J. T., DeBellis, M. D. and Leibowitz, S. F. (1984). Clonidine-induced feeding: analysis of central sites of action and fiber projections mediating this response. *Brain Res.* **309**, 85–104.

Majeed, N. H., Mohammad, F. K. and Ayoub, R. S. (1991). Stimulation of food intake in rats by the alpha 2-adrenoceptor agonists xylazine and detomidine. *Pharmacol. Res.* **23**, 415–419.

Martin, K. F. and Marsden, C. A. (1985). *In vivo* diurnal variations of 5-HT release in hypothalamic nuclei. In *Circadian Rhythms in the Central Nervous System* (P. H. Redfern, I. C. Campbell, J. A. Davies and K. F. Martin, eds), pp. 81–92. Macmillan Press, London.

Mason, R. (1986). Circadian variation in sensitivity of suprachiasmatic and lateral geniculate neurons to 5-hydroxytryptamine in the rat. *J. Physiol.* **377**, 1–13.

Neill, J. C. and Cooper, S. J. (1989). Evidence that D-fenfluramine anorexia is mediated by 5-HT₁ receptors. *Psychopharmacology* **97**, 213–218.

Paez, X., Stanley, B. G. and Leibowitz, S. F. (1993). Microdialysis analysis of norepinephrine levels in the paraventricular nucleus in association with food intake at dark onset. *Brain Res.* **606**, 167–170.

Pazos, A. and Palacios, J. M. (1985). Quantitative autoradiographic mapping of serotonin receptors in the rat brain. I. Serotonin-1 receptors. *Brain Res.* **346**, 205–230.

Rockhold, R. W., Acuff, C. G. and Clower, B. R. (1990). Excitotoxic lesions of the paraventricular hypothalamus: metabolic and cardiac effects. *Neuropharmacology* **29**, 663–673.

Rogacki, N., Weiss, G. F., Fueg, A., Suh, J. S., Pal, S. and Leibowitz, S. F. (1989). Impact of hypothalamic serotonin on macronutrient intake. *Ann. N. Y. Acad. Sci.* **575**, 619–621.

Roland, C. R., Oppenheimer, R. L., Chang, K. and Leibowitz, S. F. (1985). Hypophysectomy disturbs noradrenergic feeding system of the paraventricular nucleus. *Psychoneuroendocrinology* **10**, 109–120.

Roland, C. R., Bhakthavatsalam, P. and Leibowitz, S. F. (1986). Interaction between corticosterone and alpha-2-noradrenergic system of the paraventricular nucleus in relation to feeding behavior. *Neuroendocrinology* **42**, 296–305.

Rowland, N. and Carlton, J. (1986). Neurobiology of an anorectic drug: fenfluramine. *Prog. Neurobiol.* **27**, 13–62.

Samanin, R. and Garattini, S. (1989). Serotonin and the pharmacology of eating disorders. *Ann. N. Y. Acad. Sci.* **575**, 194–208.

Sanger, D. J. (1983). An analysis of the effects of systemically administered clonidine on the food and water intake of rats. *Br. J. Pharmacol.* **78**, 159–164.

Sawchenko, P. E., Gold, R. M. and Leibowitz, S. F. (1981). Evidence for vagal involvement in the eating elicited by adrenergic stimulation of the paraventricular nucleus. *Brain Res.* **225**, 249–269.

Sawchenko, P. E., Swanson, L. W., Steinbusch, H. W. M. and Verhofsted, A. A. J. (1983). The distribution of cells of origin of serotonergic input to the paraventricular and supraoptic nuclei of the rat. *Brain Res.* **277**, 355–360.

Schwartz, D. H., Hernandez, L. and Hoebel, B. G. (1990). Serotonin release in lateral and medial hypothalamus during feeding and its anticipation. *Brain Res. Bull.* **25**, 797–802.

Shor-Posner, G., Azar, A. P., Jhanwar-Uniyal, M., Filart, R. and Leibowitz, S. F. (1986a). Destruction of noradrenergic innervation to the paraventricular nucleus: deficits in food intake, macronutrient selection, and compensatory eating after food deprivation. *Pharmacol. Biochem. Behav.* **25**, 381–392.

Shor-Posner, G., Grinker, J. A., Marinescu, C., Brown, O. and Leibowitz, S. F. (1986b). Hypothalamic serotonin in the control of meal patterns and macronutrient selection. *Brain Res. Bull.* **17**, 663–671.

Shor-Posner, G., Azar, A. P., Volpe, M., Grinker, J. A. and Leibowitz, S. F. (1988). Clonidine hyperphagia: neuroanatomical substrates and specific function. *Pharmacol. Biochem. Behav.* **30**, 925–932.

Stanley, B. G., Schwartz, D. H., Hernandez, L., Hoebel, B. G. and Leibowitz, S. F. (1989a). Patterns of extracellular norepinephrine in the paraventricular hypothalamus: relation to circadian rhythm and deprivation-induced eating behavior. *Life Sci.* **45**, 275–282.

Stanley, B. G., Schwartz, D. H., Hernandez, L., Leibowitz, S. F. and Hoebel, B. G.

(1989b). Patterns of extracellular 5-hydroxyindoleacetic acid (5-HIAA) in the paraventricular hypothalamus (PVN): relation to circadian rhythm and deprivation-induced eating behavior. *Pharmacol. Biochem. Behav.* **33**, 257–260.

Steinbusch, H. W. M. (1981). Distribution of serotonin-immunoreactivity in the central nervous system of the rat-cell bodies and terminals. *Neuroscience* **6**, 557–618.

Sugrue, M. F. (1987). Neuropharmacology of drugs affecting food intake. *Pharmacol. Ther.* **32**, 145–182.

Tempel, D. L. and Leibowitz, S. F. (1990). Diurnal variations in the feeding responses to norepinephrine, neuropeptide Y and galanin in the PVN. *Brain Res. Bull.* **25**, 821–825.

Tempel, D. L., Shor-Posner, G., Dwyer, D. and Leibowitz, S. F. (1989). Nocturnal patterns of macronutrient intake in freely feeding and food-deprived rats. *Am. J. Physiol.* **256**, R541–R548.

Tian, Y., Eaton, M. J., Goudreau, J. L., Lookingland, K. L. and Moore, K. E. (1993). Neurochemical evidence that 5-hydroxytryptaminergic neurons tonically inhibit noradrenergic neurons terminating in the hypothalamus. *Brain Res.* **607**, 215–221.

Touzani, K. and Velley, L. (1992). Ibotenic acid lesion of the hypothalamic paraventricular nucleus produces weight gain but modifies neither preference nor aversion for saccharin. *Physiol. Behav.* **52**, 673–678.

U'Prichard, D. C. (1981). ^{3}H-clonidine and ^{3}H-p-aminoclonidine interactions *in vitro* with central and peripheral α-2-adrenergic receptors. In *Psychopharmacology of Clonidine* (H. Lal and S. Fiedling, eds), pp. 53–74. Alan R. Liss, New York.

Weiss, G. F. and Leibowitz, S. F. (1985). Efferent projections from the paraventricular nucleus mediating α_2-noradrenergic feeding. *Brain Res.* **347**, 225–238.

Weiss, G. F., Papadakos, P., Knudson, K. and Leibowitz, S. F. (1986). Medial hypothalamic serotonin: effects on deprivation and norepinephrine-induced eating. *Pharmacol. Biochem. Behav.* **25**, 1223–1230.

Weiss, G. F., Rogacki, N., Fueg, A., Buchen, D. and Leibowitz, S. F. (1990). Impact of hypothalamic D-norfenfluramine and peripheral D-fenfluramine injection on macronutrient intake in the rat. *Brain Res. Bull.* **25**, 849–859.

Weiss, G. F., Rogacki, N., Fueg, A., Buchen, D., Suh, J. S., Wong, D. T. and Leibowitz, S. F. (1991). Effect of hypothalamic and peripheral fluoxetine injection on natural patterns of macronutrient intake in the rat. *Psychopharmacology* **105**, 467–476.

Wellman, P. J. (1992). Overview of adrenergic anorectic agents. *Am. J. Clin. Nutr.* **55**, 193S–198S.

Wellman, P. J. and Davies, B. T. (1990). Effects of paraventricular hypothalamic microinjecctions of phenylpropanolamine and D-amphetamine on mash intake in rats. *Brain Res. Bull.* **25**, 335–338.

Wellman, P. J. and Davies, B. T. (1991). Suppression of feeding induced by phenylephrine microinjections within the paraventricular hypothalamus in rats. *Appetite* **17**, 121–128.

Wellman, P. J., Davies, B. T., Morien, A. and McMahon, L. (1993). Modulation of feeding by hypothalamic paraventricular nucleus α_1- and α_2-adrenergic receptors. *Life Sci.* **53**, 669–679.

Wong, D. T., Reid, L. R. and Threlkeld, P. G. (1988). Suppression of food intake in rats by fluoxetine: comparison of enantiomers and effects of serotonin antagonists. *Pharmacol. Biochem. Behav.* **31**, 475–479.

Zhang, T. X. and Ciriello, J. (1985). Kainic acid lesions of the paraventricular nucleus reverse the elevated arterial pressure after aortic baroreceptor denervation in the rat. *Brain Res.* **358**, 334–338.

14

Glutamate and its Receptors in Lateral Hypothalamic Stimulation of Eating

B. GLENN STANLEY

Departments of Psychology and Neuroscience, University of
California, Riverside, CA 92521, USA

1 Goals and hypothesis

We have recently shown that glutamate injected into the lateral hypothalamus
(LH) elicits a robust feeding response in satiated rats (Stanley *et al.*, 1993a,b).
Conversely, injection of some glutamate receptor antagonists into the LH
produce the opposite effect, suppressing natural feeding and, when administered repeatedly, reducing body weight gain (Stanley *et al.*, in press). The
primary purpose of this chapter is to review these data and integrate them into a
hypothesis which begins to address mechanisms of action of glutamate and its
roles in the control of feeding behaviour. In brief, it is proposed that glutamate
acts via several types of glutamate receptor, including the NMDA (*N*-methyl-
D-aspartic acid) subtype, to excite LH neurons, which form a part of the
neurocircuitry controlling feeding behaviour. This emphasizes an important
role for glutamate in the LH in the neurophysiological control of feeding
behaviour and body weight regulation.

Our research was inspired by two main sources of evidence. The first
suggests that LH neurons play a part in the initiation of eating, while the second
indicates that glutamate is the principal excitatory neurotransmitter affecting
hypothalamic neurons. These sources are reviewed below.

2 The lateral hypothalamus and feeding behaviour

That LH neurons might participate in the regulation of eating behaviour and
body weight was first suggested by Anand and Brobeck (1951), who showed
that lesions within the LH resulted in dramatically reduced eating and in loss of
body weight in rats and cats. Shortly thereafter Delgado and Anand (1953)
reported a complementary finding, demonstrating that intense eating could be
elicited by electrical stimulation in the LH through chronically implanted

DRUG RECEPTOR SUBTYPES AND INGESTIVE BEHAVIOUR
ISBN 0-12-187620-9

electrodes. In work that initially appeared to support this, Grossman (1960) showed that LH application of the neurotransmitters noradrenaline or adrenaline may elicit eating in satiated animals. Finally, electrophysiological studies demonstrated that the unit activity of some LH neurons is sensitive to circulating levels of metabolic fuels, such as glucose (Anand et al., 1964) and that the activity of many of these neurons increases while animals are eating (Oomura et al., 1969). Collectively, these findings gave rise to the idea that eating behaviour was naturally triggered by heightened activity of LH neurons. Research in this area flourished for approximately two decades, largely guided by the dual-centre hypothesis of Stellar (1954).

This period ended in 1971, when two studies cast doubt on the role of the LH in feeding. In one study Marshall et al. (1971) showed that rats lesioned in the LH exhibited profound sensory neglect and motor impairments. It was suggested that the sensorimotor neglect rather than loss of a 'feeding centre' might be the major cause of the reduced eating in the LH-lesioned rats. In the other study, Ungerstedt (1971) showed that destruction of nigrostriatal dopamine neurons, which traverse the LH and points lateral, produced aphagia and body weight loss. He suggested that LH lesions might produce their effects by destruction of this pathway, rather than by destruction of neurons originating within the LH. Further doubt was cast by studies relocalizing the feeding-stimulatory effects of noradrenaline. Leibowitz (1970, 1978b) showed in extensive cannula-mapping studies that this effect was actually due to the action of noradrenaline in medial hypothalamic structures, particularly the paraventricular nucleus (PVN), not to its actions in the LH. Additionally, the significance of the eating elicited by electrical stimulation in the LH was questioned by Valenstein et al. (1970), who pointed out that LH electrodes that elicited eating could frequently yield other motivated behaviours, such as drinking or gnawing. They suggested that the elicited behaviours result from a generalized enhancement in motivational state, rather than the stimulation of neurons specific to a particular behaviour. With much of the original data suspect, many investigators questioned whether LH neurons had any role in feeding control. As a result, there has been considerable skepticism about a role for LH neurons in the control of eating behaviour, and behavioural research in this area has languished for over 20 years.

Nevertheless, numerous findings still support a role for LH neurons in the initiation of feeding. If the effectiveness of LH lesions in reducing eating was an artifact of interrupted fibres of passage, then lesions that destroyed cell bodies in the LH but spared fibres of passage should be relatively ineffective. However, numerous studies (Grossman et al., 1978; Stricker et al., 1978; Grossman and Grossman, 1982; Winn et al., 1990) have shown that LH lesions generated by injections of cytotoxins do indeed reduce eating behaviour and produce body weight loss even though they spare fibres of passage. Furthermore, animals given cytotoxic LH lesions do not exhibit significant sensorimotor deficits (Dunnett et al., 1985). These findings argue that neurons originating within the LH do contribute to the control of eating and the regulation of body weight. However, the magnitude and duration of these effects were considerably smaller than those produced by electrolytic lesions, suggesting that the effects of electrolytic lesions result from the combined destruction of LH neurons and fibres of passage.

An important role for LH neurons in eating control has also been consistently supported by numerous electrophysiological studies. For example, the work of Rolls and colleagues identified a population of neurons in primate LH which respond when the animals see food, another population that responds when the animals taste food and yet another that responds to either the sight or taste of food (Mora *et al.*, 1976; Rolls *et al.*, 1980). The specificity of these neural responses is illustrated by the failure of the sight-sensitive neurons to respond when the animals ate food in the dark. The response of LH neurons to food is modulated by hunger; as fasted animals eat to satiety, the neuronal response diminishes and is absent when the animals are completely satiated. Perhaps most interesting is that these LH neurons will *learn* to respond to a neutral object that is paired with food delivery (i.e. the neurons acquire a selective response to a syringe used to deliver oral glucose solutions) (Mora *et al.*, 1976). Across conditions, the response of these LH neurons precedes and predicts that animal's subsequent behavioural response to food, suggesting that they may actually participate in triggering the eating behaviour. Complementing these results, it has been found that some LH neurons are sensitive to olfactory cues (Oomura *et al.*, 1991), that many are directly sensitive to local application of metabolic fuels, such as glucose, and that these neurons also receive relayed information about the peripheral levels of these fuels (Oomura, 1985). More recent studies, chronically recording the unit activity of LH neurons in freely behaving rats, have shown that the majority of these neurons show sensitivity to circadian light–dark cycles, with most exhibiting high levels of activity during the dark phase when the animals normally eat (Ono *et al.*, 1986). Also, approximately 40% of the LH neurons show pronounced increases in activity at the onset of spontaneous meals. Given this rich electrophysiological evidence and the supportive data from LH cytotoxin studies, a balanced view might suggest that LH neurons do play important roles in the stimulation of feeding. However, a major deficiency was that no neurotransmitter has been shown to stimulate eating by acting specifically within the LH.

3 Glutamate as an excitatory neurotransmitter: general background

We suspected that glutamate might perform this function. L-glutamate or glutamic acid is a non-essential amino acid that does not cross the blood–brain barrier but rather is synthesized from a variety of precursors, including glucose and glutamine (Price *et al.*, 1981; Fonnum, 1984). In turn, glutamate participates in many functions: it is a constituent of many peptides and proteins; it participates in intermediary metabolism; it serves as a precursor for γ-aminobutyric acid (GABA) synthesis; and, it is now recognized as the major excitatory neurotransmitter in the mammalian brain (Fonnum, 1984). The multiple functions in which glutamate participates, along with some of its unusual properties as a neurotransmitter, may have resulted in some misconceptions about this nearly ubiquitous amino acid. One of the more cherished notions about neural function has been that neurons respond selectively to particular neurotransmitters. Yet, it has been found that the vast majority of neurons are excited by glutamate application (Curtis et al., 1960; Mayer and Westbrook, 1987b). Consequently, some investigators concluded that this responsiveness was artifactual and that glutamate's lack of specificity made it relatively uninteresting. Perhaps adding to this perception was the evidence that glutamate and most of its receptor agonists are typically neurotoxic at high concentrations (Meldrum and Garthwaite, 1990; Coyle and Puttfarcken, 1993); it might seem counterintuitive that a neurotransmitter could also be a neurotoxin. Nevertheless, accumulating evidence suggests that the ubiquitous responsiveness of neurons to glutamate is not an artifact but rather a reflection of their normal physiology: glutamate appears to stimulate most neurons when applied exogenously, precisely because most neurons express glutamate receptors and apparently receive significant synaptic or extrasynaptic input from endogenous glutamate (Monaghan et al., 1989; van den Pol and Trombley, 1993). As for the neurotoxicity, it is now accepted that endogenous glutamate, when released in unusually high amounts, is indeed neurotoxic. In fact, much of the cell death that is associated with head trauma and stroke is believed to be a result of excess glutamate released by these events (Meldrum and Garthwaite, 1990; Coyle and Puttfarcken, 1993). Convincing evidence now suggests that glutamate is not just a neurotransmitter but may indeed be the primary excitatory neurotransmitter in the mammalian brain. That neurons exhibit ubiquitous sensitivity to glutamate presents some interesting experimental challenges; however, it makes understanding glutamate's functions and mechanisms of action more, not less, important.

Several findings suggested that glutamate might act within the LH as a feeding-stimulatory neurotransmitter. Given that eating can readily be elicited in satiated animals by electrical stimulation in the LH (Delgado and Anand, 1953), this possibility seemed plausible because of glutamate's excitatory effects on most neurons. When applied to the soma or dendrites, glutamate typically causes excitatory postsynaptic potentials (EPSPs) and increases spiking; yet it is ineffective when applied to axons (Goodchild et al., 1982). Therefore, if eating elicited by electrical stimulation of the LH is due to stimulation of cell bodies rather than axons, then glutamate injected into the LH might also elicit eating. In addition to the above were findings suggesting that endogenous glutamate is actually employed by hypothalamic neurons as an excitatory neurotransmitter. Specifically, van den Pol and co-workers used immunohistochemical and electrophysiological procedures to show that *endo-*

genous glutamate exists within synaptic vesicles in the hypothalamus and that, in contrast to the excitatory effect of glutamate receptor *agonists*, glutamate receptor *antagonists* markedly and consistently suppress spontaneous and evoked EPSPs in hypothalamic slice preparations (van den Pol *et al.*, 1990; van den Pol, 1991; van den Pol and Trombley, 1993). The latter finding suggests that endogenous glutamate mediates most excitatory synaptic transmission in the hypothalamus. Taken together with the earlier findings, these data suggested that LH glutamate might act to stimulate neurons in that region to trigger eating behaviour.

4 Glutamate and feeding at sites other than the LH

There were several studies that had already examined aspects of a relationship between glutamate and feeding. Work from Ritter's laboratory has shown that eating behaviour may be stimulated in satiated rats by peripheral injection of high doses of glutamate (Reddy *et al.*, 1986). It was suggested that the locus of this eating stimulatory effect is the area postrema because the blood–brain barrier, which is impermeable to glutamate, does not exist at this site, and because lesions of the area postrema block the eating response elicited by peripherally injected glutamate (Ritter and Stone, 1987). It has also recently been shown that eating may be elicited in the rat by intracerebroventricular injection of glutamate (Stricker-Krongrad *et al.*, 1992), and that a small eating response was elicited in the sheep by ventromedial hypothalamic injection of this excitatory amino acid (Wandji *et al.*, 1989). Since GABA also elicits eating, it was noted that the eating might be due to GABA synthesized from the injected glutamate. In addition to these studies showing that eating may be elicited by injection of glutamate, Wirtshafter and Trifunovic (1988) have shown that eating, drinking and hyperactivity can be elicited by an antagonist of the NMDA glutamate receptor subtype injected into the median raphe.

5 LH glutamate and feeding stimulation: initial results

As an initial test of whether LH glutamate might elicit eating, we injected L-glutamate, in the form of monosodium glutamate, through indwelling guide cannulas directly into the LH of satiated adult male rats and measured their consequent feeding behaviour (Stanley *et al.*, 1993a). As shown in Fig. 1, when compared with the responses after vehicle, animals injected with glutamate exhibited clear dose-dependent feeding. The threshold dose was 300 nmol, and a peak effect was obtained at 900 nmol. At this high dose the animals ate an average of 5.2 g in the hour after injection but did not increase their intake further in the subsequent 3-h period.

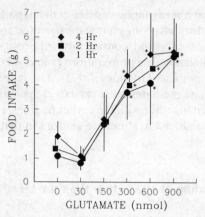

Fig. 1 Mean ± SEM cumulative food intake 1, 2 and 4 h after LH injection of various doses of glutamate or vehicle. *$P < 0.05$ *vs* vehicle at corresponding time (Duncan's multiple range test). From Stanley *et al*. (1993a), with permission.

While these data demonstrating that glutamate can elicit eating when injected into the LH were highly encouraging, the doses required to produce this effect were quite large. By comparison, other feeding-stimulatory neurotransmitters, such as noradrenaline and neuropeptide Y, have threshold doses in the low pmol range and produce peak effects at 235 pmol and 40 nmol, respectively (Leibowitz, 1978a; Stanley and Leibowitz, 1985). Therefore, we were concerned that non-specific membrane or osmotic effects rather than glutamate's receptor binding properties might mediate the eating responses. As an initial test of the chemical specificity, we examined whether LH injection of sodium chloride might also elicit eating. In contrast to glutamate, 300 nmol NaCl produced no effect and 900 nmol elicited a small eating response of 1.8 g, which was considerably smaller than the 5.2-g response produced by the equivalent dose of glutamate. These findings indicate that glutamate's effects in the LH are due to its specific binding to receptors and not to any non-specific effects. Further data supporting this conclusion are discussed below. That still leaves open the question of why such comparatively high doses of glutamate are required to elicit eating in the LH. We do not have an answer to this question, as yet, but speculate that it may be due to the combination of rapid glutamate uptake and the wide distribution of neurons in the LH. Specifically, the LH is a large and relatively cell-poor region, with neurons distributed rather widely. Therefore, the glutamate may need to spread widely to reach effective concentrations at a sufficient number of neurons. This may be particularly difficult for glutamate, because it is taken up rapidly by both neurons and glia (Nicholls and Attwell, 1990), perhaps necessitating the injection of high doses.

6 Glutamate receptor subtypes and eating stimulation

Given that LH injection of glutamate can elicit eating, a logical question is which of its receptor subtypes are involved in mediating the effect. The two currently recognized families of glutamate receptors are the metabotropic and the ionotropic receptors. The metabotropic receptors can produce long-lasting effects on enzyme pathways, gene expression and cellular growth because they activate multiple second-messenger systems via G proteins (Hollmann and Heinemann, 1994). The ionotropic subtypes can produce short (and sometimes long-lasting) effects because they consist of ion channels that permit the flux of cations when opened by glutamate or its receptor agonists. The three major subtypes are called the AMPA receptor, the kainate receptor, and the NMDA receptor, after AMPA (D,L,-α-amino-3-hydroxy-5-methyl-isoxazole propionic acid), kainic acid and NMDA (N-methyl-D-aspartic acid), respectively, the most potent and selective agonist for these subtypes (Watkins et al., 1990). Activation of kainate or AMPA receptors typically produces EPSPs and depolarization of the neuron as Na^+, and in some cases Ca^{2+}, flows into the neurons through the open ion channel (Watkins et al., 1990; Miller, 1991). The NMDA receptor, in contrast, is unique in several ways. For one, at normal resting membrane potentials, the binding of glutamate or NMDA is insufficient to open this channel effectively, in part because the pore is blocked by Mg^{2+}. Instead, the gating of this channel also requires membrane depolarization, which removes the Mg^{2+} (Mayer et al., 1987; Mayer and Westbrook, 1987a). Thus, the NMDA receptor is both ligand and voltage sensitive, requiring both for full activation. Interestingly, to open the NMDA receptor also requires binding by a second ligand, glycine (Johnson and Ascher, 1987). That is, in the absence of glycine, glutamate is completely ineffective in opening the NMDA receptor channel (Kleckner and Dingledine, 1988). Therefore the NMDA receptor acts as a coincidence detector for glutamate, glycine and depolarization. Finally, the NMDA receptor subtype is highly permeable to the Ca^{2+} ion, in addition to Na^+ and K^+, yielding not only depolarization but also increases in intracellular Ca^{2+}, which essentially acts as a second messenger (Mayer et al., 1987).

These characteristics confer Hebbian-like qualities on the NMDA receptor, suggesting its involvement in neural plasticity and neuromodulation. This involvement in various forms of learning and developmental plasticity has been supported by abundant empirical evidence (Kleinschmidt et al., 1987; Collingridge and Singer, 1990; Rabacchi et al., 1992). It may be interesting to note that, in contrast to most other receptors, each of which is apparently expressed by only a small subset of neurons, glutamate receptors are apparently expressed by the vast majority of neurons, perhaps as many as 90%. Further, evidence is beginning to suggest that many neurons typically express multiple subtypes of these receptors, with combinations of the AMPA–kainate, the NMDA and the metabotropic subtypes sometimes coexpressed at a single

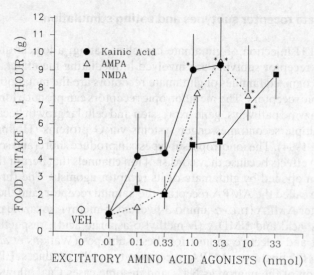

Fig. 2 Mean ± SEM cumulative food intake 1 h after LH injection of kainic acid, AMPA or NMDA. *$P < 0.05$ *vs* vehicle (VEH) (Duncan's multiple range test). From Stanley *et al.* (1993a), with permission.

postsynaptic site (Bekkers and Stevens, 1989; Nusser *et al.*, 1994). As to the functions of these multiple receptor subtypes expressed at single synaptic sites, data suggest that the AMPA–kainate receptors sometimes mediate the initial depolarization of a complex EPSP, while the NMDA receptors more frequently mediate the delayed component of the EPSP (Jones and Baughman, 1988).

As a first step in determining which glutamate receptor subtypes might be involved in LH stimulation of eating, we injected kainic acid, AMPA or NMDA into the LH of three groups of satiated adult male rats and measured the resulting food intake (Stanley *et al.*, 1993a). As shown in Fig. 2, each of these agonists elicited a strong dose-dependent eating response. In contrast to glutamate, each of these agonists was relatively potent, with threshold effects at 0.33 to 1.0 nmol and peak effects at 1–33 nmol. Also, the magnitude of the eating responses was much greater with the agonists. As shown in Fig. 2 (and in later experiments), each of these agonists is capable of inducing rats to eat an average of over 10 g food within 1 h of injection. There were no further increases after that time. As described below, the eating responses consist of a single meal beginning within 2 min of injection, and the magnitude of this effect is one of the largest yet produced by any neurotransmitter or receptor agonist. Additionally, these findings suggest that multiple glutamate receptor subtypes may participate in LH stimulation of feeding behaviour. Consistent with this possibility, receptor autoradiography suggests that each of the ionotropic glutamate receptors exists within the hypothalamus, including the LH (Meeker *et al.*, 1994). More specifically, it is suggested that AMPA and/or kainate receptors, which are sometimes collectively called non-NMDA receptors, participate as well as NMDA receptors. The qualification regarding the AMPA and kainate receptors is based on the relative lack of specificity of AMPA and kainic acid to distinguish between these two subtypes. Thus, it could be that AMPA and kainic acid elicit eating via actions on their respective receptors or, alternatively, it may be that these agonists both elicit eating by acting on only one of these two subtypes. However, the NMDA receptor is likely to participate in eating because NMDA is highly specific for its receptor and neither of the other agonists has much affinity for it (Watkins *et al.*, 1990). A secondary point of these agonist data is that they argue that eating was elicited in the previous experiment by glutamate itself, rather than by GABA to which glutamate can be converted (Fonnum, 1984; Wandjii *et al.*, 1989). This is based on the effectiveness of the glutamate receptor agonists, which are not convertible into GABA.

As noted above, glutamate in high concentrations can be neurotoxic and each of the agonists employed has been shown to be cytotoxic in the LH at some dose (Grossman *et al.*, 1978; Stricker *et al.*, 1978). In fact kainic acid was used as a neurotoxin by Grossman in studies of the LH (Grossman *et al.*, 1978; Grossman and Grossman, 1982), and NMDA was used to lesion LH neurons in the studies by Winn and colleagues (1990). Therefore, we were interested in whether the doses of these compounds that are capable of eliciting eating with injection into the LH might also be lesioning the neurons in this structure. If the agonists are killing the relevant LH neurons, one would predict that only the first injection of an agonist should elicit feeding. To examine this, we tested subjects with glutamate or kainic acid in three consecutive tests separated by 2 days (Stanley *et al.*, 1993a). For both compounds, we found that the feeding response was consistent across tests. For example, on the first test after LH injection of kainic acid (1.0 nmol) the animals ate 9.1 g in 1 h. In the second test the animals ate 8.0 g, while in the final test the subjects ate 9.7 g. Thus, it is clear that the responsiveness of these animals was maintained across repeated application of glutamate and kainic acid, arguing that the neurons survived and, by extension, that the treatments were not neurotoxic. Consistent with this, the doses of kainic acid and NMDA that are sufficient to elicit peak feeding are considerably lower than those that have been used to produce lesions in the LH and other brain areas. Finally, microscopic examination revealed no evidence of neurotoxicity around the injection site.

7 Meal patterns and behavioural specificity

We also wanted to examine the feeding patterns and behavioural specificity of some of these treatments. In particular, we were interested in: (1) whether the animals begin to eat very soon after the injections or following a delay; (2) whether the eating occurs in normally sized meals or in small bouts; (3) if the

Table 1   Patterns of eating following injection of glutamate or kainic acid

	Vehicle (0.3 µl)	Glutamate (600 nmol)	Kainic acid (1.0 nmol)
Latency to eat (min)	25.7 ± 7.9 (18.0)	9.6 ± 4.8* (2.5)	8.0 ± 6.7 (2.0)
Meals eaten	1.0 ± 0.4 (1.0)	0.7 ± 0.2 (1.0)	1.3 ± 0.4 (1.0)
Meal size (g)	1.2 ± 0.6 (0.6)	3.0 ± 1.2 (2.1)	5.1 ± 0.9† (6.0)
Meal duration (min)	2.8 ± 0.8 (2.5)	3.9 ± 0.9 (3.0)	4.2 ± 1.0* (5.0)

Values are mean ± SEM, with median in parentheses.
$P < 0.05$, †$P < 0.01$ vs vehicle (paired t tests). From Stanley et al. (1993a), with permission.

intake occurs in meals, whether there is a single meal or multiple meals; and
(4) whether the effects are specific to eating or the animals also engage in
other behaviours, like drinking or gnawing. To answer these questions we
gave rats LH injections of glutamate at 600 nmol, kainic acid at 1.0 nmol or
vehicle, and observed their eating and behavioral patterns before and for 60
min after these injections (Stanley et al., 1993a). Meal patterns were obtained
by an automated meal-pattern analysis system and the animals' behaviours
were observed and categorized each minute by an observer blind to the
treatment conditions.

As shown in Table 1, rats injected with glutamate or kainic acid typically
began to eat 2–2.5 min after the injection, and they ate a single meal averaging
3.0–5.1 g. These values are typical of rats eating spontaneously. Analysis of
the behavioural observations revealed that all the eating occurred within 10
min of injection and that there was no unusual drinking, gnawing of available
wood blocks, grooming or rearing. For animals injected with glutamate there
was a delayed increase in sleeping, beginning about 50 min after the injection.
As rats normally exhibit increased sleeping after a meal (Antin et al., 1975),
this effect may be secondary to the increased food intake, rather than to a
direct effect of glutamate. For the rats injected with kainic acid the opposite
effect occurred. They actually showed marked behavioural hyperactivity and
increased locomotion, starting 20 min after injection, accompanied by a
decrease in the amount of time spent resting (lying down but not asleep).
Collectively, these findings show that LH injection of glutamate and kainic
acid produces an immediate and intense but transient eating response. The
eating pattern appears normal in that the animals consume food in a single
normally sized meal, following which they engage in postprandial behaviours
typical of rats. Although the effects are not specific to eating, there are no
unusual behaviours and the animals do not engage in other oral or motivated
behaviours. These findings are consistent with glutamate and its agonists
acting on LH neurons involved in feeding stimulation, rather than the eating
being secondary to a general increase in motivational state, or to a non-
specific enhancement of an oral behaviour like gnawing, or to some other

behaviourally non-specific effect. Not surprisingly, given that glutamate and its agonists have excitatory effects on most neurons, other effects are produced, specifically hyperactivity after kainic acid injection. Similarly, we have noted that behavioural hyperactivity is typically exhibited after LH injection of either AMPA or NMDA, and have occasionally seen evidence of seizures (unpublished observations).

8 Site of action

One of the major concerns we had initially was whether or not the injected glutamate and its agonists were eliciting eating by actually acting in the LH, as opposed to acting after diffusion to another brain site, or possibly even after entry into the cerebral ventricles or peripheral circulation. This is not a trivial concern, as studies by Myers and colleagues, examining the fate of centrally injected radiolabelled neurotransmitters, have shown that they may diffuse in significant amounts as much as several millimetres away from the site of injection. Further, significant amounts of label were also found in cerebrospinal fluid and in blood after hypothalamic injection (Myers *et al.*, 1971; Myers and Hoch, 1978). That actions at sites remote from the site of application may affect behaviour is suggested by the evidence that noradrenaline and adrenaline, which were originally reported to elicit eating after application in the LH, were actually producing their eating-stimulatory effects after diffusion to the medial hypothalamus, particularly the PVN (Leibowitz, 1978b). Likewise, injection of angiotensin II, which was originally reported to elicit intense drinking after hypothalamic injection, was later found actually to produce its effect by actions in extrahypothalamic sites (Johnson and Epstein, 1975). These sites were reached by the angiotensin II because much of it refluxed up the outside of the cannula shaft and entered the cerebral ventricles, through which the guide cannulas passed.

For eating elicited by LH injection of glutamate these concerns were heightened by the previously described evidence that peripheral or intracerebroventricular or ventromedial hypothalamic injection of glutamate may elicit eating (Ritter and Stone, 1987; Wandji *et al.*, 1989; Stricker-Krongrad *et al.*, 1992).

To determine whether the LH is an actual locus of action for glutamate and its receptor agonists to elicit eating, we conducted a cannula-mapping study comparing the effectiveness of these compounds in eliciting eating when injected into the LH, as opposed to when injected into a variety of nearby limbic sites (Stanley *et al.*, 1993b). The seven sites tested were: the LH; the anterior LH (ALH); the posterior LH (PLH); the perifornical hypothalamus (PFH), which is just medial to the LH; the PVN, which is slightly more medial; the amygdala (AMY), immediately lateral to the LH; and finally the thalamus (THL), immediately dorsal to the LH. Thus the LH site was bracketed anteriorly, posteriorly, medially, laterally and dorsally by sites that ranged

EATING ELICITED BY GLUTAMATE

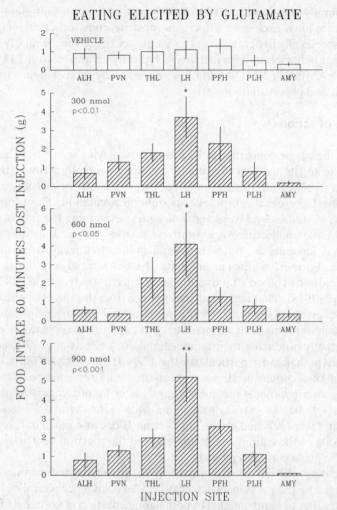

Fig. 3 Mean ± SEM food intake as a function of injection site (ALH, anterior lateral hypothalamus; PVN, paraventricular hypothalamus; THL, thalamus; LH, lateral hypothalamus; PFH, perifornical hypothalamus; PLH, posterior lateral hypothalamus; AMY, amygdala) and dose of glutamate (vehicle is shown in the top panel, with increasing dose in each successive panel). *$P < 0.05$, **$P < 0.01$ vs vehicle (Duncan's multiple range test). The P value beneath the dose in nmol reflects the significant main effect of injection site at that dose, by one-way analysis of variance. From Stanley et al. (1993b), with permission.

from 0.5 to 2 mm from the LH injection site. In one group the animals were injected with vehicle and various doses of glutamate, while the other group was injected in different tests with kainic acid, AMPA and NMDA. Food intake was measured 1 h postinjection.

of the agonists elicited 7–14 g of food intake with injection into the LH. Again, injections into other sites were usually ineffective, with sporadic eating elicited in rare cases with injection into some animals, most commonly those with PFH injection sites.

Collectively, these findings argue that the LH is an actual locus of action for glutamate, NMDA, AMPA and kainic acid in the stimulation of eating behaviour. Conversely, they argue that the elicited feeding was not due to diffusion of glutamate or its receptor agonists to nearby brain sites, to reflux up the cannula track into the cerebral ventricles, or to entry into the peripheral circulation. The argument for action in the LH rather than diffusion to a distant site is based on the ineffectiveness of injections bracketing the LH in all directions. Had a site other than the LH mediated the effect, then this site should have produced the largest response. The argument against reflux into the ventricles is based on the ineffectiveness of injections through cannulas that traversed the ventricles en route to various terminal sites other than the LH. For example, the stereotactic coordinates for the LH and thalamic sites were identical, except that the thalamic coordinates were 1.5 mm dorsal to those in the LH. Thus, the thalamic cannulas penetrated the ventricles at the same point as the LH cannulas but were 1.5 mm closer to the lateral ventricles. Nevertheless, thalamic injections were ineffective. The final argument for a LH, rather than ventricular or peripheral, mode of action is that the doses of glutamate needed to elicit eating with injection into the LH are 50–1000-fold less than those needed with intracerebroventricular or peripheral injection (Wandji *et al.*, 1989; Stricker-Krongrad *et al.*, 1992). It should be noted that the LH may not be the exclusive site of action for glutamate to influence eating behaviour. It is possible that it may also act at sites such as the area postrema to stimulate eating, as suggested by Ritter and Stone (1987), and at midbrain sites such as the medial raphe to inhibit eating, as suggested by Wirtshafter and Trifunovic (1988). While glutamate may act in multiple sites by many modes of action to influence eating, our data suggest that the LH is an important site of action for glutamate to stimulate eating. This is the first neurotransmitter that has been demonstrated to stimulate eating by its action within the LH.

9   Implications for LH neuronal involvement in feeding stimulation

While these data may be significant in various ways, one is that they provide strong support for the once-discredited 'classical' view that LH neurons are critically involved in the initiation of eating. As previously discussed, this theory was questioned because: (1) lesions and electrical stimulation in the LH might have produced their effects via actions on fibres of passage rather than on LH cell bodies. Yet, glutamate and its agonists, which should act on dendrites and cell bodies but not axons, elicit eating specifically by their actions within the LH; (2) lesions and electrical stimulation might produce their effects on feeding by behaviourally non-specific means. Yet, glutamate and its agonists injected into the LH are behaviourally selective in that they elicit intense eating, without stimulating drinking or gnawing of wood blocks. In fact, the only apparent effect of LH glutamate injection was a delayed increase in sleeping. That any neurotransmitter is capable of acting specifically within the LH to elicit eating, and that its effect is receptor mediated and does not generalize to other ingestive behaviours, strongly argues that LH neurons are indeed capable of participating in the control of eating behaviour.

10   Antagonist data suggesting involvement of NMDA receptors

While the demonstrations that eating can be elicited by LH glutamate in an anatomically, behaviourally and receptor-specific manner are important, they do not show that *endogenous* LH glutamate actually participates in the regulation of natural eating. That additionally requires the demonstration that blocking the actions of endogenous glutamate suppresses natural eating under some circumstances. We have begun to address this for glutamate and the NMDA receptor by determining whether LH injection of an NMDA receptor antagonist can suppress natural eating, specifically that occurring at the onset of the nocturnal feeding period and after fasting (Stanley *et al.*, in press). First, we needed to determine whether the eating produced by LH injection of NMDA itself could be suppressed by pretreatment with LH injection of the highly potent and specific NMDA receptor antagonist, D(-)-2-amino-5-phosphonopentanoic acid (D-AP5) (Watkins *et al.*, 1990). We found that pretreatment with D-AP5 produces a dose-related suppression of eating produced by LH injection of NMDA, with 10 nmol suppressing NMDA-elicited eating by at least 70%. In contrast, the eating responses produced by LH injection of either kainic acid or AMPA were unaffected by pretreatment with this dose of D-AP5. There are two major points made by these data. Firstly, that NMDA- but not kainic acid- or AMPA-elicited eating is suppressed by this NMDA receptor antagonist, demonstrates that the NMDA and non-NMDA receptor agonists act via different mechanisms to elicit eating. Specifically, they suggest that eating produced by NMDA is actually due to its action on this receptor subtype rather than to possible cross-over effects. Similarly, that the NMDA receptor antagonist did not suppress eating elicited by kainic acid or AMPA suggests that these agonists actually elicit eating by acting on non-NMDA receptors rather than by possible cross-over effects on NMDA receptors. These antagonist data support the agonist data, with both suggesting that NMDA and non-NMDA glutamate receptors are capable of mediating feeding stimulation. Secondly, because D-AP5 did not suppress eating elicited by either kainic acid or AMPA, there is a strong argument that its reversal of NMDA-elicited eating is behaviourally selective rather than due to possible malaise or other general behavioural effects. This conclusion about behavioural selectivity is strengthened by the similarity of the effects produced by NMDA, AMPA and kainic acid injection. All were injected into the same site, the LH, and all produced eating behaviour of approximately the same magnitude, latency and duration. Yet D-AP5 suppressed NMDA-, but not AMPA- or kainic acid-, elicited eating. Thus, D-AP5 effects are both receptor and behaviourally selective, suggesting that it is a good probe for examining the role of endogenous LH glutamate and NMDA receptors in the control of natural eating.

11 Endogenous LH glutamate, NMDA receptors and natural eating

To examine whether endogenous glutamate and NMDA receptors might participate in the mediation of natural eating behaviour, we first determined whether blocking the actions of endogenous glutamate on the NMDA receptor in the LH with D-AP5 would attenuate eating elicited by either food deprivation or by the onset of the nocturnal eating period (Stanley et al., in press). One group of rats was fasted for 24 h and then given bilateral LH injections of D-AP5 just before refeeding. The other group was not food deprived, but was given bilateral LH injections of D-AP5 just before the onset of the dark phase of the light–dark cycle. It was found that bilateral LH injection of the NMDA receptor antagonist suppressed food deprivation-induced eating by as much as 61%, and eating at the onset of the dark phase of the light–dark cycle by as much as 40%. Given the behavioural selectivity suggested by the previously described lack of effect of D-AP5 on eating elicited by AMPA or kainic acid, these powerful suppressions argue that endogenous LH glutamate and the NMDA receptor participate in the regulation of natural eating. More specifically, these findings suggest that endogenous glutamate released in the LH acts on NMDA receptors to participate in producing both the spontaneous eating that occurs in rats at the onset of the nocturnal eating period and the intense eating that occurs after food deprivation.

12 Endogenous LH glutamate, NMDA receptors and body weight

Given the evidence that LH glutamate and the NMDA receptor may participate in the short-term regulation of feeding behaviour, might they also play a role in the long-term regulation of eating behaviour and body weight? To begin answering this question, we investigated whether blocking the NMDA receptor with repeated LH injections of D-AP5 could suppress daily food intake and body weight gain (Stanley et al., in press). More specifically, 50 nmol D-AP5 or vehicle was injected bilaterally into the LH twice daily for 8 consecutive days, and daily food intake and body weight were measured. The results showed that the LH treatment with D-AP5 reduced daily food intake by 40% or more, and that this suppression was maintained throughout the 8-day test period. The D-AP5 injected group also lost weight rapidly, and had a total body weight loss of

over 50 g during the 8-day test period. The vehicle-injected subjects also
showed some reduced eating and weight loss. However, these were not
apparent until at least 4 days into the test period and were considerably less
than those in the treatment group. Food intake and body weight gain normalized as soon as the antagonist injections were stopped. These findings suggest
that, in addition to a possible role in the short-term regulation of feeding,
endogenous LH glutamate and the NMDA receptor may participate in the
long-term regulation of eating behaviour and body weight control.

13   Conclusions and perspectives

The findings described above collectively suggest the hypothesis that glutamate
acts as a neurotransmitter which influences the activity of LH neurons that
participate in the expression of natural feeding. The nature of the influence on
these neurons has not been established but it is most likely to be excitatory,
based on glutamate's usual electrophysiological effects. Likewise, there is
accumulating, though not definitive, evidence that the NMDA receptor subtype mediates a portion of glutamate's stimulatory effects on natural feeding.
There is less substantial evidence suggesting that activation of non-NMDA
receptors, perhaps of the AMPA and/or kainate subtypes, may also stimulate
feeding. While these receptors would seem likely to participate in natural
feeding, there is no evidence yet on this point. Further, evidence suggests that
LH glutamate and the NMDA receptor participate in the regulation of body
weight. If true, manipulations of this system might prove to be therapeutically
useful.

Given the evidence for involvement of LH glutamate in natural feeding, in
which specific aspects of eating might it participate, and what might be the
mechanisms of its effects? A problem in answering these questions is that this
area of research is in its infancy and there are few data from which to derive
answers. For example, the origins of glutamatergic neurons terminating in the
LH are unknown. Likewise, there are no data on the release patterns of
endogenous glutamate in the LH; thus it is not known whether glutamate
release actually increases in association with food deprivation, the onset of the
nocturnal eating period, or with spontaneous meals. Further, there is little
evidence on the contributions of non-NMDA receptors to natural eating, and
no evidence on whether or not the metabotropic glutamate receptors participate in eating stimulation. These and many other questions need to be resolved
before the roles of LH glutamate in eating control can be established in detail
and with confidence. Nevertheless, as discussed previously, it may be note-
worthy that behaviourally relevant forms of plasticity are exhibited by LH
neurons and that NMDA receptors participate in mediating neural plasticity in
a wide range of conditions. A most intriguing possibility is that the NMDA
receptors in the LH may mediate some of the neuronal plasticity that is
intimately involved in neurophysiological control of feeding.

Acknowledgement

This work was supported by NIH grant NS24268.

References

Anand, B. K. and Brobeck, J. R. (1951). Hypothalamic control of food intake in rats and cats. *Yale J. Biol. Med.* **24**, 123–140.

Anand, B. K., Chhina, G. S., Sharma, K. N., Dua, S. and Singh, B. (1964). Activity of single neurons in the hypothalamic feeding centers: effects of glucose. *Am. J. Physiol.* **207**, 1146–1154.

Antin, J., Gibbs, J., Holt, J., Young, R. C. and Smith, G. P. (1975). Cholecystokinin elicits the complete behavioral sequence of satiety in rats. *J. Comp. Physiol. Psychol.* **87**, 784–790.

Bekkers, J. M. and Stevens, C. F. (1989). NMDA and non-NMDA receptors are co-localized at individual excitatory synapses in cultured rat hippocampus. *Nature* **341**, 230–233.

Collingridge, G. L. and Singer, W. (1990). Excitatory amino acid receptors and synaptic plasticity. *Trends Pharmacol. Sci.* **11**, 290–296.

Coyle, J. T. and Puttfarcken, P. (1993). Oxidative stress, glutamate, and neurodegenerative disorders. *Science* **262**, 689–695.

Curtis, D. R., Phillis, J. W. and Watkins, J. C. (1960). The excitation of spinal neurones by certain acidic amino acids. *J. Physiol.* **150**, 656–682.

Delgado, J. and Anand, B. K. (1953). Increases in food intake induced by electrical stimulation of the lateral hypothalamus. *Am. J. Physiol.* **172**, 162–168.

Dunnett, S. B., Lane, D. M. and Winn, P. (1985). Ibotenic acid lesions of the lateral hypothalamus: comparison with 6-hydroxydopamine-induced sensorimotor deficits. *Neuroscience* **14**, 509–518.

Fonnum, F. (1984). Glutamate: a neurotransmitter in mammalian brain. *J. Neurochem.* **42**, 1–11.

Goodchild, A. K., Dampney, R. A. L. and Bandler, R. (1982). A method for evoking physiological responses by stimulation of cell bodies, but not axons of passage, within localized regions of the central nervous system. *J. Neurosci. Methods* **6**, 351–363.

Grossman, S. P. (1960). Eating or drinking by direct adrenergic or cholinergic stimulation of the hypothalamus. *Science* **132**, 301–302.

Grossman, S. P. and Grossman, L. (1982). Iontophoretic injections of kainic acid into the rat lateral hypothalamus: effects on ingestive behavior. *Physiol. Behav.* **29**, 553–559.

Grossman, S. P., Dacey, D., Halaris, A. E., Collier, T. and Routtenberg, A. (1978). Aphagia and adipsia after preferential destruction of nerve cell bodies in hypothalamus. *Science* **202**, 537–539.

Hollmann, M. and Heinemann, S. (1994). Cloned glutamate receptors. *Ann. Rev. Neurosci.* **17**, 31–108.

Johnson, A. K. and Epstein, A. N. (1975). The cerebral ventricles as the avenue for the dipsogenic action of intracranial angiotensin. *Brain Res.* **86**, 399–418.

Johnson, J. W. and Ascher, P. (1987). Glycine potentiates the NMDA response in cultured mouse brain neurons. *Nature* **325**, 529–531.

Jones, K. A. and Baughman, R. W. (1988). NMDA- and non-NMDA-receptor components of excitatory synaptic potentials recorded from cells in layer V of rat visual cortex. *J. Neurosci.* **8**, 3522–3534.

Kleckner, N. W. and Dingledine, R. (1988). Requirement for glycine in activation of *N*-methyl-D-aspartate receptors expressed in *Xenopus* oocytes. *Science* **241**, 835–837.

Kleinschmidt, A., Bear, M. F. and Singer, W. (1987). Blockade of 'NMDA' receptors disrupts experience-dependent plasticity of kitten striate cortex. *Science* **238**, 355–358.

Leibowitz, S. F. (1970). Reciprocal hunger-regulating circuits involving alpha- and beta-adrenergic receptors located, respectively, in the ventromedial and lateral hypothalamus. *Proc. Natl. Acad. Sci. USA* **67**, 1063–1070.

Leibowitz, S. F. (1978a). Adrenergic stimulation of the paraventricular nucleus and its effects on ingestive behaviour as a function of drug dose and time of injection in the light–dark cycle. *Brain Res. Bull.* **3**, 357–363.

Leibowitz, S. F. (1978b). Paraventricular nucleus: a primary site mediating adrenergic stimulation of feeding and drinking. *Pharmacol. Biochem. Behav.* **8**, 163–175.

Marshall, J. F., Turner, B. H. and Teitelbaum, P. (1971). Sensory neglect produced by lateral hypothalamic damage. *Science* **174**, 523–525.

Mayer, M. L. and Westbrook, G. L. (1987a). Permeation and block of *N*-methyl-D-aspartic acid receptor channels by divalent cations in mouse central neurons. *J. Physiol.* **394**, 501–527.

Mayer, M. L. and Westbrook, G. L. (1987b). The physiology of excitatory amino acids in the vertebrate central nervous system. *Prog. Neurobiol.* **28**, 197–276.

Mayer, M. L., MacDermott, A. B., Westbrook, G. L., Smith, S. J. and Barker, J. L. (1987). Agonist- and voltage-gated calcium entry in cultured mouse spinal cord neurons under voltage. *J. Neurosci.* **7**, 3230–3244.

Meeker, R. B., Greenwood, R. S. and Hayward, J. N. (1994). Glutamate receptors in the rat hypothalamus and pituitary. *Endocrinology.* **134**, 621–629.

Meldrum, B. and Garthwaite, J. (1990). Excitatory amino acid neurotoxicity and neurodegenerative disease. *Trends Pharmacol. Sci.* **11**, 379–387.

Miller, R. J. (1991). The revenge of the kainate receptor. *Trends Neurosci.* **14**, 477–479.

Monaghan, D. T., Bridges, R. J. and Cotman, C. W. (1989). The excitatory amino acid receptors: their classes, pharmacology and distinct properties in the function of the central nervous system. *Ann. Rev. Pharmacol. Toxicol.* **29**, 365–402.

Mora, F., Rolls, E. T. and Burton, M. J. (1976). Modulation during learning of the responses of neurons in the lateral hypothalamus to the sight of food. *Exp. Neurol.* **53**, 508–519.

Myers, R. D. and Hoch, D. B. (1978). ^{14}C-dopamine microinjected into the brain-stem of the rat: dispersion kinetics, site content and functional dose. *Brain Res. Bull.* **3**, 601–609.

Myers, R. D., Tytell, M., Kawa, A. and Rudy, T. (1971). Micro-injection of ^{3}H-acetylcholine, ^{14}C-serotonin and ^{3}H-norepinephrine into the hypothalamus of the rat: diffusion into tissue and ventricles. *Physiol. Behav.* **7**, 743–751.

Nicholls, D. and Attwell, D. (1990). The release and uptake of excitatory amino acids. *Trends Pharmacol. Sci.* **11**, 462–468.

Nusser, Z., Mulvihill, E., Streit, P. and Somogyi, P. (1994). Subsynaptic segregation of metabotropic and ionotropic glutamate receptors as revealed by immunogold localization. *Neuroscience* **61**, 421–427.

Ono, T., Sasaki, K., Nishino, H., Fukuda, M. and Shibata, R. (1986). Feeding and diurnal related activity of lateral hypothalamic neurons in freely behaving rats. *Brain Res.* **373**, 92–102.

Oomura, Y. (1985). Feeding control through bioassay of body chemistry. *Jpn. J. Physiol.* **35**, 1–19.

Oomura, Y., Ooyama, H., Naka, F., Yamamoto, T., Ono, T. and Kobayashi, N.

(1969). Some stochastical patterns of single unit discharges in the cat hypothalamus under chronic conditions. *Ann. N.Y. Acad. Sci.* **157**, 666–689.

Oomura, Y., Nishino, H., Karadi, Z., Aou, S. and Scott, T. R. (1991). Taste and olfactory modulation of feeding related neurons in behaving monkey. *Physiol. Behav.* **49**, 943–950.

Price, M. T., Olney, J. W., Lowry, O. H. and Bachsbaum, S. (1981). Uptake of exogenous glutamate and aspartate by circumventricular organs but not other regions of brain. *J. Neurochem.* **36**, 1774–1780.

Rabacchi, S., Bailly, Y., Delhaye-Bouchaud, N. and Mariani, J. (1992). Involvement of the N-methyl D-aspartate (NMDA) receptor in synapse elimination during development. *Science* **256**, 1823–1825.

Reddy, V. M., Meharg, S. S. and Ritter, S. (1986). Dose-related stimulation of feeding by systemic injections of monosodium glutamate. *Physiol. Behav.* **38**, 465–469.

Ritter, S. and Stone, S. L. (1987). Area postrema lesions block feeding induced by systemic injections of monosodium glutamate. *Physiol. Behav.* **41**, 21–24.

Rolls, E. T., Burton, M. J. and Mora, F. (1980). Neurophysiological analysis of brain-stimulation reward in the monkey. *Brain Res.* **194**, 339–357.

Stanley, B. G. and Leibowitz, S. F. (1985). Neuropeptide Y injected in the paraventricular hypothalamus: a powerful stimulant of feeding behavior. *Proc. Natl. Acad. Sci. USA* **82**, 3940–3943.

Stanley, B. G., Ha, L. H., Spears, L. C. and Dee, M. G. II (1993a). Lateral hypothalamic injections of glutamate, kainic acid, D,L-α-amino-3-hydroxy-5-methyl-isoxazole propionic acid or N-methyl-D-aspartic acid rapidly elicit intense transient eating in rats. *Brain Res.* **613**, 88–95.

Stanley, B. G., Willett, V. L. III, Donias, H. W., Ha, L. H. and Spears, L. C. (1993b). The lateral hypothalamus: a primary site mediating excitatory amino acid-elicited eating. *Brain Res.* **630**, 41–49.

Stanley, B. G., Willett, V. L. III, Donias, H. W., Dee, M. G. II and Duva, M. A. (1996). Lateral hypothalamic NMDA receptors and glutamate as physiologic mediators of eating and body weight control. *Am. J. Physiol.* (in press).

Stellar, E. (1954). The physiology of motivation. *Psychol. Rev.* **61**, 5–22.

Stricker, E. M., Swerdloff, A. F. and Zigmond, M. J. (1978). Intrahypothalamic injections of kainic acid produce feeding and drinking deficits in rats. *Brain Res.* **158**, 470–473.

Stricker-Krongrad, A., Beck, B., Nicholas, J. P. and Burlet, C. (1992). Central effects of monosodium glutamate on feeding behavior in adult Long-Evans rats. *Pharmacol. Biochem. Behav.* **43**, 881–886.

Ungerstedt, U. (1971). Adipsia and aphagia after 6-hydroxydopamine induced degeneration of the nigro-striatal dopamine system. *Acta Physiol. Scand.* **367**, 95–121.

Valenstein, E. S., Cox, V. C. and Kakolewski J. W. (1970). Re-examination of the role of the hypothalamus in motivation. *Psychol. Rev.* **77**, 16–31.

van den Pol, A. (1991). Glutamate and aspartate immunoreactivity in hypothalamic presynaptic axons. *J. Neurosci.* **11**, 2087–2101.

van den Pol, A. N. and Trombley, P. Q. (1993). Glutamate neurons in hypothalamus regulate excitatory transmission. *J. Neurosci.* **13**, 2829–2836.

van den Pol, A., Wuarin, J.-P. and Dudek, F. E. (1990). Glutamate, the dominant excitatory transmitter in neuroendocrine regulation. *Science* **250**, 1276–1278.

Wandji, S. A., Seoane, J. R., Roberge, A. G., Bedard, L. and Thibault, L. (1989). Effects of intrahypothalamic injections of GABA, muscimol, pentobarbital, and L-glutamic acid on feed intake of satiated sheep. *Can. J. Physiol. Pharmacol.* **67**, 5–9.

Watkins, J. C., Krogsgaard-Larsen, P. and Honore, T. (1990). Structure–activity relationships in the development of excitatory amino acid receptor agonists and competitive antagonists. *Trends Pharmacol. Sci.* **11**, 25–33.

Winn, P., Clark, A., Hastings, M., Clark, J., Latimer, M., Rugg, E. and Brownlee, B. (1990). Excitotoxin lesions of the lateral hypothalamus made by *N*-methyl-D-aspartate in the rat: behavioural, histological and biochemical analyses. *Exp. Brain. Res* **82**, 628–636.

Wirtshafter, D. and Trifunovic, R. (1988). Stimulation of ingestive behaviors following injections of excitatory amino acid antagonists into the median raphe nucleus. *Pharmacol. Biochem. Behav.* **30**, 529–533.

15

The Receptor Basis of Neuropeptide Y-induced Food Intake

ERIC S. CORP

Department of Psychiatry, Cornell University Medical College and The Edward W. Bourne Behavioral Research Laboratory, The New York Hospital–Cornell Medical Center, 21 Bloomingdale Road, White Plains, NY 10605, USA

1 Overview of neuropeptide Y receptor pharmacology

Neuropeptide Y (NPY) and peptide YY (PYY) are structurally similar members of the pancreatic polypeptide (PP) family of peptides (Tatemoto *et al.*, 1982). Defining features of peptides in this family include a hairpin-like folded structure and *C*-terminal amidation. Both of these features are necessary for binding and activity (Fuhlendorff *et al.*, 1990; Schwartz *et al.*, 1990; Wahlestedt *et al.*, 1990). Unlike PP, however, NPY and PYY are potent as agonists in their stimulant effects on feeding when administered centrally (Clark *et al.*, 1984; Morley *et al.*, 1985, 1987; Stanley *et al.*, 1985b; Corp *et al.*, 1990b).

Receptors for NPY and PYY have been classified as one of three subtypes based on physiology, ligand binding and biochemical characteristics. These have been designated NPY-Y_1, -Y_2 and -Y_3 (Grundemar *et al.*, 1993; Wahlestedt *et al.*, 1991; Wahlestedt and Reis, 1993). Of these subtypes, only the NPY-Y_1 receptor has been cloned (Larhammar *et al.*, 1992). All three NPY receptor subtypes are members of the superfamily of G protein-coupled receptors, which typically have seven transmembrane domains of similar structure (Grundemar *et al.*, 1993; Wahlestedt and Reis, 1993).

Characterization of NPY receptors in the brain by Unden and colleagues (1984) followed closely on the isolation of NPY and PYY from porcine tissues by Tatemoto and co-workers (1982). All three NPY receptor subtypes are found in the brain (Inui *et al.*, 1989; Grundemar *et al.*, 1991; Dumont *et al.*, 1992), and in this chapter all three subtypes will be discussed with regard to their possible contribution to NPY-stimulated feeding behaviour.

DRUG RECEPTOR SUBTYPES AND INGESTIVE BEHAVIOUR
ISBN 0-12-187620-9

Table 1 Rank order of potency of NPY-related peptides for NPY receptor subtypes and regional concentrations in rat brain. See text for references.

Receptor	Rank order of potency	Brain localization
Y_1	$PYY \geq NPY \geq Leu^{31}$, $Pro^{34}NPY > NPY2\text{–}36 >>>$ NPY13–36	*High*: cerebral cortex, dentate gyrus, cerebral arteries, thalamus *Low*: hypothalamus, medulla, dorsal pons
Y_2	$PYY > NPY \geq NPY2\text{–}36 >$ NPY13–36 $>>> Leu^{31},Pro^{34}NPY$	*High*: hypothalamus, ventrolateral medulla, dorsal pons *Low*: cerebral cortex
Y_3	$NPY \geq Leu^{31}$, $Pro^{34}NPY > NPY13\text{–}36 >>>$ PYY	*High*: NTS None detected in the forebrain

To a large extent, definition of NPY receptor subtypes has relied on the relative agonist potencies of NPY-related peptides, fragments and analogues in ligand binding and physiological experiments (Fuhlendorff *et al.*, 1990; Grundemar *et al.*, 1993; Wahlestedt and Reis, 1993). Furthermore, central administration of these same agonists has been used to draw inferences on the NPY receptor substrate involved in feeding behaviour (Kalra *et al.*, 1991; Stanley *et al.*, 1992). Table 1 shows the relative potencies of ligands that distinguish each of the three NPY receptor subtypes and where they are concentrated in rat brain.

Throughout this chapter the potency of centrally administered NPY and PYY will be discussed in an attempt to identify the receptor subtypes that mediate their behavioural effects. It is important to note, however, that only modest concentrations of PYY have been detected in brain (Bromme *et al.*, 1985; Ekman *et al.*, 1986). NPY, on the other hand, is abundant in neurons within regions where injections of NPY-related peptides elicit feeding (O'Donohue *et al.*, 1985). This is particularly true in the hypothalamus and strongly suggests that NPY is the natural ligand for NPY receptors in this region (Sawchenko *et al.*, 1985). Small concentrations of PYY have been localized within neurons in the hindbrain, but here too NPY is the more abundant of the two transmitters (Bromme *et al.*, 1985; Ekman *et al.*, 1986).

NPY-Y_1 and -Y_2 receptors recognize their natural ligands, NPY and PYY, with high affinity, and both peptides are full agonists at both receptor subtypes (Grundemar *et al.*, 1993). In ligand binding studies, however, PYY is slightly more potent than NPY at Y_2 receptor binding sites in neural tissue, including rat vagus nerve (Corp and Smith, 1991) and human neuroblastoma cell lines (Wahlestedt *et al.*, 1991). A difference in binding affinities for NPY and PYY is less marked in regions of the central nervous system richly endowed with Y_1 receptors (Corp and McQuade, 1992; Grundemar *et al.*, 1993).

Modification of NPY by truncation and substitutions in the amino acid composition of NPY and PYY has produced agonists with preference or selectivity for differing NPY receptor subtypes (Wahlestedt *et al.*, 1986; Fuhlendorff *et al.*, 1990; Schwartz *et al.*, 1990). Some general properties of the receptor recognition sites can be inferred from binding and functional studies with these fragments and substitutions. One principal feature of NPY-Y$_1$ receptors that distinguishes this subtype from NPY-Y$_2$ receptors is their stringent requirement for integrity of the *N*-terminus for full potency and efficacy (Fuhlendorff *et al.*, 1990). The loss of a single *N*-terminal amino acid (tyrosine to produce NPY2–36) results in significant loss of biological potency and binding affinity at Y$_1$ receptors (Larhammar *et al.*, 1992; Dumont *et al.*, 1993; Grundemar *et al.*, 1993; Wahlestedt and Reis, 1993). *C*-terminal fragments of NPY and PYY, such as NPY18–36, NPY13–36 and PYY13–36, which are active at Y$_2$ receptors are more than 100 times less active at Y$_1$ receptors than native NPY, PYY or the Y$_1$ (and Y$_3$) receptor agonist [Leu^{31},Pro^{34}]NPY (Wahlestedt *et al.*, 1986; Fuhlendorff *et al.*, 1990; Schwartz *et al.*, 1990; Grundemar *et al.*, 1993; Wahlestedt and Reis, 1993).

In the *C*-terminal region, requirements for binding to NPY-Y$_1$ receptors are less stringent. In fact, amino acid substitutions of leucine at position 31 and of proline at position 34 of NPY produce an analogue, [Leu^{31}, Pro^{34}]NPY, that binds with high affinity and activity to NPY-Y$_1$ receptors (Fuhlendorff *et al.*, 1990; Schwartz *et al.*, 1990). [Leu^{31} Pro^{34}]NPY is inactive at NPY-Y$_2$ receptors (Fuhlendorff *et al.*, 1990; Gehlert *et al.*, 1992; Dumont *et al.*, 1993; Larsen *et al.*, 1993).

NPY-Y$_2$ receptors, unlike Y$_1$ receptors, do recognize *C*-terminal fragments of NPY and PYY with nanomolar affinity. Some *C*-terminal fragments with reported activity at NPY-Y$_2$ receptors include NPY2–36, PYY3–36, NPY18–36 and the prototypical Y$_2$ receptor agonists PYY13–36 and NPY13–36 (Wahlestedt *et al.*, 1986, 1991; Quirion *et al.*, 1990; Schwartz *et al.*, 1990; Dumont *et al.*, 1993). In rat brain, binding affinities for these fragments vary depending on the length of the *C*-terminus. NPY2–36 is 5–10 times more potent than NPY13–36 in competing for [^{125}I]PYY binding in regions where binding sites fit a Y$_2$ binding profile (Grundemar *et al.*, 1993; Wahlestedt and Reis, 1993). The possibility that central peptidases may degrade *N*-terminal amino acids of NPY to produce *C*-terminal forms has been suggested by recent studies showing *N*-terminal processing of PYY and NPY by dipeptidyl peptidase IV in human serum (Mentlein *et al.*, 1993) and an abundance of PYY3–36 in extracts from canine colon (Grandt *et al.*, 1992).

NPY-Y$_3$ receptors exhibit high affinity for NPY and very low affinity for PYY (Grundemar *et al.*, 1991; Wahlestedt *et al.*, 1991). This insensitivity to PYY distinguishes Y$_3$ receptors from Y$_1$ and Y$_2$ receptors. Since PYY potently stimulates food intake when administered in the hindbrain or hypothalamus (Morley *et al.*, 1985; Stanley *et al.*, 1985b; Corp *et al.*, 1990b), it seems unlikely that Y$_3$ receptors are involved in the *enhancement* of feeding associated with

NPY-related peptides. The possible influence of NPY-Y_3 on feeding-related behaviour is discussed below. Centrally, Y_3 receptors are found in the region of the nucleus of the solitary tract (NTS), where they are implicated in cardiovascular regulation (Grundemar *et al.*, 1991, 1993).

1.1   *Functional role of NPY receptors in peripheral tissue*

In peripheral tissue, NPY-Y_1 receptors are found at neuroeffector sites in vascular smooth muscle postjunctional to sympathetic nerves where they mediate NPY's vasoconstrictor effects (Lundberg *et al.*, 1982; Wahlestedt *et al.*, 1986, 1987; Larhammar *et al.*, 1992). NPY-Y_2 receptors are present presynaptically in sympathetic neurons which co-localize NPY and noradrenaline. In these sympathetic neurons, Y_2 receptors mediate an inhibitory action of NPY on noradrenaline release (Lundberg *et al.*, 1982; Wahlestedt *et al.*, 1986, 1987). NPY-Y_2 receptors have been found in other peripheral tissue including platelets, kidney and small intestine (Myers *et al.*, 1990; Dumont *et al.*, 1992; Sheikh *et al.*, 1992; Grundemar *et al.*, 1993). NPY-Y_2 receptors are also present in parasympathetic nerves (Stjernquist and Owman, 1990), and Y_2 receptor binding sites have been shown to be axonally transported in the vagus nerve (Corp and Smith, 1991).

But do NPY and PYY receptors in peripheral nerves participate directly in the control of food intake? Recent evidence indicates that peripheral injection of PYY results in expression of c-*fos* in the NTS (Bonaz *et al.*, 1993). Since c-*fos* is a marker of neural activity, and Y_2 binding sites are present on vagus nerve, it is possible that Y_2 receptors on primary vagal afferent may be involved in peripheral–central signalling. There is, however, no evidence supporting a role for peripheral PYY or NPY in the stimulation or control of food intake. In fact, McLaughlin and colleagues (1991) have shown that peripheral injection of NPY fails to affect feeding even at doses 500–1000-fold greater than those delivered centrally.

1.2   *Location of NPY receptors in the brain*

In the brain Y_2 receptors represent perhaps the most abundant subtype and are particularly concentrated in CA1–CA3 of the hippocampus, and in other subcortical regions including the hypothalamus and hindbrain (Corp *et al.*, 1991, Dumont *et al.*, 1992, 1993). NPY-Y_2 receptors have been identified in synaptosomal preparations (Walker and Miller, 1988) and NPY-Y_1 receptors are concentrated in several areas of rat brain including the thalamus, dentate gyrus of the hippocampus, cerebral cortex, and basilar and cerebral arteries and arterioles (Colmers *et al.*, 1991; Corp and McQuade, 1992; Gehlert *et al.*, 1992; Dumont *et al.*, 1993; Larsen *et al.*, 1993). NPY-Y_1 receptors have recently been cloned and Y_1 receptor messenger RNA has been localized in neurons in the arcuate, dorsal medial and paraventricular nuclei of the hypothalamus, and in the cerebral cortex (Larhammar *et al.*, 1992; Larsen *et al.*, 1993). Overall, however, Y_2 receptors are the most abundant subtype in regions such as the hypothalamus and hindbrain where NPY-related peptides act to stimulate feeding (Harfstrand *et al.*, 1986; Nakajima *et al.*, 1986; Dumont *et al.*, 1993). Fig. 1 illustrates the distribution of Y_1 and Y_2 binding sites across a coronal section of forebrain at the level of the hypothalamic paraventricular nucleus (PVN) and also in a section of hindbrain at the level of the pons.

Despite the considerable heterogeneity in the respective distribution of Y_1 and Y_2 receptors, low concentrations of Y_1 receptors can be detected with autoradiographic methods in regions predominantly enriched with Y_2 receptors. In the medial and lateral divisions of hypothalamus, to take an example relevant to feeding, both Y_1 and Y_2 receptor binding sites are distributed diffusely (Gehlert *et al.*, 1992; Corp *et al.*, 1993; Dumont *et al.*, 1993; Larsen *et al.*, 1993) (Fig. 1 and Plate 1).

Additionally, we have found a small and diffuse population of Y_1 receptors within the Y_2 receptor-enriched area of the dorsal pons (Fig. 1 and Plate 2). A population of Y_1 receptors can be resolved in the pontine central grey (CGPn) and adjacent sphenoid nuclei. There is a marked similarity between the profile of agonist binding in the hypothalamus and the profile of agonist binding in these nuclei: Y_1 receptors account for 15–25% while Y_2 receptors account for 75–85% of the saturable $[^{125}I]PYY$ binding sites in both regions (Corp *et al.*, 1990a, 1993; Dumont *et al.*, 1993) (Figs. 3A and 4A). The apparent co-distribution of Y_1 and Y_2 receptors may be of some importance in understanding the receptor basis of feeding behaviour.

2 NPY-induced feeding: forebrain sites of action

Clark and co-workers (1984) were the first to provide evidence that members of the PP family of peptides could stimulate feeding when administered centrally to ovariectomized and intact female rats. Using forebrain ventricular injections, they showed that NPY acted with greater potency than PP, confirming that the receptor mediating the response was distinct from PP receptors. Levine and Morley (1984) demonstrated that the stimulatory effect of NPY on food intake was dose related and long lasting. In non-food-deprived male rats they observed a tenfold increase in total intake that was maximal at 2 h and sustained for 4 h after lateral ventricle injection. In addition to the profound stimulant effect of NPY on feeding, both groups noted that the average latency to initiate eating was long, approximately 20 min after ventricular injection (Clark *et al.*, 1984; Levine and Morley, 1984). The delay to the onset of action may result from slow diffusion of the peptide from the ventricle, across the ependyma to neural sites of action. This hypothesis, however, has not been tested directly.

In the first of a comprehensive set of experiments to specify the locus for NPY's action, Stanley and Leibowitz (1984) showed that injections of NPY into

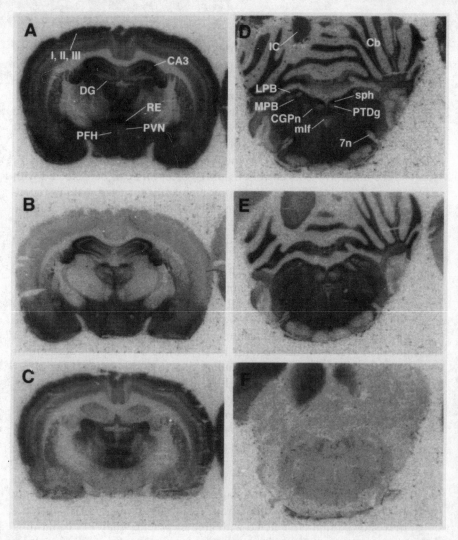

Fig. 1 Film autoradiograms of [^{125}I]PYY binding to coronal sections made through the forebrain at the level of the paraventricular nucleus of the hypothalamus (PVN) and perifornical region (PFH) (A–C), and through the hindbrain at the level of the pons (D–F). (A) and (D) show total [^{125}I]PYY binding (0.04 nM). (B) and (E) reveal optical densities associated with Y_2 receptor binding by inclusion of unlabelled [Leu^{31},Pro^{34}]NPY (30 nM), a Y_1 receptor agonist, with [^{125}I]PYY. (C) and (F) reveal optical densities associated with Y_1 receptor binding by inclusion of unlabelled NPY13–36 (200 nM), a Y_2 receptor agonist, with [^{125}I]PYY. In the forebrain, high levels of Y_2-like receptor binding sites are seen in the hypothalamus and CA3 region of the hippocampus (B). High levels of Y_1 receptor binding are seen in the lamina of the cerebral cortex (I, II and III) dentate gyrus (DG) and the reuniens nucleus of the thalamus (Re), with a low level of Y_1 binding in the PFH (C). In the pons, most NPY receptor binding is of the Y_2 receptor subtype (E). Y_1 binding can be seen in the inferior colliculus (IC) with a smaller concentration in the CGPn and sphenoid nucleus (Sph) (F). Little or no specific [^{125}I]PYY binding is present in the seventh cranial nerve (7n), dorsal pontine tegmental nuclei (PTDg) or medial longitudinal fasciculus (mlf) (D). Other regions in the pons with moderate to high levels of Y_2 binding include the lateral parabrachial nucleus (LPB), medial parabrachial nucleus (MPB) and cerebellum (Cb) (D and E).

the hypothalamic PVN were very potent in stimulating food intake. In rats, the PVN was already well established as a critical site in the regulation of food intake (Stanley, 1993). Follow-up studies indicated that the ventromedial nucleus of the hypothalamus (VMN) was as sensitive as the PVN to NPY, while extrahypothalamic regions were largely insensitive to the orexigenic effects of NPY (Stanley *et al.*, 1985a). Morley and colleagues (1987) confirmed these studies and further demonstrated that injection of NPY into the anterior ventromedial hypothalamus (at the level of the PVN) was more potent and efficacious in eliciting feeding than injection into the posterior ventromedial hypothalamus. Recently, one extrahypothalamic forebrain site has been shown to be sensitive to the effects of NPY on ingestion. McGregor and colleagues (1990) showed that a small dose of NPY injected into the sulcal prefrontal cortex enhanced food intake and produced an increase in the respiratory quotient. Overall, administration of NPY into other forebrain regions in rats, including the globus pallidus, striatum, amygdala and thalamus, did not elicit significant intake (Stanley *et al.*, 1985a; Morley *et al.*, 1987).

Using precise injection of small doses of NPY in nanolitre volumes, Stanley and colleagues (1993) determined that a hypothalamic locus adjacent to the PVN and medial to the fornix is the most sensitive site for NPY-stimulated food intake. This sensitive region, designated the perifornical hypothalamus (PFH), encompasses the caudal extension of anterior hypothalamic nucleus (Paxinos and Watson, 1986). It is perhaps significant that this region of the hypothalamus appears to express a higher density of NPY receptor binding sites than adjacent hypothalamic areas (Fig. 1 and Plate 1). The PFH is richly innervated with NPY immunoreactive fibres (O'Donohue *et al.*, 1985).

2.1 Pharmacology of feeding and NPY receptor subtypes in the PFH

Stanley and co-workers (1985b) have shown that PYY is 2–5 times as potent as NPY in stimulating food intake following PVN injection. Similarly, Morley and colleagues (1985) demonstrated that PYY is more potent than NPY following lateral ventricular infusion. Furthermore, Morley *et al.* (1985) found that PYY produced a larger maximal response than NPY. In contrast to these data, Stanley and colleagues (1985b) demonstrated equivalent maximal effects of NPY and PYY following PVN administration. Although these two data sets differ with regard to maximal response, or efficacy between NPY and PYY, both are consistent in showing that PYY is more potent than NPY when administered in the region of the hypothalamus. It should be noted that Clark and co-workers (1987) found NPY to be slightly more potent than PYY in stimulating food intake after third ventricular administration. Although there is some inconsistency between studies from different laboratories, all reports support the potency of PYY in feeding and thus tend to rule out the direct participation of NPY-Y_3 receptors in NPY-induced feeding behaviour.

Following hypothalamic injection, the Y_1 agonist [Leu^{31},Pro^{34}]NPY

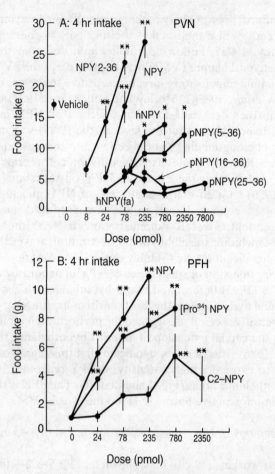

Fig. 2 Dose–effect of NPY-related peptides on total 4-h intake after injection of NPY fragments into the PVN (A) and receptor-selective agonists into the PFH (B). Note the potency of NPY2–36 in relation to NPY (A) and the potencies of [Pro^{34}]NPY and C2-NPY relative to NPY (B). [Pro^{34}]NPY has activity comparable with [Leu^{31},Pro^{34}]NPY at Y_1 receptors. Values are mean ± SEM. *$P < 0.05$, **$P < 0.01$, relative to vehicle. From Stanley et al. (1992), with permission from Elsevier Science Ltd.

stimulates food intake with a potency approaching that of NPY (Stanley et al., 1992). At comparable doses, the prototypical Y_2 receptor agonist NPY13–36 and the related analogue [Cys^2,8-aminooctanoic acid$^{5-24}$, D-Cys^{27}]NPY (C2-NPY) are only weakly potent or impotent in stimulating food intake. Fig. 2 shows the dose–response effects, reported by Stanley and co-workers (1992), for NPY-related peptides after administration into the PVN and PFH. Their results, and similar findings from Kalra and co-workers (1991), strongly suggest that activation of Y_1 receptors in the hypothalamus are involved in NPY's stimulant effect on food intake. Based on the ineffectiveness of short C-terminal fragments, Y_2 receptors have not been considered as important in feeding. This conclusion, however, is tempered by evidence showing that the C-terminal peptide NPY2–36 is more potent in stimulating feeding than NPY or [Leu^{31},Pro^{34}]NPY (Fig. 2) (Kalra *et al.*, 1991; Stanley *et al.*, 1992).

Recall that a stringent requirement of Y_1 receptors for full binding potency is the integrity of the N-terminus (Fuhlendorff *et al.*, 1990; Schwartz *et al.*, 1990). Deletion of the N-terminal tyrosine from NPY creates a ligand with a significant loss of binding potency at Y_1 receptors. At Y_2 receptors, however, NPY2–36 is roughly equipotent with NPY, while NPY13–36 is about 5–10 times less potent than NPY (Grundemar *et al.*, 1993).

Thus, there is an apparent paradox in the relative potencies of NPY-related peptides in feeding and the reported pharmacology of NPY receptors. Based on the selectivity of the Y_1 agonist [Leu^{31},Pro^{34}]NPY and the potency of the C-terminal fragment NPY2–36, Stanley and associates (1992) have proposed that a variant of the Y_1 receptor ([Leu^{31},Pro^{34}]NPY-sensitive and NPY2–36-preferring) may mediate the orexigenic effects of NPY-related peptides. This is an attractive hypothesis for several reasons. The relative potencies of NPY and [Leu^{31},Pro^{34}]NPY at Y_1 receptors is in good agreement with their relative potencies for feeding (Grundemar *et al.*, 1993); and [Leu^{31},Pro^{34}]NPY does not cross-react significantly with Y_2 receptors (Schwartz *et al.*, 1990). Additionally, and consistent with their relative potencies for feeding, NPY2–36 is more potent than [Leu^{31},Pro^{34}]NPY in competing for specific [^{125}I]PYY binding sites in the PFH (Fig. 3A, Plate 1) (Corp *et al.*, 1993).

There is, however, a problem with the hypothesis proposed by Stanley and co-workers (1992). A single receptor exhibiting a pharmacological profile similar to that of feeding elicited by NPY-related peptides has not been characterized in any other system (Dumont *et al.*, 1993; Grundemar *et al.*, 1993). Furthermore, examining the binding potencies of NPY agonists in the PFH, it can be seen that [Leu^{31},Pro^{34}]NPY produces a concentration-dependent inhibition of only a fraction of the sites occupied by [^{125}I]PYY, while NPY2–36 almost completely inhibits [^{125}I]PYY-specific binding (Fig. 3A and Plate 1). This difference in the maximal inhibition produced by NPY2–36 and [Leu^{31},Pro^{34}]NPY suggests the possibility that these two ligands are binding to two or more NPY receptors.

If NPY is acting to stimulate food intake at a single receptor where the relative potencies of NPY2–36 and [Leu^{31},Pro^{34}]NPY are similar (NPY2–36 > [Leu^{31},Pro^{34}]NPY), then blockade or masking of Y_2 receptors in a competitive binding experiment by the inclusion of a high concentration of NPY 13–36 with [^{125}I]PYY should reveal a parallel leftward shift of competitive inhibition curves produced by [Leu^{31},Pro^{34}]NPY and NPY2–36. This parallel shift, however, is not seen (compare Figs 3A and 3B). With Y_2 receptor blockade, the competition curve for [Leu^{31},Pro^{34}]NPY is shifted to the left, compared with that without blockade, and the maximal inhibition produced by

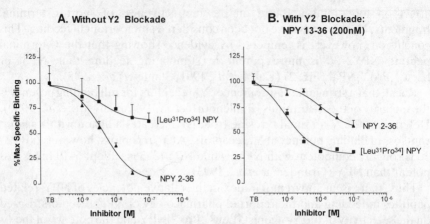

Fig. 3 Competition of specific [^{125}I]PYY binding in the PFH by agonists that are potent in feeding under standard binding conditions (A), and under conditions where Y$_2$ receptors are masked by inclusion of a high concentration of NPY13–36 with the radioligand (B). Data are normalized to the percentage of maximal specific binding (n = 2–4 rats per point in three experiments). Non-specific binding was defined as binding remaining in the presence of NPY2–36 (100 nM) plus [Leu^{31},Pro^{34}]NPY (100 nM) and was typically less than 10% of total binding. Slide-mounted tissues were incubated for 4 h in standard buffer (Corp *et al.*, 1991) containing approximately 0.04 nM [^{125}I]PYY plus inhibitors and blockers.

[Leu^{31},Pro^{34}]NPY is greater than that produced by [Leu^{31},Pro^{34}]NPY without Y$_2$ receptor blockade. On the other hand, the competitive potency of NPY2–36 is reduced under conditions where Y$_2$ receptor binding is masked, particularly at low concentrations (compare Figs 3A and 3B). Accordingly, the competition curve for NPY2–36 is shifted to the right of the curve for [Leu^{31},Pro^{34}]NPY (Fig. 3B). These binding experiments indicate NPY2–36 and [Leu-^{31},Pro^{34}]NPY bind to different NPY–PYY receptor populations in the PFH. Furthermore, under conditions of Y$_2$ receptor blockade, the failure of NPY2–36 to inhibit specific [^{125}I]PYY binding suggests that NPY2–36 is binding principally to Y$_2$ receptors.

Extending this conclusion to the behavioural domain, the results suggest that the feeding potency of NPY2–36 involves a receptor that is distinct from the receptor mediating [Leu^{31}Pro^{34}]NPY's feeding potency. Since blockade of Y$_2$ receptors reduces the binding potency of NPY2–36, the feeding potency of NPY2–36 is most likely mediated by a Y$_2$ receptor. The feeding potency of [Leu^{31},Pro^{34}]NPY is most likely mediated by a Y$_1$ receptor.

A problem with the interpretation that two receptors (one NPY2–36-sensitive and the other [Leu^{31},Pro^{34}]NPY-sensitive) participate in feeding is that the maximal responses produced by [Leu^{31},Pro^{34}]NPY, NPY2–36 and NPY are approximately equal after injection into the PFH (Fig. 2) (Stanley *et al.*, 1992). Since NPY binds to both Y$_1$ and Y$_2$ receptors, it would be predicted that NPY2–36 and [Leu^{31},Pro^{34}]NPY would be only partial agonists for feeding, while NPY and PYY would be fully efficacious. In contrast to the report by Stanley and co-workers (1992), showing equal efficacy between [Leu^{31},Pro^{34}]NPY and NPY2–36, Kalra and colleagues (1991) showed that the maximal response produced by [Leu^{31},Pro^{34}]NPY after PVN injection is significantly less than that elicited by NPY. In the same experiment, however, NPY2–36 was more effective than NPY.

An additional problem with the interpretation that both Y_1 and Y_2 receptors are involved in mediating NPY-induced effects on feeding resides is the failure of prototypical Y_2 receptor ligands such as NPY13–36 or C2-NPY to stimulate more than a marginal feeding response (Fig. 2) (Kalra et al., 1991; Stanley et al., 1992). Because NPY13–36 and C2–NPY are less potent than NPY2–36 at Y_2 receptors, it is possible that their low potency may be responsible for their poor effects in feeding. There may be more than one class of Y_2 receptor. Evidence for the existence of multiple receptors within the Y_2 receptor class is suggested from functional and binding studies. In rat colon, for instance, NPY13–36 is more efficacious than NPY and NPY2–36 in producing contractions (Quirion et al., 1990). In the rat brain, however, the competitive potency of NPY13–36 at [^{125}I]PYY-occupied binding sites is less relative to that of NPY2–36. The relative difference in binding potential can be seen, for example, in the pontine central grey (Fig. 4A).

3   NPY and feeding: hindbrain sites of action

In addition to the PFH, an additional locus for the action of NPY-related agonists in feeding may exist in the hindbrain. We have shown that both NPY and PYY administered into the fourth ventricle stimulate large increases in food intake (Corp et al., 1990b). Steinman and co-workers (1994) demonstrated comparable efficacy of NPY administered into the third or fourth ventricle. Based on evidence that India ink injected into the fourth ventricle does not pass in a retrograde fashion through the cerebral aqueduct into the forebrain ventricles, it appears likely that delivery of NPY-related peptides into the fourth ventricle restricts their distribution to the medullary–pontine–caudal midbrain area.

But where within this broad region do NPY-related peptides act to stimulate feeding? The precise site of action is not yet known. Some direction as to where a site of action may lie can be gained from several lines of evidence. Since PYY acts with a short latency when given into the fourth ventricle (average of 4 min at a maximally effective dose), it is more likely that a site of action for NPY-related peptides lies in the dorsal areas of hindbrain adjacent to the fourth ventricle (Corp et al., 1990b). Furthermore, results from two groups suggest that the hindbrain site is closely associated with pathways that project and receive projections from the medial hypothalamus. Sahu and co-workers (1988) have shown that bilateral neural transection at the midbrain dorsal tegmental level results in a large reduction in NPY levels in the hypothalamic

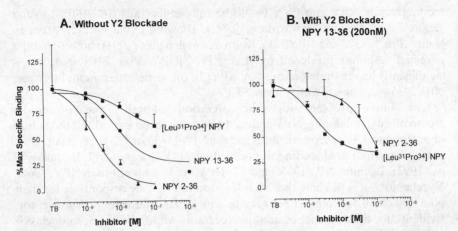

Fig. 4 Competition of specific [^{125}I]PYY binding in the CGPn by agonists that are potent in feeding, NPY2–36 and [Leu^{31}Pro^{34}]NPY, under standard binding conditions (A), and under conditions where Y$_2$ receptors are masked by inclusion of a high concentration of NPY13–36 with the radioligand (B). Data are normalized to percentage of maximal specific binding ($n = 2$–3 rats per point in four experiments). In A, competitive inhibition with NPY13–36 is shown. NPY2–36 was five to 20 times as potent as NPY13–36 (IC$_{50}$ = 1.7 nM for NPY2–36 and 28 nM for NPY13–36). General binding conditions were as described in Fig. 3.

PVN, and in enhanced potency of NPY to stimulate feeding after third ventricular administration (Sahu *et al.*, 1989). Steinman and colleagues (1994) showed that laterally placed midbrain knife cuts reduce the potency of third and fourth ventricularly administered NPY to increase feeding. Although these studies used different lesions and had divergent results, they suggest that hindbrain sites with afferent and efferent connections to the hypothalamus are good candidates as sites of action for NPY-related peptides administered into the fourth ventricle. Finally, the site of action for NPY-related peptides in hindbrain should exhibit a profile of agonist binding that is in good agreement with the pharmacology for agonists in feeding. The rank order of potency for agonists to stimulate feeding following fourth ventricular administration is similar to that after injection into the PFH (Fig. 5). Therefore, a hindbrain region would be of interest if the binding potencies of [^{125}I]PYY and receptor-selective agonists were comparable with those of the same ligands in the PFH.

Based on the criteria outlined above, the pontine central grey is a candidate as a site of action for NPY. In this nucleus, as in the PFH, both Y$_1$ and Y$_2$ receptor binding sites can be resolved (Fig. 4; discussed below). Moreover, this region is proximal to the sphenoid nucleus, locus ceruleus and parabrachial nuclei; all these sites have extensive neural connections with the hypothalamus (Andrezik and Beitz, 1985; Loughlin and Fallon, 1985). The pontine central grey also contains a population of NPY-immunoreactive cell bodies (O'Donohue *et al.*, 1985).

3.1   Pharmacology of feeding and NPY receptor subtypes in the dorsal pons

In general, PYY is approximately 2–4 times as potent as NPY in stimulating feeding, based on comparison of doses that elicit a half-maximal response (Corp *et al.*, 1990b). This relative potency is in good agreement with the relative potencies of these two peptides after hypothalamic injection (Stanley *et al.*, 1985b) and is consistent with competitive binding data showing that PYY is more potent than NPY in inhibiting [^{125}I]PYY binding in nerve and other tissues (Inui *et al.*, 1989; Corp and Smith, 1991). In addition to differences in potency between NPY and PYY, we have also shown a difference in the maximal response elicited by the NPY and PYY in some, but not all, of our experiments (Corp *et al.*, 1990b). In rats fed powdered chow (90-min test), PYY was approximately 1.5 times more efficacious than NPY based on parameters of total intake and the amount of time rats were observed to be eating (Corp *et al.*, 1990b). More recent studies show that the maximal response produced by PYY in 2-h tests with lab chow is approximately twofold larger than that elicited by NPY (Fig. 5). This difference in maximal response, or efficacy, is surprising in light of binding and functional studies showing that both NPY and PYY are full competitor–agonists at NPY-Y_1 and Y_2 receptors

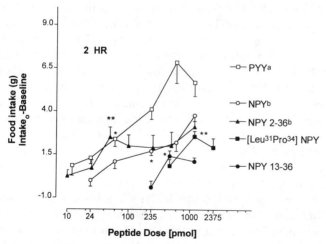

Fig. 5   Dose–effect of NPY-related peptides on cumulative intake following fourth ventricular administration ($n = 6$–7 per peptide group). Values are mean ± SEM intake measured 2 h after injection. Intake was calculated by subtracting the average baseline intake for each rat from the intake observed (intake$_o$) at each dose of peptide tested. Based on one-way ANOVA (repeated measures on dose), all peptides stimulated food intake. *Post-hoc* comparisons were made using the Tukey–Kramer test. The lowest dose of peptide eliciting a significant increase above baseline intake is indicated by *$P < 0.05$ or **$P < 0.01$. Comparison of the numerically maximal effects were made between peptides using one-way ANOVA with *post-hoc* comparisons using the Tukey–Kramer test. [a]$P < 0.05$ compared with all other peptides; [b]$P < 0.05$ compared with NPY13–36.

and that NPY and PYY are equally efficacious injected into the PVN (Stanley *et al.*, 1992).

Our results with fourth ventricular injection are similar to reports showing that PYY is more potent and efficacious than NPY injected into the lateral ventricle (Morley *et al.*, 1985). Therefore, a possible explanation for the difference in efficacy between NPY and PYY is that diffusion and distribution of peptides to receptors in sensitive sites of action is less efficient for NPY than PYY. Alternatively, it may be that activation of NPY-Y_3 receptors in the hindbrain produces physiological or motivational effects that effectively antagonize feeding behaviour. Y_3 receptors are present in the NTS of the hindbrain medulla where they participate in cardiovascular regulation (Barraco *et al.*, 1990; Grundemar *et al.*, 1991; Wahlestedt and Reis, 1993). PYY is impotent at Y_3 receptors and it is possible that the cardiovascular effects of NPY may effectively antagonize feeding behaviour. Indeed, we have observed that high doses of NPY administered into the fourth ventricle produce long-lasting ataxia and catalepsy (unpublished results).

More selective NPY receptor agonists act with varying potencies and efficacy to stimulate food intake (Fig. 5). The prototypical Y_2 receptor agonist NPY13–36 is only a weak agonist for feeding. This fits well with the low potency observed for similar fragments following hypothalamic administration (Fig. 2) (Kalra *et al.*, 1991; Stanley *et al.*, 1992).

Compared with its effect on feeding following hypothalamic injection (Kalra *et al.*, 1991; Stanley *et al.*, 1992), the effect of [Leu^{31},Pro^{34}]NPY after fourth ventricular injection appears blunted (Fig. 5): relatively high doses of [Leu^{31},Pro^{34}]NPY are required to elicit feeding following fourth ventricular injection, the dose–response range is narrow, and the maximal effect on intake produced [Leu^{31},Pro^{34}]NPY is less than that produced by PYY. This disparity between forebrain and hindbrain results with the selective Y_1 agonist may arise because distribution of [Leu^{31},Pro^{34}]NPY to hindbrain sites of action is slow or impeded. It is significant, however, that both NPY and [Leu^{31},Pro^{34}]NPY are potent at Y_3 receptors (Wahlestedt and Reis, 1993). Thus, it is possible that the reduced efficacy of [Leu^{31},Pro^{34}]NPY, as well as that of NPY, in comparison to PYY arises from its activation of NPY-Y_3 receptors.

Administered into the fourth ventricle, NPY2–36 displays an unusual dose–response profile. At low doses, NPY2–36 elicits feeding with a potency comparable to that of PYY. Similar to its effect in the hypothalamus (Stanley *et al.*, 1992), NPY2–36 is more potent than the parent molecule NPY. The feeding response to NPY2–36 after fourth ventricular injection, however, asymptotes at a dose of 50 pmol and no greater increase in food intake is observed across a tenfold range of doses (Fig. 5). The dose–response effect for PYY, on the other hand, increases through a broad range of doses and the maximal effect is observed at a dose of 600 pmol. Furthermore, a dose of 1175 pmol PYY elicits twice the ingestive response produced by NPY2–36 at the same dose.

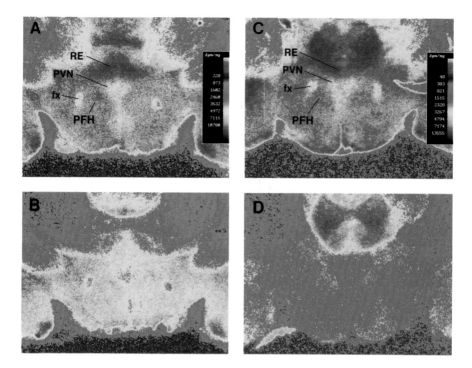

Plate 1 Colour-enhanced photomicrographs of coronal sections through the hypothalamus at the level of the PVN and PFH. (A) and (C) show total [^{125}I]PYY binding. (B) shows [^{125}I]PYY binding remaining in the presence of [Leu^{31},Pro^{34}]NPY (100 nM). Approximately 25% of the specific binding is inhibited by this Y$_1$ receptor-specific ligand. (D) shows [^{125}I]PYY binding in the presence of NPY2–36 (100 nM). At this concentration of NPY2–36, a small amount of specific binding remains in the PFH.

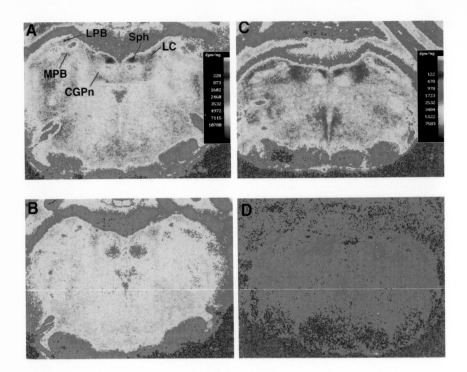

Plate 2 Colour-enhanced photomicrographs of coronal sections through the pons at the level of the central grey pontine nucleus (CGPn) and locus ceruleus (LC). (A) and (C) show total [125I]PYY binding. (B) shows [125I]PYY binding remaining in the presence of [Leu31,Pro34]NPY (100 nM). Approximately 25% of the specific binding is inhibited by this Y_1 receptor-specific ligand. (D) shows [125I]PYY binding in the presence of NPY2–36 (100 nM). At this concentration of NPY2–36, a small amount of specific binding remains in the region of the CGPn and sphenoid nucleus (Sph).

The reduced efficacy of NPY2–36 cannot be explained by any apparent non-specific effects of the peptide, i.e. abnormal or competing behaviours that might antagonize the feeding response are not observed following NPY2–36 administration. Moreover, at maximally effective doses, the latencies for NPY2–36 and PYY to initiate eating are similar (4 ± 1 min and 8 ± 5 min, respectively). It is also unlikely that the comparatively reduced efficacy of NPY2–36 at higher doses can be explained by degradation of the peptide since low doses of NPY2–36 which should be more affected by degradative processes, appear to be very potent. Moreover, in plasma, the rates of metabolism and clearance of a related truncated C-terminal peptide, PYY3–36 have been shown to be comparable with those of PYY (Grandt et al., 1992).

The rank order of potency for NPY-related peptides to stimulate feeding after hypothalamic or hindbrain administration is similar (compare Figs 2 and 5). Potencies and efficacies relative to PYY, however, differ considerably between the agonists. In the hindbrain, a stronger case can be made for the participation of two NPY receptor subtypes in the feeding response because of the comparatively similar potency (at low doses) but reduced efficacy of NPY2–36 (at high doses) compared with PYY. This evidence, and the partial agonistic activity of [Leu^{31}Pro^{34}]NPY, is consistent with the participation of both Y_1 and Y_2 receptors in the full expression of the feeding response. The greater efficacy of PYY arises, in this formulation, from action at both Y_1 and Y_2 receptors. This conclusion is tentative, pending future experiments with more selective agonists–antagonists under conditions where distribution of peptides to targets and counteractive Y_3 receptor effects are under control.

As noted, the pontine central grey (CGPn) is a candidate as a possible site for the action of NPY in feeding. Moderate levels of [^{125}I]PYY-specific binding are present in this loci and this binding is sensitive to competition by both NPY2–36 and [Leu^{31},Pro^{34}]NPY (Plate 2 and Fig. 4). (By contrast [Leu^{31},Pro^{34}]NPY does not effectively compete for [^{125}I]PYY in the area postrema and NTS of the dorsal medulla (unpublished results).)

In particular, [^{125}I]PYY-specific binding in the pontine central grey exhibits sensitivity to NPY2–36 and [Leu^{31},Pro^{34}]NPY that is comparable to the binding potencies for these ligands in the hypothalamus (compare Figs 4A, B and 3A,B). Furthermore, under conditions where Y_2 receptors are masked, or blocked, by NPY13–36, there is an increase in the maximal inhibition produced by [Leu^{31},Pro^{34}]NPY in comparison with that of [Leu^{31},Pro^{34}]NPY in the unblocked condition (Fig. 4A,B). As in the PFH, under conditions of Y_2 receptor blockade, the potency of NPY2–36 to inhibit [^{125}I]PYY binding is radically shifted to the right (Fig. 4B). These results suggest that in the pontine central grey, as in the PFH, NPY2–36 and [Leu^{31},Pro^{34}]NPY-sensitive binding sites are independent. In the unblocked condition, NPY2–36 is significantly more potent than the prototypical Y_2 receptor agonist, NPY13–36 (Fig. 4A). This is consistent with the relative potencies of these two agonists in feeding after fourth ventricular administration (Fig. 5).

While the pontine central grey is an attractive candidate as a site of action for NPY-related peptides in feeding because binding profiles in this region are similar to those obtained in the PFH, direct evidence of its role in NPY-induced feeding is lacking. Other nuclei within the region of the dorsal pons cannot be ruled out as possible sites of action. For instance, NPY is expressed in high concentrations within cell bodies in the locus ceruleus, from where efferents project extensively to the hypothalamus (Loughlin and Fallon, 1985). But while NPY2–36-sensitive, Y_2 receptor binding sites are present in the locus ceruleus, $[^{125}I]PYY$ binding is less sensitive to $[Leu^{31},Pro^{34}]NPY$ than $[^{125}I]PYY$ binding in the hypothalamus and pontine central grey (Plate 2A,B). The medial and lateral parabrachial nuclei are two other possible sites of action within this region. Both are enriched with Y_2 receptors, contain NPY-immunoreactive fibres and are intimately involved in sensory control of feeding (Norgren, 1983; Andrezik and Beitz, 1985; Herbert et al., 1990). Again, as in the locus ceruleus, few Y_1 binding sites can be detected in the medial and lateral parabrachial nuclei. The highest levels of $[^{125}I]PYY$-specific binding in the dorsal pons is detected in the sphenoid nucleus; the binding here is both NPY2–36 and $[Leu^{31},Pro^{34}]NPY$ sensitive (Plate 2). The critical experiments that will determine whether these loci, or others in the hindbrain, are important as sites of action for NPY's stimulating effect on food intake are yet to be performed.

To summarize, administration of NPY-related peptides into the fourth ventricle in rats elicits feeding with marked differences in potency and efficacy. The relative differences in potency and efficacy between the agonists suggests that, in the hindbrain, receptors of both the NPY-Y_1 and -Y_2 class may be involved in the full feeding effect produced by PYY. A precise site of action for NPY-related peptides in the hindbrain is not yet known; however, based on latencies required to initiate eating, a site proximal to the fourth ventricle is most likely involved. Based on the sensitivity of $[^{125}I]PYY$ binding in the dorsal pons to NPY2–36 and $[Leu^{31},Pro^{34}]NPY$, this region is attractive as a possible site of action. In particular, the pontine central grey is interesting because the binding of NPY-related peptides here is comparable to that measured in the PFH, the most sensitive site of action for NPY in the hypothalamus.

4 NPY receptor coupling and signal transduction

NPY receptor subtypes have not been well differentiated based on coupling and second messenger systems. All three subtypes share similar intracellular trafficking pathways and are coupled to inhibition of adenylate cyclase through linkage to G proteins in brain, as well as and other tissues (Westlind-Danielsson et al., 1987; Aakerlund et al., 1990; Wahlestedt et al., 1991; Herzog et al., 1992; Wahlestedt and Reis, 1993). Additionally, activation of all three receptors is coupled to elevated intracellular Ca^{2+} levels in many cell types (Aakerlund et al., 1990; Herzog et al., 1992; Wahlestedt and Reis, 1993). In some brain regions, G protein-coupled activation of phosphoinositide hydrolysis has been demonstrated (Hinson *et al.*, 1988).

Chance and co-workers (1989) have shown that NPY-induced feeding in rats is inhibited by pertussis toxin. This suggests that NPY receptors mediating ingestion link to G proteins through G_i or G_o α subunits. Evidence, however, has not been shown that NPY receptors in the hypothalamus modulate feeding through inhibition of adenylate cyclase and a coupled decrease in the production of cyclic adenosine monophosphate (cAMP). On the contrary, in rats treated centrally with cobalt protoporphyrin, a haem analogue that induces anorexia, weight loss and insensitivity to the orexigenic effects of NPY (Galbraith and Kappas, 1989), Turner *et al.* (1994) found no change in hypothalamic concentrations of cAMP, or in NPY receptor binding parameters, in response to ventricularly administered NPY.

Indeed, there is evidence that food intake is stimulated by increasing the intracellular cAMP concentrations in the hypothalamus. Gillard and co-workers (1994), in a preliminary communication, found that administration of the membrane-permeable cAMP analogue 8-bromoadenosine 3′,5′-cyclic monophosphate (8-BR-cAMP) into the PFH stimulated robust feeding responses. Moreover, coadministration of NPY and 8-BR-cAMP appears to have an additive effect on stimulating feeding (B.G. Stanley, personal communication).

Within rat brain, the sensitivity of [^{125}I]PYY binding to NPY receptors varies considerably in the presence of the non-hydrolysable analogue of guanosine triphosphate (GTP), Gpp(NH)p. In the Y_1 receptor-enriched areas, such as the cerebral cortex and basilar artery, Gpp(NH)p at a concentration of $100\,\mu\text{M}$ almost completely inhibits [^{125}I]PYY binding (Fig. 6). In some Y_2 receptor-enriched regions, however, including those implicated in NPY-stimulated feeding, [^{125}I]PYY binding is nearly insensitive to Gpp(NH)p at concentrations as high as $100\,\mu\text{M}$ (Fig. 6). These regions include the medial hypothalamus and the dorsal tegmentum of the midbrain and pons. Other Y_2 receptor-enriched regions that exhibit GTP insensitivity include the pyriform cortex, CA1–CA3 of the hippocampus (Fig. 6 and unpublished observations). [^{125}I]PYY binding in other Y_2-enriched regions appears to be more sensitive to Gpp(NH)p, particularly in the ventrolateral hindbrain regions (Fig. 6). One implication of these data is that Y_2 receptors in brain loci that are sites of action for NPY in feeding may belong to a subclass of Y_2 receptors that are distinct from Y_2 receptors showing GTP sensitivity. GTP sensitivity is a typical feature of Y_2 receptors characterized in cultured cell lines (Wahlestedt *et al.*, 1991). Alternatively, Y_2 receptors may couple to G proteins through unique, and as yet poorly understood, subunits in regions of the hypothalamus and hindbrain where NPY-related peptides act to stimulate food intake.

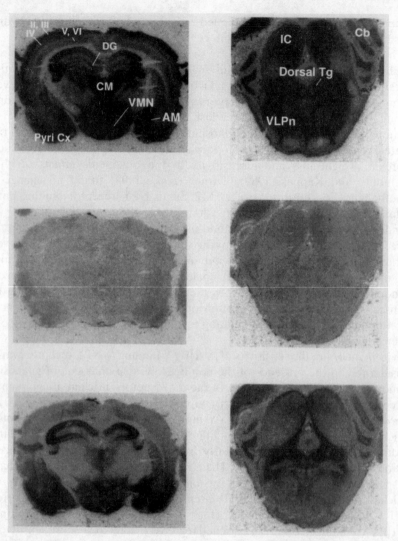

Fig. 6 Photomicrographs of coronal sections through the forebrain (left) and hindbrain (right) showing the regional sensitivity of [^{125}I]PYY binding to Gpp(NH)p (100 μM). Top panels show total [^{125}I]PYY without inhibitors. Middle panels show non-specific binding remaining in the presence of Gpp(NH)p (100 μM) and NPY (100 nM). Bottom panels show the inhibition of binding by Gpp(NH)p (100 μM). Y_1- receptor-enriched regions such as the cerebral cortex (lamina I, II, III and IV) were extremely sensitive to Gpp(NH)p. Some Y_2 receptor-enriched areas such as the ventrolateral pons (VLPn) are sensitive to Gpp(NH)p while Y_2-enriched regions in the dorsal tegmentum (Dorsal Tg) are largely insensitive to Gpp(NH)p. DG, dentate gyrus; CM, central medial nucleus of the thalamus; VMN, ventral medial nucleus of the hypothalamus; AM, anteromedial nucleus of the thalamus; Pyri Cx, pyriform cortex; Ic, inferior colliculus.

5 Summary

In this chapter I have attempted to summarize the research relevant to the putative NPY receptors involved in feeding. Based on the potencies of NPY2–36 and [Leu^{31},Pro^{34}]NPY in behavioural and binding experiments, a two-receptor hypothesis is advanced for the action of NPY-related peptides in stimulating feeding. I consider this more likely than the alternative hypothesis that NPY–PYY acts at a single feeding receptor to stimulate food intake. However, a strong conclusion about the specific receptor, or receptors, involved in the feeding effects of NPY cannot be made at this time.

Certainly, the development of selective and potent NPY receptor antagonists will provide the tools necessary to determine the specific role of NPY receptor subtypes in feeding behaviour. A recently developed drug antagonist, BIBP3226, exhibits high affinity and selectivity for Y_1 receptors in rat cerebral cortex (Rudolf et al., 1994). Use of this antagonist in feeding experiments may help resolve questions concerning the contribution of typical Y_1 receptors to NPY-related feeding phenomenon. In the absence of drug antagonists for Y_2 receptors, a new and promising strategy for studying specific receptor contributions to behaviour is the in vivo use of antisense oligonucleotide sequences which block translation of messenger RNA coding for specific receptor protein. Already, Wahlestedt and co-workers (1995) have used an antisense oligomer effectively to interrupt synthesis of Y_1 receptors and have examined the effect of this receptor antagonism on NPY-induced anxiolysis. The application of antisense technology to the study of ingestive behaviours, using new oligonucleotides that will be developed as the cloning of NPY receptors progresses, promises an exciting avenue for the advancement of research aimed at understanding the receptor basis of NPY-induced feeding.

Acknowledgements

The author thanks Dr Gerard Smith for reviewing this manuscript and making useful suggestions, Dietrich Conze for technical assistance, and Terri Popiel and Jane Magnetti for help with preparation of the manuscript. The author's research on NPY receptors was supported by The Whitehall Foundation.

References

Aakerlund, L., Gether, U., Fuhlendorff, J., Schwartz, T. W. and Thastrup, O. (1990). Y_1 receptors for neuropeptide Y are coupled to mobilization of intracellular calcium and inhibition of adenylate cyclase. FEBS Lett. **260**, 73–78.

Andrezik, J. A. and Beitz, A. J. (1985). Reticular formation, central gray and related tegmental nuclei. In The Rat Nervous System. Vol. 2. Hindbrain and Spinal Cord (G. Paxinos, ed.), pp. 1–28. Academic Press, New York.

Barraco, R. A., Ergene, E., Dunbar, J. C. and El-Ridi, M. R. (1990). Cardiorespiratory response patterns elicited by microinjections of neuropeptide Y in the nucleus tractus solitarius. Brain Res. Bull. **24**, 465–485.

Bonaz, B., Taylor, T. and Tache, T. (1993). Peripheral peptide YY induces c-*fos*-like immunoreactivity in the rat brain. *Neurosci. Lett.* **163**, 77–80.

Bromme, M., Hokfelt, T. and Terenius, L. (1985). Peptide YY (PYY)-immunoreactive neurons in the lower brainstem and spinal cord of rat. *Acta Physiol. Scand.* **125**, 349–352.

Chance, W. T., Sheriff, S., Foley-Nelson, T., Fisher, J. E. and Balasubramaniam, A. (1989). Pertussis toxin inhibits neuropeptide Y-induced feeding in rats. *Peptides* **10**, 1283–1286.

Clark, J. T., Kalra, P. S., Crowley, W. R. and Kalra, S. P. (1984). Neuropeptide Y and human pancreatic polypeptide stimulate feeding behaviour in rats. *Endocrinology* **115**, 427–429.

Clark, J. T., Sahu, A., Kalra, P. S., Balasubramaniam, A. and Kalra, S. P. (1987). Neuropeptide Y (NPY)-induced feeding behavior in female rats: comparison with human NPY ([Met^{17}]NPY), NPY analog ([norLeu4]NPY) and peptide YY. *Regul. Pept.* **17**, 31–39.

Colmers, W. F., Klapstein, G. J., Fournier, A., St-Pierre, S. and Treherne, K. A. (1991). Presynaptic inhibition by neuropeptide Y in rat hippocampal slice *in vitro* is mediated by a Y_2 receptor. *Br. J. Pharmacol.* **102**, 41–44.

Corp, E. S. and McQuade, J. A. (1992). Detection of Y_1-neuropeptide Y binding sites in rat basilar artery by quantitative receptor autoradiography. *Soc. Neurosci. Abstr.* **18**, 1467.

Corp, E. S. and Smith, G. P. (1991). Characterization of axonally transported [^{125}I]PYY binding sites in rat vagus nerve. *Brain Res.* **553**, 175–179.

Corp, E. S., Curcio, M. and Smith, G. P. (1990a). Potency of peptide YY analogues for stimulation of feeding and in competition for [^{125}I]-PYY binding sites in the hindbrain. *Soc. Neurosci. Abstr.* **16**, 978.

Corp, E. S., Melville, L. D., Greenberg, D., Gibbs, J. and Smith, G. P. (1990b). Effect of fourth ventricular neuropeptide Y and peptide YY on ingestive and other behaviors. *Am. J. Physiol.* **259**, R317–R323.

Corp, E. S., Curcio, M. and Smith, G. P. (1991). Competition by Y_1 and Y_2 receptor agonists for ^{125}I-peptide YY binding sites in rat hindbrain. *Int. J. Obes.* **15** (**supplement 3**), 42.

Corp, E. S., McQuade, J. A. and Smith, G. P. (1993). Localization of NPY-Y_1 binding sites in the rat medial hypothalamus. *Appetite* **21**, 169.

Dumont, Y., Martel, J., Fournier, A., St-Pierre, S. and Quirion, R. (1992). Neuropeptide Y and neuropeptide Y receptor subtypes in brain and peripheral tissues. *Prog. Neurobiol.* **38**, 125–167.

Dumont, Y., Fournier, A., St-Pierre, S. and Quirion, R. (1993). Comparative characterization and autoradiographic distribution of neuropeptide Y receptor subtypes in the rat brain. *J. Neurosci.* **13**, 73–86.

Ekman, R., Wahlestedt, C., Bottcher, G., Sundler, F., Hakanson, R. and Panula, P. (1986). Peptide YY-like immunoreactivity in the central nervous system of the rat. *Regul. Pept.* **16**, 157–168.

Fuhlendorff, J., Gether, U., Aakerlund, L., Langeland-Johansen, N., Thogersen, H., Melberg, S. G., Olsen, U. B., Thastrup, O. and Schwartz, T. W. (1990). [Leu^{31},Pro^{34}]neuropeptide Y: a specific Y_1 receptor agonist. *Proc. Natl. Acad. Sci.* **87**, 182–186.

Galbraith, R. A. and Kappas, A. (1989). Regulation of food intake and body weight by cobalt porphyrins in animals. *Proc. Natl. Acad. Sci.* **86**, 7653–7657.

Gehlert, D. R., Gackenheimer, S. L. and Schober, D. A. (1992). [Leu^{31}-Pro^{34}]neuropeptide Y identifies a subtype of ^{125}I labeled peptide YY binding sites in the rat brain. *Neurochem. Int.* **21**, 45–67.

Gillard, E. R., Khan, A. M., Haq, A. U., Grewal, R. S. and Stanley, B. G. (1994). Stimulation of feeding behavior in the rat by intrahypothalamic injection of 8-BR-cAMP. *Soc. Neurosci. Abstr.* **20**, 1680.

Grandt, D., Teyssen, S., Schimiczek, M., Reeve, J. R., Jr., Feth, F., Rascher, W., Hirche, H., Singer, M. V., Layer, P., Goebell, H., Ho, F. J. and Eysselein, V. E. (1992). Novel generation of hormone receptor specificity by amino terminal processing of peptide YY. *Biochem. Biophys. Res. Commun.* **186**, 1299–1306.

Grundemar, L., Wahlestedt, C. and Reis, D. J. (1991). Neuropeptide Y acts at an atypical receptor to evoke cardiovascular depression and to inhibit glutamate responsiveness in the brainstem. *J. Pharmacol. Exp. Ther.* **258**, 633–638.

Grundemar, L., Sheikh, S. P. and Wahlestedt, C. (1993). Characterization of receptor types for neuropeptide Y and related peptides. In *The Biology of Neuropeptide Y and Related Peptides* (W. F. Colmers and C. Wahlestedt, eds), pp. 197–239. Humana Press, Totowa, NJ.

Harfstrand, A., Fuxe, K., Agnati, L. F., Benefenati, F. and Goldstein, M. (1986). Receptor autoradiographical evidence for high densities of ^{125}I-neuropeptide Y binding sites in the nucleus tractus solitarius of the normal male rat. *Acta Physiol. Scand.* **128**, 195–200.

Herbert, H., Moga, M. M. and Saper, C. B. (1990). Connections of the parabrachial nucleus with the nucleus of the solitary tract and the medullary reticular formation in the rat. *J. Comp. Neurol.* **293**, 540–580.

Herzog, H., Hort, Y. J., Ball, H. J., Hayes, G., Shine, J. and Selbie, L. A. (1992). Cloned human neuropeptide Y receptor couples to two different second messenger systems. *Proc. Natl. Acad. Sci.* **89**, 5794–5798.

Hinson, J., Rauh, C. and Coupet, J. (1988). Neuropeptide Y stimulates inositol phospholipid hydrolysis in rat brain microprisms. *Brain Res.* **446**, 379–382.

Inui, A., Okita, M., Inoue, T., Sakatani, N., Oya, M., Moribka, H., Shii, K., Yokono, K., Mizuno, N. and Baba, S. (1989). Characterization of peptide YY receptors in the brain. *Endocrinology* **124**, 402–409.

Kalra, S. P., Dube, M., Fournier, A. and Kalra, P. S. (1991). Structure–function analysis of stimulation of food intake by neuropeptide Y: effects of receptor agonists. *Physiol. Behav.* **50**, 5–9.

Larhammar, D., Blomqvist, A. G., Yee, F., Jazin, E., Yoo, H. and Wahlestedt, C. (1992). Cloning and functional expression of a human neuropeptide Y/peptide YY receptor of the Y_1 type. *J. Biol. Chem.* **267**, 10 935–10 938.

Larsen, P. J., Sheikh, S. P., Jakobsen, C. R., Schwartz, T. W. and Mikkelsen, J. D. (1993). Regional distribution of putative NPY Y_1 receptors and neurons expressing Y_1 mRNA in forebrain areas of the rat central nervous system. *Eur. J. Neurosci.* **5**, 1622–1637.

Levine, A. S. and Morley, J. E. (1984). Neuropeptide Y: a potent inducer of consummatory behaviour in rats. *Peptides* **5**, 1025–1030.

Loughlin, S. E. and Fallon, J. H. (1985). Locus coeruleus. In *The Rat Nervous System. Vol. 2. Hindbrain and Spinal Cord* (G. Paxinos, ed.), pp. 79–93. Academic Press, New York.

Lundberg, J. M., Terenius, L., Hokfelt, T., Tatemoto, K., Mutt, V., Polak, J. and Goldstein, M. (1982). Neuropeptide Y (NPY)-like immunoreactivity in peripheral noradrenergic neurons and effects of NPY on sympathetic function. *Acta Physiol. Scand.* **116**, 477–480.

McGregor, I. S., Menendez, J. A. and Atrens, D. M. (1990). Metabolic effects of neuropeptide Y injected into the sulcal prefrontal cortex. *Brain Res. Bull.* **24**, 363–367.

McLaughlin, C. L., Tou, J. S., Rogan, G. J. and Baile, C. A. (1991). Full amino acid sequence of centrally administered NPY required for maximal food intake response. *Physiol. Behav.* **49**, 521–526.

Mentlein, R., Dahms, P., Grandt, D. and Kruger, R. (1993). Proteolytic processing of the neuropeptide Y and peptide YY by dipeptidyl peptidase IV. *Regul. Pept.* **49**, 133–144.

Morley, J. E., Levine, A. S., Grace, M. and Kneip, J. (1985). Peptide YY (PYY), a potent orexigenic agent. *Brain Res.* **341**, 200–203.

Morley, J. E., Levine, A. S., Gosnell, B. A., Kneip, J. and Grace, M. (1987). Effect of neuropeptide Y on ingestive behaviors in the rat. *Am. J. Physiol.* **252**, R599–R609.

Myers, A. K., Farhat, M. Y., Shen, G. H., Debinski, W., Wahlestedt, C. and Zukowska-Grojec, Z. (1990). Platelets as a source and site of action for neuropeptide Y. *Ann. N. Y. Acad. Sci.* **611**, 408–411.

Nakajima, T., Yashima, Y. and Nakamura, K. (1986). Quantitative autoradiographic localization of neuropeptide Y receptors in the rat lower brainstem. *Brain Res.* **380**, 144–150.

Norgren, R. (1983). Afferent interactions of cranial nerves involved in ingestion. In *Vagal Nerve Function: Behavioral and Methodological Considerations* (J. G. Kral, T. L. Powley, and C. McC. Brooks, eds), pp. 67–77. Elsevier Science, Amsterdam.

O'Donohue, T. L., Chronwall, B. M., Pruss, R. M., Mezey, E., Kiss, J. Z., Eiden, L. E., Massari, V. J., Tessel, R. E., Pickel, V. M., DiMaggio, D. A., Hotchkiss, A. J., Crowley, W. R. and Zukowska-Grojec, Z. (1985). Neuropeptide Y and peptide YY neuronal and endocrine systems. *Peptides* **6**, 755–768.

Paxinos, G. and Watson, C. (1986). *The Rat Brain in Stereotaxic Coordinates*. Academic Press, Orlando.

Quirion, R., Martel, J.-C., Dumont, Y., Jolicouer, F., St-Pierre, S., and Fournier, A. (1990). Neuropeptide Y receptors: autoradiographic distribution in the brain and structure–activity relationships. *Ann. N. Y. Acad. Sci.* **611**, 58–72.

Rudolf, K., Eberlein, W., Engel, W., Wieland, H. A., Willim, K. D., Entzeroth, M., Wienen, W., Beck-Sickinger, A. G. and Doods, H. N. (1994). The first highly potent and selective non-peptide neuropeptide YY_1 receptor antagonist: BIBP3226. *Eur. J. Pharmacol.* **271**, R11–R13.

Sahu, A., Kalra, S. P., Crowley, W. R. and Kalra, P. S. (1988). Evidence that NPY-containing neurons in the brainstem project into selected hypothalamic nuclei: implication in feeding behavior. *Brain Res.* **457**, 376–378.

Sahu, A., Dube, M. G., Kalra, S. P. and Kalra, P. S. (1989). Bilateral neural transections at the level of mesencephalon increase food intake and reduce latency to onset of feeding in response to neuropeptide Y. *Peptides* **9**, 1269–1273.

Sawchenko, P. E., Swanson, L. W., Grzanna, R., Howe, P. R. C., Bloom, S. R. and Polak, J. M. (1985). Colocalization of neuropeptide Y immunoreactivity in brainstem catecholaminergic neurons that project to the paraventricular nucleus of the hypothalamus. *J. Comp. Neurol.* **241**, 138–153.

Schwartz, T. W., Fuhlendorff, J., Kjems, L. L., Kristensen, M. S., Vervelde, M., O'Hare, M., Kretenansky, J. L. and Bjornholm, B. (1990). Signal epitopes in the three-dimensional structure of NPY interaction with Y_1, Y_2 and PP receptors. *Ann. N. Y. Acad. Sci.* **611**, 35–47.

Sheikh, S. P., Hansen, A. P. and Williams, J. A. (1992). Solubilization and affinity purification of the Y_2 receptor for neuropeptide Y and peptide YY from rabbit kidney. *J. Biol. Chem.* **266**, 23 959–23 966.

Stanley, B. G. (1993). Neuropeptide Y in multiple hypothalamic sites controls eating behavior, endocrine, and autonomic systems for body energy balance. In *The Biology of Neuropeptide Y and Related Peptides* (W. F. Colmers and C. Wahlestedt, eds), pp. 457–509. Humana Press, Totowa, NJ.

Stanley, B. G. and Leibowitz, S. F. (1984). Neuropeptide Y: stimulation of feeding and drinking by injection into the paraventricular nucleus. *Life Sci.* **35**, 2635–2642.

Stanley, B. G., Chin, A. S. and Leibowitz, S. F. (1985a). Feeding and drinking elicited by central injection of neuropeptide Y: evidence for a hypothalamic site(s) of action. *Brain Res. Bull.* **14**, 521–524.

Stanley, B. G., Daniel, D. R., Chin, A. S. and Leibowitz, S. F. (1985b). Paraventricular nucleus injections of peptide YY and neuropeptide Y preferentially enhance carbohydrate ingestion. *Peptides* **6**, 1205–1211.

Stanley, B. G., Magdalin, W., Seirafi, A., Nguyen, M. M. and Leibowitz, S. F. (1992). Evidence for neuropeptide Y mediation of eating produced by food deprivation and for a variant of the Y_1 receptor mediating this peptide's effect. *Peptides* **13**, 581–587.

Stanley, B. G., Magdalin, W., Seirafi, A., Thomas, W. J. and Leibowitz, S. F. (1993). The perifornical area: the major focus of (a) patchily distributed hypothalamic neuropeptide Y-sensitive feeding system(s). *Brain Res.* **604**, 304–317.

Steinman, J. L., Gunion, M. S. and Morley, J. E. (1994). Forebrain and hindbrain involvement of neuropeptide Y in ingestive behaviors of rats. *Acta Neurobiol. Exp. (Warsz.)* **47**, 207–214.

Stjernquist, M. and Owman, C. (1990). Further evidence for a prejunctional action of neuropeptide Y on cholinergic motor neurons in the rat uterine cervix. *Acta Physiol. Scand.* **138**, 95–96.

Tatemoto, K., Carlquist, M. and Mutt, V. (1982). Neuropeptide Y—a novel brain peptide with structural similarities to peptide YY and pancreatic polypeptide. *Nature* **296**, 659–660.

Turner, M. B., Corp, E. S. and Galbraith, R. A. (1994). Lack of NPY-induced feeding in cobalt protoporphyrin-treated rats is a postreceptor defect. *Physiol. Behav.* **56**, 1009–1014.

Unden, A., Tatemoto, K., Mutt, V. and Bartfai, T. (1984). Neuropeptide Y receptors in the rat brain. *Eur. J. Biochem.* **125**, 525–530.

Wahlestedt, C. and Reis, D. J. (1993). Neuropeptide Y-related peptides and their receptors—are the receptors potential therapeutic drug targets? *Annu. Rev. Pharmacol. Toxicol.* **32**, 309–352.

Wahlestedt, C., Yanaihara, N. and Hakanson, R. (1986). Evidence for different pre- and post-junctional receptors for neuropeptide Y and related peptides. *Regul. Pept.* **13**, 307–318.

Wahlestedt, C., Edvinsson, L., Ekblad, E. and Hakanson, R. (1987). Effects of neuropeptide Y at sympathetic neuroeffector junctions: existence of Y_1- and Y_2-receptors. In *Neuronal Messengers in Vascular Function* (A. Nobin, C. Owman and B. Arneklo-Nobin, eds), pp. 231–242. Elsevier, Amsterdam.

Wahlestedt, C., Grundemar, L., Hakanson, R., Heilig, M., Shen, G. H., Zukowska-Grojec, Z. and Reis, D. J. (1990). Neuropeptide Y receptor subtypes, Y_1 and Y_2. *Ann. N. Y. Acad. Sci.* **611**, 7–26.

Wahlestedt, C., Regunathan, S. and Reis, D. (1991). Identification of cultured cells selectively expressing Y_1-, Y_2-, or Y_3-type receptors for neuropeptide Y/peptide YY. *Life Sci.* **50**, PL-7–PL-12.

Wahlestedt, C., Pich, E. M., Koob, G. F., Yee, F. and Heilig, M. (1995). Modulation of anxiety and neuropeptide Y-Y_1 receptors by antisense oligodeoxynucleotides. *Am. Assoc. Adv. Sci.* **259**, 528–531.

Walker, M. W. and Miller, R. J. (1988). ^{125}I-neuropeptide Y and ^{125}I-peptide YY bind to multiple receptor sites in rat brain. *Mol. Pharmacol.* **34**, 779–792.

Westlind-Danielsson, A., Undden, A., Abens, J., Andell, S. and Bartfai, T. (1987). Neuropeptide Y receptors and the inhibition of adenylate cyclase in the human frontal and temporal cortex. *Neurosci. Lett.* **74**, 237–242.

16

Benzodiazepine Receptors and the Determination of Palatability

STEVEN J. COOPER and SUZANNE HIGGS

Department of Psychology, University of Durham, South Road, Durham DH1 3LE, UK

1 Introduction

Benzodiazepines (prototypic compounds being chlordiazepoxide and diazepam) have been used extensively as therapeutic agents, specifically as anxiolytics, anticonvulsants and hypnotics. They act as agonists at specific benzodiazepine receptors, which are present throughout the brain (Bosmann *et al.*, 1977; Möhler and Okada, 1977; Squires and Braestrup, 1977; Young and Kuhar, 1980). These receptors are closely associated with γ-aminobutyric acid $(GABA)_A$ receptors, which regulate the chloride conductance of postsynaptic membranes (Macdonald and Twyman, 1991). Benzodiazepines act to enhance the inhibitory effects of GABA, and do so by modulating $(GABA)_A$ receptor-mediated transmission (Ticku, 1991). Hence, ultimately, the behavioural effects of the benzodiazepines have to be understood in terms of augmented GABAergic inhibitory neurotransmission at central synapses.

The starting point for the present chapter is the simple observation that benzodiazepines exert a strong effect to increase food consumption (Randall *et al.*, 1960; Niki, 1965; Bainbridge, 1968; Iwahara and Iwasaki, 1969; Wise and Dawson, 1974; Fratta *et al.*, 1976). This led to ideas that benzodiazepines increase food intake by inhibiting satiety (Margules and Stein, 1967), by enhancing hunger (Wise and Dawson, 1974) or by increasing appetite (Cooper, 1980a). Analysis of the hyperphagic effect of benzodiazepines may provide important clues concerning the behavioural and neural (and neurochemical) mechanisms involved in the control of appetite and the expression of feeding behaviour. This chapter will consider: (i) behavioural processes underlying benzodiazepine-induced hyperphagia; (ii) the detailed pharmacology of this and related effects; and (iii) the possible neural mechanisms that may be critically involved in the changes in ingestive behaviour brought about by these drugs. Finally, it will consider the implications of the discovery of subunits, and

DRUG RECEPTOR SUBTYPES AND INGESTIVE BEHAVIOUR
ISBN 0-12-187620-9

their different combinations, comprising $GABA_A$ receptor–chloride channel complexes.

2 Behavioural processes in benzodiazepine-induced hyperphagia

2.1 Increases in food ingestion

Benzodiazepines increase food consumption in food-deprived animals (Bainbridge, 1968; Fratta *et al.*, 1976) and in satiated animals (Wise and Dawson, 1974). If food-deprived rats are presented with a choice between a familiar laboratory diet and a selection of novel foods, then treatment with a benzodiazepine can lead to an increase in the choice of the familiar food, but not of the unfamiliar foods (Cooper and Crummy, 1978; Cooper, 1980b). Hence, in this case, the drug treatment does not act to overcome any food neophobic response, as suggested by some (e.g. Poschel, 1971). Instead, it potentiates the response to the familiar food, implying a relatively direct effect on feeding motivation.

One of the more striking effects of benzodiazepines is that they considerably increase the consumption of a familiar, sweetened mash in non-deprived rats (Cooper, 1986b; Cooper and Gilbert, 1985; Cooper and Moores, 1985; Cooper *et al.*, 1985a). This effect arises because the drug treatments increase the duration of eating, which, in turn, depends on increases in the lengths of individual bouts of feeding (Cooper and Yerbury, 1986). Pre-satiating the animals, by allowing them to feed before the test meal, has little effect on the hyperphagic response to benzodiazepine treatment (Cooper *et al.*, 1985a). Hence, it is unlikely that the increased food consumption is a consequence of overcoming the inhibitory effect of satiety. Cooper and Estall (1985) proposed that benzodiazepine-induced hyperphagia depends, to some degree at least, on oropharyngeal stimulation during food ingestion.

2.2 Palatability: its representation and expression

In this section, we shall put forward a model of processes involved in the control of food ingestion, with an emphasis on the role of palatability. Then, we shall indicate the means by which we think that benzodiazepines bring about increases in food consumption. Following this, we shall consider the relevant evidence in favour of benzodiazepine-induced enhancement of palatability.

Fig. 1 provides the outlines of the model. In terms of behaviour, it preserves the distinction between appetitive or approach responses to food on the one hand, and the consummatory phase of food ingestion on the other. Taste and other sensory factors contribute strongly to evaluation of the palatability of food, in conjunction with previous experience and conditioning history. We assume a 'memory' for palatability (representation, in Fig. 1), against which current evaluations are made. We propose that benzodiazepines act directly on

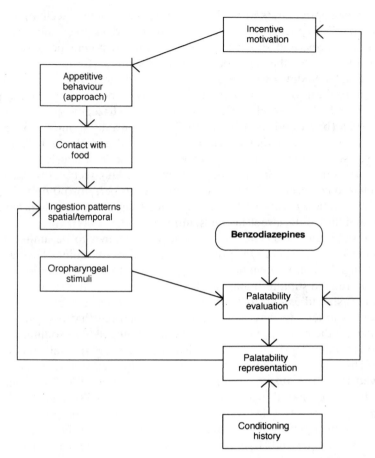

Fig. 1 Model indicating the behavioural means by which benzodiazepines influence ingestive behaviour. The central feature of the model is that benzodiazepines enhance the positive hedonic quality of food-related stimuli (e.g. taste). This helps to determine patterns of ingestion which can lead to hyperphagia.

the processes involved in the evaluation of palatability, specifically to enhance positive hedonic evaluation (cf. Berridge and Treit, 1986). In consequence, benzodiazepines will affect patterns of ingestion and incentive factors to cause approach to food.

Part of the evidence for this way of viewing the effects of benzodiazepines derives from taste-preference tests, using two sources of fluid (usually a tastant *vs* water). Maickel and Maloney (1974) reported that chlordiazepoxide enhanced the consumption of a 'pleasant-tasting saccharin solution', while Roache and Zabik (1986) noted that benzodiazepines (diazepam and chlordiazepoxide) preferentially enhanced the consumption of a saccharin solution when water-deprived rats were given a choice between the saccharin solution and water. We explicitly tested the idea that benzodiazepines enhance sweet-taste preferences, and showed that clonazepam, a potent benzodiazepine, selectively increased the ingestion of saccharin solution (Cooper and Yerbury, 1988). Similar findings were reported for chlordiazepoxide (Parker, 1991), abecarnil (a β-carboline which acts as an agonist at benzodiazepine receptors (Cooper and Greenwood, 1992) and two benzodiazepine partial agonists Ro 16-6028 (bretazenil) and Ro 17-1812 (Cooper and Green, 1993). Separately, we have shown that abecarnil, Ro 16-6028 and Ro 17-1812 reliably increase the consumption of highly palatable food in non-deprived rats (Yerbury and Cooper, 1987; Cooper and Greenwood, 1992). Hence, drugs active at benzodiazepine receptors appear to share the property of potentiating saccharin preferences in rats, and this, in turn, may depend on an enhancement of the palatability of the sweet-tasting solution (Cooper, 1989).

We should not expect the effects of benzodiazepines to be limited to the responses to sweet taste. Our proposal is that benzodiazepines have a direct impact on palatability evaluation (Fig. 1), and therefore the evaluation of other ingestion-related stimuli should also be affected. Hence, the effects of benzodiazepines should extend to the preference rats exhibit for moderately salty solutions. Earlier, we described results which showed that benzodiazepines will increase the consumption of a palatable isotonic (0.9%) sodium chloride solution in water-deprived rats (Turkish and Cooper, 1984; Estall and Cooper, 1987). This led us to evaluate their effects on salt-taste preferences in water-deprived rats. The results confirmed our expectation. We found that the benzodiazepine partial agonists bretazenil (Ro 16-6028) and Ro 17-1812 (Cooper et al., 1987b) selectively enhanced the intake of the preferred 0.9% saline without significantly affecting concurrent water consumption in a two-choice test (Cooper and Barber, 1993). Furthermore, the β-carboline abecarnil, which acts as a benzodiazepine receptor agonist, produced the same pattern of results: a selective enhancement of saline drinking (Cooper and Greenwood, 1992). Hence, we can see that effects of drugs acting as agonists of benzodiazepine receptors are not limited to the evaluation of sweet taste stimuli, but generalize to include salty taste too.

If benzodiazepines enhance the palatability of ingested solutions, what do they do if animals are presented with an aversive taste in food or fluids? Early studies showed that the benzodiazepine, oxazepam, overcame the suppressant effect of quinine adulteration (Margules and Stein, 1967), while, conversely, quinine adulteration blocked the hyperphagic effect of chlordiazepoxide (Niki, 1965). In more recent work, we demonstrated that benzodiazepine partial agonists Ro 16-6028 and Ro 17-1812 completely abolished the aversion to a dilute quinine solution in a two-choice test (Cooper and Green, 1993). One interpretation that could be placed on these data is that the effect reflects a disinhibitory or anti-aversive action of the benzodiazepines. However, an alternative we should like to propose is that the drug treatments enhance the evaluation of palatability and, therefore, as a secondary consequence, enhance the consumption of the bitter-tasting quinine solution.

We should like to avoid giving the impression that benzodiazepine-induced changes in palatability and ingestion are related solely to changes in taste evaluation. Recently, we have begun to make comparisons between non-deprived rats drinking sucrose solutions and those drinking lipid emulsions.

First, an analysis of cumulative curves for licking reveals that there is a close similarity in terms of concentration-dependent effects on licking behaviour (Fig. 2). Second, midazolam (0.3–3.0 mg/kg intraperitoneally) significantly and dose-dependently enhanced the consumption of a 3% sucrose solution and of a 1% lipid emulsion (Fig. 3). Other concentrations were little affected (except for a single dose effect on intake of 10% sucrose), which may have been due to ceiling effects at higher concentrations. In terms of ingestive behaviour, therefore, effects of benzodiazepines are not limited to sweet, caloric solutions like sucrose, but also extend to include lipid emulsions. Benzodiazepine-induced hyperphagia is not restricted to foods that are sweet-tasting, but can also apply to lipid consumption. As yet, we do not know the basis for the ingestive response to the lipid, but our results imply that, if benzodiazepines potentiate palatability, then the sources of the palatability most probably extend beyond the evaluation of specific taste stimuli.

2.3 Taste reactivity studies

A powerful approach to the study of taste palatability, together with its neural and neurochemical basis, is a methodology that relies on taste reactivity measures (Grill and Berridge, 1985). In this approach, a flavoured solution is introduced into a rat's mouth via a permanently implanted intraoral cannula. Tastes that are preferred elicit a pattern on ingestive reactions such as tongue protrusion, mouth movement and paw licking (Grill and Norgren, 1978a,b). However, tastes that are normally avoided elicit a different set of reactions (gaping, chin rubbing, paw treading, forelimb flailing and head shaking) (Grill and Norgren, 1978a,b).

If benzodiazepines do act to enhance palatability, then it should be possible to see this effect reflected in changes in the pattern of taste reactivity measures. Indeed, Berridge and Treit (1986) first demonstrated that chlordiazepoxide selectively enhanced the positive ingestive reactions, while leaving aversive reactions substantially unaltered. These authors interpreted their data as showing that benzodiazepines 'enhance the positive evaluation of palatability while having little or no effect on the aversive evaluation'. Results confirming this conclusion have been provided by Treit et al. (1987), Treit and Berridge (1990), Parker (1994) and Gray and Cooper (1995).

It appears, therefore, that benzodiazepines enhance palatability, as indexed by taste reactivity tests, and this selective effect may satisfactorily account for the enhanced taste preference and increased food consumption that are typical

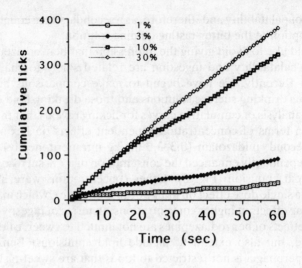

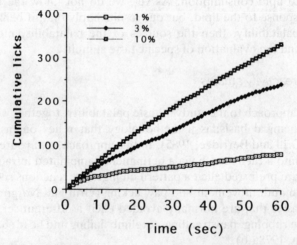

Fig. 2 Cumulative licking curves for non-deprived rats consuming sucrose solutions (above) and lipid (below), at several concentrations in a 60-s short-exposure test. The cumulative lick functions are clearly concentration dependent; note the close similarity between curves for the two situations, for example at 10% sucrose and 10% lipid. (S. Higgs and S. J. Cooper, unpublished results.)

effects of these drugs on ingestive behaviour. We shall consider, later in the chapter, evidence which identifies possible sites of action of benzodiazepines in the brainstem for their selective effects in the taste reactivity test and also for their effects on food consumption.

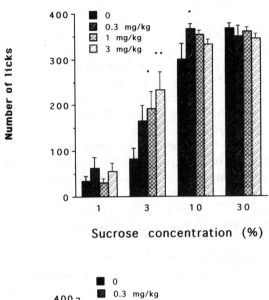

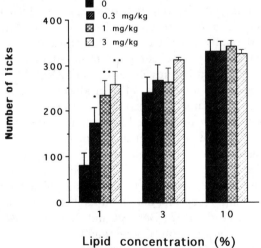

Fig. 3 Midazolam (0.3–3.0 mg/kg) significantly enhanced the number of licks in a 60-s short-exposure test, both for the consumption of sucrose (above) and for lipid (below). Ceiling effects may have intervened to prevent significant effects at higher concentrations, but it is striking that the effects of midazolam were very similar for 3% sucrose and 1% lipid. Hence, midazolam's effects are detectable within the first minute of licking, and are not limited to sweet solutions. These data suggest that benzodiazepines may have an immediate effect, within a meal, in enhancing palatability, which depends not only on taste stimuli but also on other characteristics of food. (S. Higgs and S. J. Cooper, unpublished results.)

3 Pharmacology of benzodiazepine receptor-mediated changes in food intake

3.1 Increases in food ingestion

When benzodiazepine receptors were discovered, a distinction was drawn between *central* and *peripheral* receptors (Richards and Möhler, 1984). The receptor subtypes exhibited pharmacological specificity, such that clonazepam is a selective ligand for the latter. We found that clonazepam, but not Ro 5-4864, induced a robust hyperphagic effect in non-deprived rats consuming a palatable sweetened diet (Cooper and Gilbert, 1985). Hence the hyperphagic effect of benzodiazepines depends on actions at the central-type receptor. Moreover, we demonstrated in the same work that clonazepam-induced hyperphagia could be blocked by Ro 15-1788 (flumazenil), a selective benzodiazepine receptor antagonist (Cooper and Gilbert, 1985). An atypical 1,4-benzodiazepine, Ro 5-3663, which is thought to *antagonize* GABAergic inhibitory neurotransmission (Olsen, 1981), produced an anorectic effect which could be completely overcome by clonazepam (Cooper and Gilbert, 1985).

It is not only benzodiazepines, which act as agonists at benzodiazepine receptors (clonazepam, midazolam, diazepam, chlordiazepoxide), that stimulate food consumption, but also *non*-benzodiazepines, which nevertheless exhibit agonist properties at these receptors. Thus, we showed that zopiclone (a pyrrolopyrazine derivative) and CL 218 872 (a triazolopyridazine derivative) significantly increased food consumption in non-deprived rats (Cooper and Moores, 1985). Two β-carbolines ZK 93423 and ZK 91296, which act as agonists at benzodiazepine receptors, also produced hyperphagic effects (Cooper, 1986b). Hence, it is not the benzodiazepine structure of the drugs, as such, which is responsible for the induced hyperphagic effect, but rather the agonist activity by any type of drug at benzodiazepine receptors.

Even this latter assertion has to be modified, however, if a distinction is drawn between *full* and *partial* agonists. This first became apparent when we tested the pyrazoloquinoline derivatives CGS 9896, which binds with high affinity to benzodiazepine receptors, and exhibits anxiolytic and anticonvulsant effects (Goldberg et al., 1983; Bennett and Petrack, 1984). It did not increase palatable food consumption (Cooper and Gilbert, 1985), and nor did the closely related compound CGS 9895 (Cooper and Yerbury, 1986). Instead, both CGS 9895 and CGS 9896 completely antagonized the hyperphagic effect produced by clonazepam (Cooper and Yerbury, 1986).

In non-derived animals eating a palatable diet, the pyrazoloquinolines behaved as benzodiazepine receptor antagonists. However, under certain restricted conditions, it may be possible to detect a pyrozoloquinoline-induced hyperphagic effect. Recently, Chen and colleagues (1995) showed that CGS 9896 significantly increased food consumption in non-deprived rats eating a palatable diet and in 16-h food-deprived rats eating a standard diet. However, it was ineffective in 24-h food-deprived rats or in food-deprived animals eating the palatable diet. These new data suggest that, with certain drugs at least (including weak partial agonists), hyperphagic effects can be demonstrated in some but not all experimental conditions. In addition, they effectively antagonize the hyperphagic effect of a full agonist, such as clonazepam (Cooper and Yerbury, 1986).

There are other partial agonists for which we have good evidence that they produce a hyperphagic effect. We have documented this with respect to ZK 91296, a β-carboline partial agonist at benzodiazepine receptors (Cooper, 1986b), Ro 16-6028 (bretazenil), Ro 17-1812 and Ro 23-0364, which are imidazobenzodiazepine partial agonists at these receptors (Yerbury and Cooper, 1987), and CGS 17867A, a pyrazoloquinoline (Yerbury and Cooper, 1989). An important feature of these partial agonists, in rats, is that they produce little sedation or muscle relaxation (Cooper et al., 1987a), and therefore the hyperphagic effect in which we are interested can be pharmacologically dissociated from behaviourally depressant effects (Cooper et al., 1987b).

In this way, we can envisage a continuum of drugs, from full agonists acting at benzodiazepine receptors (e.g. diazepam, midazolam) at one extreme, to partial agonists such as bretazenil and Ro 17-1812 which elicit hyperphagia in the absence of prominent side-effects, and to antagonists like flumazenil (Ro 15-1788) which will not induce hyperphagia but can block hyperphagic effects due to agonist activity at benzodiazepine receptors.

3.2   Decreases in food ingestion

So far, we have dealt exclusively with the idea that drug actions at benzodiazepine receptors result in hyperphagia. It was naturally surprising, therefore, when we discovered that a pyrazoloquinoline, CGS 8216, which binds to benzodiazepine receptors, produced a significant reduction in food intake in non-deprived rats (Cooper and Moores, 1985). This appeared to be an example of the effects of a recently described category of drugs: benzodiazepine receptor *inverse* agonists (see Sarter et al., 1995, for a complete review of these drugs). These compounds act at benzodiazepine receptors, but produce effects that oppose those of classical benzodiazepine agonists.

Hence, benzodiazepine receptor *inverse* agonists should be anorectic agents, and this is what we set out to demonstrate. Not only CGS 8216 but also the β-carbolines FG 7142 and DMCM (methyl-6,7-dimethoxy-4-ethyl-β-carboline-3-carboxylate), each of which is an inverse agonist, produced very substantial decreases in palatable food consumption (Cooper et al., 1989). In addition, in contrast to benzodiazepine receptor agonists, the inverse agonists reduce or abolish sweet-taste preferences (Cooper, 1986a; Kirkham and Cooper, 1986; Cooper et al., 1989). These data gave rise to the idea that, at benzodiazepine receptors, *bidirectional* control of either food consumption (Cooper, 1985) or taste preferences (Cooper, 1989) could be achieved. This is a fundamental idea, and directs our attention to the possibility of two-way modulation of behaviour through a single receptor type. Following our earlier discussion that benzodiazepines enhance palatability, we can now be more precise and suggest that palatability evaluation can be *bidirectionally* controlled by drugs active at benzodiazepine receptors.

4 Neural substrates

Despite such behavioural and pharmacological advances, there has been little progress to date in identifying the neural substrates for the effect of benzodiazepine receptors on ingestive behaviour. However, recent work in our laboratory has begun to identify potential central sites of action for benzodiazepine-induced hyperphagia. The focus for these studies has been on brainstem structures, which, given the fairly sparse distribution of benzodiazepine receptors in this area, may seem somewhat surprising. Nevertheless, there is evidence to suggest that brainstem sites, although often neglected in the study of ingestive behaviour, may have an important role to play. For example, using a taste reactivity paradigm, Berridge (1988) has shown that the increase in positive ingestive responses that occurs following administration of chlordiazepoxide can still be observed in the decerebrate rat. This result is important because it indicates that the neural circuitry necessary for the effects of benzodiazepine receptor agonists in the taste reactivity test may reside within the lower brainstem. Since taste is an important determinant of ingestive behaviour it is possible that benzodiazepines might increase food intake by acting on neural systems involved in the processing of taste information. According to this argument, if benzodiazepine hyperphagia is dependent on a change in the response to taste properties of ingested materials, then brainstem mechanisms may be involved in both the effects of benzodiazepines in the taste reactivity paradigm and also in intake tests.

4.1 Hyperphagia

We set out to test directly the hypothesis that brainstem structures are involved in benzodiazepine-induced hyperphagia by microinjecting the water-soluble benzodiazepine receptor agonist midazolam directly into the fourth ventricle of the rat, and then measuring the effect on intake of a palatable diet.

As Fig. 4 indicates, microinjection of 30 μg/μl midazolam into the fourth ventricle induced a significant increase in the intake of the palatable diet. Midazolam's central hyperphagic effect could be blocked by the specific benzodiazepine receptor antagonist flumazenil, administered systemically. Hence, the midazolam effect was due to action at specific benzodiazepine receptors. Although not sufficient to identify the precise structures involved in the effects of benzodiazepines on ingestion, these data suggest that receptors in

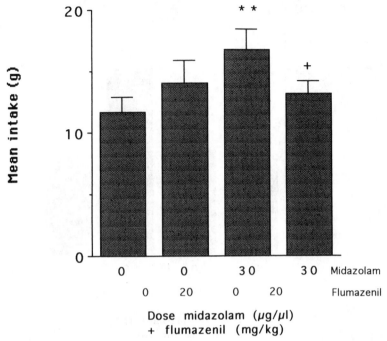

Fig. 4 The selective benzodiazepine receptor antagonist flumazenil blocked the hyperphagic effect of midazolam, which had been injected directly into the fourth ventricle. Values are mean + SEM intake for non-deprived rats eating a palatable diet in a 30-min test. $**P < 0.01$ vs baseline intake; $^+P < 0.01$ vs midazolam alone. (S. Higgs and S. J. Cooper, unpublished results.)

the brainstem, located in the proximity of the fourth ventricle, could mediate the effect.

To investigate further which brainstem structures might be involved, it was necessary to inject benzodiazepines into specific sites close to the fourth ventricle. For a number of reasons the parabrachial nucleus (PBN) was selected as a possible candidate (Cooper and Higgs, 1994a). Significantly, an autoradiographic binding study identified a population of benzodiazepine receptors in the region of the PBN (Higgs *et al.*, 1993). The PBN is the second relay in the gustatory pathway (Norgren and Leonard, 1973; Norgren and Pfaffman, 1975) and, given the hypothesis outlined above that benzodiazepines may act on components of the taste system, this nucleus was a natural choice. The nucleus of the solitary tract (NTS), which is the first relay in the taste pathway and is also located close to the fourth ventricle, was a less obvious candidate given that the autoradiographic binding study (Higgs *et al.*, 1993) failed to identify benzodiazepine receptors in a region corresponding to the NTS. Additional evidence pointing to a role for the PBN comes from anatomical data showing that the PBN makes extensive reciprocal connections with

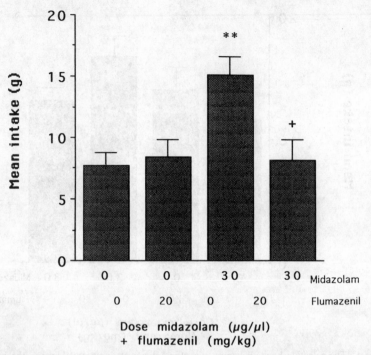

Fig. 5 Flumazenil blocked the hyperphagic effect of midazolam, which had been injected directly into the parabrachial nucleus. Values are mean + SEM intake for non-deprived rats eating a palatable diet in a 30-min test. **$P < 0.01$ vs baseline intake; +$P < 0.01$ vs midazolam alone. (S. Higgs and S. J. Cooper, unpublished results.)

other regions of the brain such as the hypothalamus (Norgren, 1976; Saper and Loewy, 1980; Krukoff et al., 1993) and amygdala (Norgren, 1976), which have previously been implicated in the control of ingestive behaviour. The results from various behavioural studies involving lesions of the PBN also strongly suggest a role for this nucleus in the control of feeding. Lesions of the PBN have been shown to cause a hyperphagic response (Nagai et al., 1987) and to disrupt the formation of conditioned taste aversions (Flynn et al., 1991b; Spector et al., 1992; Aguero et al., 1993a,b). Finally, lesioning the PBN also alters taste preferences, taste reactivity responses and the expression of sodium appetite (Flynn et al., 1991a,b).

Direct injection of midazolam ($30\,\mu g/\mu l$) into the PBN produced a significant increase in the consumption of a palatable mash (Fig. 5). The hyperphagic effect was blocked by flumazenil, indicating that the effect was mediated by specific benzodiazepine receptors.

4.2 Taste reactivity

To assess the role of brainstem structures in the increase in ingestive responding brought about the benzodiazepines, Peciña and Berridge (1992) microinjected the benzodiazepine receptor agonist diazepam directly into the fourth ventricle. They found that hedonic reactions to a palatable 7% sucrose solution were greatly enhanced in animals receiving diazepam injections as opposed to a vehicle control injection. The authors argued for a brainstem site of action specifically, as opposed to an action in forebrain areas occurring as a result of diffusion throughout the ventricular system, based on experiments that compared the relative efficacy of fourth *vs* lateral ventricle injection. The threshold dose required for lateral ventricle enhancement of ingestive reactions is much greater than that for fourth ventricular injections. This comparison suggests that the primary site of action is located in the brainstem.

Therefore, evidence from the experiments described above seems to suggest that brainstem structures may be important in mediating both the hyperphagic and hedonic-enhancing effects of the benzodiazepines (Berridge and Peciña, 1995). The results from the intake studies and the taste reactivity studies outlined here may be combined to suggest a common theory accounting for the effects of benzodiazepines on ingestive behaviour. It seems likely that benzodiazepine receptor agonists acting at receptors located within the taste pathway, specifically in the PBN, may alter the hedonic assessment of tastants, leading to an increase in the consumption of the associated food or fluid (Cooper and Higgs, 1994a,b).

4.3 Interactions with opioid mechanisms

It is striking that the effects of benzodiazepines on food intake are very similar to the effects of opioid agonists on ingestion. For example, morphine brings about a significant increase in food consumption when administered systemically (Sanger and McCarthy, 1980; Kavaliers and Hirst, 1985). Various κ (Cooper *et al.*, 1985b) and σ (Gosnell *et al.*, 1983) opioid agonists also bring about reliable increases in feeding (see Chapter 7). In addition, opioid agonists like benzodiazepines increase the preference for saccharin in water-deprived rats (Calcagnetti and Reid, 1983). Importantly, for any hypothesis claiming similarity of effects between the benzodiazepines and opioids, Doyle and co-workers (1993) have shown that morphine, in a manner analogous to that of chlordiazepoxide, enhances positive taste reactions. The parallels being so clear, it has been suggested that benzodiazepine and opioid effects on ingestion may be interrelated (Cooper, 1983; Reid, 1985). This hypothesis is supported by the finding that opioid antagonists will block benzodiazepine-induced hyperphagia (Birk and Noble, 1981; Britton *et al.*, 1981; Jackson and Sewell, 1985).

An examination of the neurochemistry of the PBN raises the interesting possibility that the postulated interaction between benzodiazepines and opioids on feeding behaviour may occur in this area. Analysis of the distribution of the opioid receptor subtypes in the rat and human brain has revealed that μ and κ receptors are localized in the PBN (Mansour *et al.*, 1988). There is also some evidence which points to a connection between the PBN and the lateral hypothalamus, which could exert some control over ingestive behaviour. For example, Touzani *et al.* (1993) have demonstrated that a projection from the lateral hypothalamus to the PBN is immunoreactive to α-neoendorphin antisera. Feeding elicited by electrical stimulation of the lateral hypothalamus can be affected by opioid microinjection of the μ opioid antagonist naloxone into the PBN (Carr *et al.*, 1991). Direct injection of morphine into the PBN has also been shown to alter saccharin preference, which in turn is affected by lesions of the lateral hypothalamus (Moufid-Bellancourt and Velley, 1994). Although the possibility that the PBN is intimately involved in interactions between benzodiazepines and opioids still remains to be tested thoroughly, further research may prove useful in bringing together much neuropharmacological data on taste preferences and taste reactivity.

5   Receptor subtypes

5.1 GABA$_A$ receptor subtypes

It was mentioned earlier in this chapter that benzodiazepine ligands exert their pharmacological effects through allosteric modulation of the GABA$_A$ receptor protein (Haefely *et al.*, 1985; Polc, 1988). Recent advances in molecular biology have greatly increased our understanding of the structural characteristics of the GABA$_A$–receptor complex, including the requirements for drug actions at the benzodiazepine receptor site located on the complex (Lüddens *et al.*, 1995). The GABA$_A$–receptor complex comprises five subunits, which are currently grouped into five classes, with up to six variants in each (i.e. $\alpha1$–6, β–3, $\gamma1$–3, δ and $\rho1$–2). As we shall see below, the variants within subunits help determine the pharmacological characteristics of the assembled receptor complex.

The amazing molecular diversity that has been revealed has mainly been the result of the application of biochemical and complementary DNA (cDNA) cloning techniques. The first evidence suggesting GABA$_A$ receptor multiplicity came from selective photoaffinity labelling studies in which one subunit was irreversibly labelled by [^{3}H]flunitrazepam and another was labelled by [^{3}H]muscimol (Sigel *et al.*, 1983). Improvements in the resolution of gel electrophoresis techniques then revealed that these subunits consisted of several different proteins (Fuchs and Seighart, 1989). Molecular biological cloning techniques, involving the screening of cDNA libraries with oligonucleotide probes, have since allowed the identification of novel subunits and many more structural isoforms of the $GABA_A$ receptor. As mentioned above, five different subunits have been identified in all, the α, β, γ, δ and ρ subunits (Olsen and Tobin, 1990; Lüddens and Wisden, 1991). Each, apart from the δ and ρ subunits, exists in multiple isoforms. In the rodent brain six α subunits have currently been identified ($\alpha1$–$\alpha6$), four β subunits ($\beta1$–$\beta4$), three γ subunits ($\gamma1$–$\gamma3$), a δ subunit, and ρ subunits which are located in the retina.

5.2   Subunit functions

The discovery of multiple receptor subunits does not in itself allow the composition of functional receptors to be identified. To establish which subunits need to be assembled to form a functional receptor, and what the specific functional contribution of each subunit might be, recombinant $GABA_A$ receptors have been expressed in the *Xenopus* oocyte cells. A combination of α and β subunits expressed in *Xenopus* oocytes has been found successfully to mimic $GABA_A$-induced chloride ion flux. However, receptors composed only of α and β subunits have not been shown to be pharmacologically identical to the native $GABA_A$ receptor, because benzodiazepine potentiation is not observed (Levitan *et al.*, 1988). This result implies that other subunits are required for benzodiazepine activity. The critical subunit was isolated by Pritchett and co-workers (1989), and is referred to as the γ subunit. The majority of studies have reported expression of the $\gamma2$ subunit because it was the first to be cloned, but limited studies with the $\gamma1$ subunit (Ymer *et al.*, 1990) suggest that it produces unusual responses. When the $\gamma1$ subunit is combined with $\alpha1$ or $\alpha5$, and $\beta1$ subunits in oocytes, a reduced potentiation is observed following flunitrazepam administration. In addition, the response to inverse agonists such as DMCM is either reduced or unexpectedly potentiated (von Blankenfield *et al.*, 1990). Consequently, it has been suggested that this particular receptor subunit combination may not occur *in vivo* (Ymer *et al.*, 1990). The novel $\gamma3$ subunit recently isolated by Herb and colleagues (1992) also appears to confer benzodiazepine responsivity and has been shown to be able functionally to replace the $\gamma2$ subunit (Knoflach *et al.*, 1991).

Although it appears that the γ subunit is required to obtain a benzodiazepine response, studies in which the effects of different combinations of α subunit have been investigated indicate that it is the α subunit which determines the type of benzodiazepine pharmacology, and that the type of α subunit affects both the efficacy and affinity of benzodiazepine binding (Siegel *et al.*, 1990; von Blankenfield, 1990).

Substitution of a δ subunit for a γ subunit in recombinant receptors results in a loss of benzodiazepine sensitivity (Shivers *et al.*, 1989), suggesting that receptors containing a δ subunit may constitute $GABA_A$ receptors that are not modulated by benzodiazepines.

5.3 Multiple benzodiazepine receptor subtypes

No selective drugs are available at present with which to probe the function of different $GABA_A$ receptors, but two benzodiazepine receptor subtypes have been distinguished on the basis of binding studies. Some receptors have greater affinity for benzodiazepines such as CL 218 872 and β-carbolines, and have been referred to as type 1 receptors. They are distributed ubiquitously in the brain but are particularly abundant in the cerebellum. Alternatively, type II receptors have a high affinity for benzodiazepines but a reduced affinity for other compounds, and are more selectively located in the hippocampus, striatum and spinal cord.

The molecular basis for this receptor heterogeneity has been examined once again by expression of recombinant receptors in cell lines. Receptors composed of the $\alpha 1$, $\beta 1$ and $\gamma 2$ subunits have a high affinity for CL 218 872 (Pritchett *et al.*, 1989). The distribution of $\alpha 1$ subunits is high in the cerebellum (Lüddens *et al.*, 1990), suggesting that this subunit confers type I receptor pharmacology. Evidence indicates that several α subunits may be responsible for type II receptor pharmacology, because receptors expressing the $\alpha 1$ and $\alpha 2$ subunits show lower affinity for benzodiazepine receptor-selective ligands (Pritchett *et al.*, 1989; Pritchett and Seeburg, 1990). Substitution of the $\alpha 5$ subunit results in type II-like pharmacology but with a reduced affinity for the benzodiazepine ligand zolpidem (Pritchett and Seeburg, 1990).

The inverse agonist Ro 15-4513 has been shown to bind not only to sites that can be competitively labelled with [^{3}H]flunitrazepam but also to cerebellar granule sites that are not labelled by [^{3}H]flunitrazepam. These sites, first described by Turner *et al.* (1991), have been described as diazepam-insensitive sites because diazepam fails to displace a significant proportion of bound [^{3}H]Ro 15-4513 at these sites. A number of other inverse agonists, including CGS 8216, also bind to diazepam-insensitive sites. However, the site does not uniquely bind inverse agonists, since two other compounds observed to bind to the site are the β-carbolines ZK 912216 and ZK 94323, which have agonist properties. The diazepam-insensitive binding site may represent a novel class of $GABA_A$ receptor subtype. Turner and colleagues (1991) found that antagonism of Ro 15-4513 binding by CGS 8216 could be modulated by GABA. This conclusion is reinforced by molecular cloning results from Lüddens *et al.* (1990), who found that diazepam-insensitive-like properties were exhibited by human embryonic kidney cells transfected with $\alpha 6$, $\beta 2$, $\gamma 2$ $GABA_A$ receptor subunits' (but not other subunits) cDNAs. The distribution of the $\alpha 6$ subunit also quite conveniently corresponds to the distribution of diazepam-insensitive sites, since it is almost exclusively expressed in the cerebellum (Lüddens *et al.*, 1990). Ro 15-4513, as well as having inverse benzodiazepine properties, behaves as an ethanol antagonist, and it has been suggested that the diazepam-insensitive sites may mediate the ethanol-antagonistic properties of this compound.

5.4 Significance of benzodiazepine-induced hyperphagia

We have reached an interesting stage in studies of benzodiazepine receptor mechanisms and pharmacology, and molecular biology has revealed a hitherto unsuspected complexity in the structural characteristics of the $GABA_A$ receptor complex. For a considerable period of time, we have been aware of the many and varied behavioural effects of benzodiazepines, and we are now reaching a position where the neural basis of these effects can be analysed in some detail. Not only are the regions of the brain in which benzodiazepine receptors are located highly relevant to the effects these drugs produce, but also there is a strong likelihood that subunit composition of assembled $GABA_A$ receptors may be an important determinant of the effects.

This leads us to anticipate a richer future pharmacology, which may allow us to dissect the several important consequences of benzodiazepine action. In this chapter, we have provided a behavioural account of benzodiazepine modulation of ingestive responses, and directed attention to the possible importance of the PBN in the lower brainstem as an important site of action. What lies before us is the problem of explaining how the effects of benzodiazepines at a molecular level lead to changes in neuronal activity within identified systems in the brain, which in turn bring about the selective behavioural changes that we and others have sought to identify.

New drug developments, exploiting either agonist or inverse agonist properties at newly characterized benzodiazepine receptor subtypes, may hold the key for important therapeutic developments in relation to obesity and eating disorders. The $GABA_A$–receptor complex is attracting a great deal of attention, and this may lead to quite novel pharmacological advances. In addition, continued study of benzodiazepines and their effects on ingestive responses may bring us closer to an understanding of the neural mechanisms responsible for taking important evaluative decisions about the foods we choose to ingest.

Acknowledgements

The authors wish to express our sincere thanks to Mrs Margaret Hall for her help in the preparation of this chapter.

References

Aguero, A., Arnedo, M., Gallo, M. and Puerto, P. (1993a). Lesions of the lateral parabrachial nuclei disrupt aversion learning induced by electrical stimulation of the area postrema. *Brain Res. Bull.* 30, 585–592.

Aguero, A., Arnedo, M., Gallo, M. and Puerto, A. (1993b). The functional relevance of the lateral parabrachial nucleus in lithium chloride-induced aversion learning. *Pharmacol. Biochem. Behav.* 45, 973–978.

Bainbridge, J. G. (1968). The effect of psychotropic drugs on food reinforced behaviour and on food consumption. *Psychopharmacology (Berl.)* 12, 204–213.

Bennett, D. A. and Petrack, B. (1984). CGS 9896: a nonbenzodiazepine, nonsedating potential anxiolytic. *Drug Rev. Res.* **4**, 75–82.

Berridge, K. C. (1988). Brain stem systems mediate the enhancement of palatability by chlordiazepoxide. *Brain Res.* **447**, 262–268.

Berridge, K. C. and Peciña, S. (1995). Benzodiazepines, appetite and taste palatability. *Neurosci. Biobehav. Rev.* **19**, 121–131.

Berridge, K. C. and Treit, D. (1986). Chlordiazepoxide directly enhances positive ingestive reactions in rats. *Pharmacol. Biochem. Behav.* **24**, 217–221.

Birk, J. and Noble, R. G. (1981). Naloxone antagonism of diazepam-induced feeding in the Syrian hamster. *Life Sci.* **29**, 1297–1302.

Bosmann, H. B., Case, R. and DiStefano, P. (1977). Diazepam receptor characterization: specific binding of a benzodiazepine to macromolecules in various areas of rat brain. *FEBS Lett.* **82**, 368–372.

Britton, D. R., Britton, K. T., Dalton, D. and Vale, W. (1981). Effects of naloxone on anti-conflict and hyperphagic actions of diazepam. *Life Sci.* **29**, 1297–1302.

Calcagnetti, D. J. and Reid, L. D. (1983). Morphine and acceptability of putative reinforcers. *Pharmacol. Biochem. Behav.* **5**, 495–497.

Carr, K. D., Aleman, D. O., Bak, T. H. and Simon, E. J. (1991). Effects of parabrachial opioid antagonism on stimulation-induced feeding. *Brain Res.* **545**, 283–286.

Chen, S.-W., Davies, M. F. and Loew, G. H. (1995). Food palatability and hunger modulated effects of CGS 9896 and CGS 8216 on food intake. *Pharmacol. Biochem. Behav.* **51**, 499–503.

Cooper, S. J. (1980a), Benzodiazepines as appetite-enhancing compounds. *Appetite* **1**, 7–19.

Cooper, S. J. (1980b). Effects of chlordiazepoxide and diazepam on feeding performance in a food-preference test. *Pharmacology* **69**, 73–78.

Cooper, S. J. (1983). Benzodiazepine–opiate interactions in relation to feeding and drinking. *Neuropharmacology* **21**, 483–486.

Cooper, S. J. (1985). Bidirectional control of palatable food consumption through a common benzodiazepine receptor: theory and evidence. *Brain Res. Bull.* **15**, 397–410.

Cooper, S. J. (1986a). Effects of the beta-carboline FG 7142 on saccharin preference and quinine aversion in water-deprived rats. *Neuropharmacology* **25**, 213–216.

Cooper, S. J. (1986b). Hyperphagic and anorectic effects of β-carbolines in a palatable food consumption test: comparisons with triazolam and quazepam. *Eur. J. Pharmacol.* **120**, 257–265.

Cooper, S. J. (1989). Benzodiazepine receptor-mediated enhancement and inhibition of taste reactivity, food choice and intake. *Ann. N.Y. Acad. Sci.* **575**, 321–337.

Cooper, S. J. and Barber, D. J. (1993). The benzodiazepine receptor partial agonist bretazenil and the partial inverse agonist Ro 15-4513: effects on salt preference and aversion in the rat. *Brain Res.* **612**, 313–318.

Cooper, S. J. and Crummy, Y. M. T. (1978). Enhanced choice of familiar food in a food preference test after chlordiazepoxide administration. *Psychopharmacology* **59**, 51–56.

Cooper, S. J. and Estall, L. B. (1985). Behavioural pharmacology of food, water and salt intake in relation to drug actions at benzodiazepine receptors. *Neurosci. Biobehav. Rev.* **9**, 5–19.

Cooper, S. J. and Gilbert, D. B. (1985). Clonazepam-induced hyperphagia in non-deprived rats: tests of pharmacological specificity with Ro 5-4864, Ro 5-3663, Ro 15-1788 and CGS 9896. *Pharmacol. Biochem. Behav.* **22**, 753–760.

Cooper, S. J. and Green, A. E. (1993). The benzodiazepine receptor partial agonists bretazenil (Ro 16-6028) and Ro 17-1812, affect saccharin preference and aversion in the rat. *Behav. Pharmacol.* **4**, 81–85.

Cooper, S. J. and Greenwood, S. E. (1992). The β-carboline abecarnil, a novel agonist at central benzodiazepine receptors, influences saccharin and salt preference in the rat. *Brain Res.* **59**, 144–147.

Cooper, S. J. and Higgs, S. (1994a). The benzodiazepine agonist midazolam microinjected into the rat parobrachial nucleus produces hyperphagia. *Soc. Neurosci. Abstr.* **20**, 1285.

Cooper, S. J. and Higgs, S. (1994b). Neuropharmacology of appetite and taste preferences. In *Appetite: Neural and Behavioural Bases* (C. R. Legg and D. A. Booth, eds), pp. 212–216. Oxford University Press, Oxford.

Cooper, S. J. and Moores, W. R. (1985) Benzodiazepine-induced hyperphagia in the nondeprived rat: comparisons with CL 218 872, zopiclone, tracazolate and phenobarbital. *Pharmacol. Biochem. Behav.* **23**, 169–172.

Cooper, S. J. and Yerbury, R. E. (1986). Benzodiazepine-induced hyperphagia: stereospecificity and antagonism by pyrazoloquinolines, CGS 9895 and CGS 9896. *Psychopharmacology* **89**, 462–466.

Cooper, S. J. and Yerbury, R. E. (1988). Clonazepam selectively increases saccharin consumption in a two choice test. *Brain Res.* **456**, 173–176.

Cooper, S. J., Barber, D. J., Gilbert, D. B. and Moores, W. R. (1985a). Benzodiazepine receptor ligands and the consumption of a highly palatable diet in non-deprived male rats. *Psychopharmacology* **86**, 348–355.

Cooper, S. J., Moores, W. R., Jackson, A. and Barber, D. J. (1985b). Effects of tifluadom on food consumption compared with chlordiazepoxide and κ agonists in the rat. *Neuropharmacology* **24**, 877–883.

Cooper, S. J., Kirkham, T. C. and Estall, L. B. (1987a). Pyrazoloquinolines: second generation benzodiazepine receptor ligands have heterogeneous effects. *Trends Pharmacol. Sci.* **8**, 180–184.

Cooper, S. J., Yerbury, R. E., Neill, J. C. and Desa, A. (1987b). Partial agonists acting as benzodiazepine receptors can be differentiated in tests of ingestional behaviour. *Physiol. Behav.* **41**, 247–255.

Cooper, S. J., Bowyer, D. M. and van der Hoek, G. (1989). Effects of the imidabenzodiazepine Ro 15-4513 on saccharin choice and acceptance in the rat. *Brain Res.* **494**, 172–174.

Doyle, T. G., Berridge, K. C. and Gosnell, B. A. (1993). Morphine enhances hedonic taste palatability in rats. *Pharmacol. Biochem. Behav.* **12**, 195–200.

Estall, L. B. and Cooper, S. J. (1987). Differential effects of benzodiazepine receptor ligands on isotonic saline and water consumption in water-deprived rats. *Pharmacol. Biochem. Behav.* **26**, 247–252.

Flynn, F. W., Grill, H. J., Schulkin, J. and Norgren, R. (1991a). Central gustatory lesions: 2. Effects on sodium appetite, taste aversion learning and feeding behaviours. *Behav. Neurosci.* **105**, 944–954.

Flynn, F. W., Grill, H. J., Schwartz, G. J. and Norgren, R. (1991b). Central gustatory lesions: preference and taste reactivity tests. *Behav. Neurosci.* **105**, 933–943.

Fratta, W., Mereu, G., Chessa, P., Paglietti, E. and Gessa, G. (1976). Benzodiazepine-induced voraciousness in cats and inhibition of amphetamine-anorexia. *Life Sci.* **18**, 1157–1166.

Fuchs, K. and Sieghart, W. (1989). Evidence for the existence of several different α and β subunits of GABA/benzodiazepine receptor complex from rat brain. *Neurosci. Lett.* **97**, 329–333.

Goldberg, M. E., Salama, A. I., Patel, J. B. and Malick, J. B. (1983). Novel non-benzodiazepine anxiolytics. *Neuropharmacology* **22**, 1499–1504.

Gosnell, B. A., Levine, A. S. and Morley, J. E. (1983). N-allylnormetazocine (SKK-10 047): the induction of feeding by a putative sigma agonist. *Pharmacol. Biochem. Behav.* **19**, 737–742.

Gray, R. W. and Cooper, S. J. (1995). Benzodiazepines and palatability: taste reactivity in normal ingestion. *Physiol. Behav.* **58**, 853–859.

Grill, H. J. and Berridge, K. C. (1985). Taste reactivity as a measure of the neural control of palatability. *Prog. Psychobiol. Physiol. Psychol.* **11**, 1–16.

Grill, H. J. and Norgren, R. (1978a). The taste reactivity test. I. Mimetic responses to gustatory stimuli in neurologically normal rats. *Brain Res.* **143**, 263–279.

Grill, H. J. and Norgren, R. (1978b). The taste reactivity test. II. Mimetic responses to gustatory stimuli in neurologically normal rats. *Brain Res.* **143**, 281–297.

Haefely, W., Kyburz, E., Gerecke, M. and Möhler, H. (1985). Recent advances in the molecular pharmacology of benzodiazepine receptors and in the structure activity relationships of their agonists and antagonists. In *Advances in Drug Research* (B. Testa, ed), pp. 165–322. Academic Press, London.

Herb, A., Wisden, W., Lüddens, H., Puia, G., Vicini, S. and Seeburg, P. H. (1992). A third γ subunit of the γ-aminobutryric acid type A receptor family. *Proc. Natl. Acad. Sci.* **89**, 1433–1437.

Higgs, S., Gilbert, D. B., Barnes, N. M. and Cooper, S. J. (1993). Possible brainstem mediation of benzodiazepine-induced hyperphagia. *Appetite*, **21**, 183 (abstract).

Iwahara, S. and Iwasaki, T. (1969). Effect of chlordiazepoxide upon food-intake and spontaneous motor activity of the rat as a function of hours of deprivation. *Jpn. Psychol. Res.* **11**, 117–128.

Jackson, H. C. and Sewell, R. D. E. (1985). Involvement of endogenous enkephalins in the feeding response to diazepam. *Eur. J. Pharmacol.* **107**, 389–901.

Kavaliers, M. and Hirst, M. (1985). The influence of opiate agonists on day–night feeding rhythms in young and old mice. *Brain Res.* **326**, 160–167.

Knoflach, F., Rhyner, T., Villa, M., Kellenberger, S., Drescher, U., Malherbe, P., Sigel, E. and Möhler, H. (1991). The γ3-subunit of the $GABA_A$–receptor confers sensitivity to benzodiazepine receptor ligands. *FEBS Lett.* **293**, 191–194.

Krukoff, T. L., Harris, K. H. and Jhamandas, J. H. (1993). Efferent projections from the parabrachial nucleus demonstrated with the anterograde tracer *Phaseolus vulgaris* leucoagglutinin. *Brain Res. Bull.* **30**, 163–172.

Kirkham, T. C. and Cooper, S. J. (1986). CGS 8216, a novel anorectic agent, selectively reduces saccharin solution consumption in the rat. *Pharmac. Biochem. Behav.* **25**, 341–345.

Levitan, E. S., Blair, L. A., Dione, V. E. and Barnard, E. A. (1988). Biophysical and pharmacological properties of cloned $GABA_A$ receptor subunits expressed in *Xenopus* oocytes. *Neuron* **1**, 773–781.

Lüddens, H. and Wisden, W. (1991). Function and pharmacology of multiple $GABA_A$ receptor subunits. *TIPS* **12**, 49–51.

Lüddens, H., Pritchett, D. B., Köhler, M., Killisch, I., Keinänen, K., Monyer, H., Sprengel, R. and Seeburg, P. H. (1990). Cerebellar $GABA_A$ receptor selective for a behavioural alcohol antagonist. *Nature* **346**, 648–651.

Lüddens, H., Korpi, E. R. and Seeburg, P. H. (1995). $GABA_A$/benzodiazepine receptor heterogeneity: neurophysiological implications. *Neuropharmacology* **34**, 245–254.

Macdonald, R. L. and Twyman, R. E. (1991). Biophysical properties and regulation of $GABA_A$ receptor channels. *Semin. Neurosci.* **3**, 219–235.

Maickel, R. P. and Maloney, G. J. (1974). Taste phenomena influences on stimulation of deprivation-induced fluid consumption in rats. *Neuropharmacology* **13**, 763–767.

Mansour, A., Khachaturian, H., Lewis, M. E., Akil, H. and Watson, S. J. (1988). Anatomy of CNS opioid receptors. *TINS* **7**, 308–314.

Margules, D. L. and Stein, L. (1967). Neuroleptics *v.* tranquilizers: evidence from animal studies of mode and site of action. In *Neuropsychopharmacology* (H. Brill, J. O. Cole, P. Deniker, H. Hippius and P. B. Bradley, eds), pp. 108–120. Excerpta Medica Foundation, Amsterdam.

Möhler, H. and Okada, T. (1977). Benzodiazepine receptors: demonstration in the central nervous system. *Science* **198**, 849–851.

Moufid-Bellancourt, S. and Velley, L. (1994). Effects of morphine injection into the parabrachial area on saccharin preference: modulation by lateral hypothalamic neurons. *Pharmacol. Biochem. Behav.* **48**, 127–133.

Nagai, K., Ino, H., Nakagawa, H., Yamono, M., Toyama, M., Shiosaka, S., Shiotani, Y., Iangaki, S. and Kitoh, S. (1987). Lesions of the lateral part of the parabrachial nucleus caused hyperphagia and obesity. *J. Clin. Biochem. Nutr.* **3**, 103–112.

Niki, H. (1965). Chlordiazepoxide and food-intake in the rat. *Jpn. Psychol. Res.* **7**, 80–85.

Norgren, R. (1976). Taste pathways to hypothalamus and amygdala. *J. Comp. Neurol.* **166**, 17–30.

Norgren, R. and Leonard, C. M. (1973). Ascending central gustatory pathways. *J. Comp. Neurol.* **150**, 217–238.

Norgren, R. and Pfaffman, C. (1975). The pontine taste area in the rat. *Brain Res.* **91**, 99–117.

Olsen, R. W. (1981). GABA–benzodiazepine–barbiturate receptor interactions. *J. Neurochem.* **37**, 1–13.

Olsen, R. W. and Tobin, A. J. (1990). Molecular biology of $GABA_A$ receptors. *FASEB J.* **4**, 1469–1480.

Parker, L. A. (1991). Chlordiazepoxide nonspecifically enhances the consumption of a saccharin solution. *Pharmacol. Biochem. Behav.* **38**, 374–377.

Parker, L. A. (1994). Chlordiazepoxide enhances the palatability of lithium-, amphetamine-, and saline-paired saccharin solution. *Pharmacol. Biochem. Behav.* **38**, 375–377.

Peciña, S. and Berridge, K. C. (1992). Fourth ventricle microinjections of diazepam enhance hedonic reactions to taste. *Soc. Neurosci. Abstr.* **18**, 1231.

Polc, P. (1988). Electrophysiology of benzodiazepine receptor ligands and sites of action. *Prog. Neurobiol.* **31**, 349–424.

Poschel, B. P. H. (1971). A simple and effective screen for benzodiazepine-like drugs. *Psychopharmacologia* **19**, 193–198.

Pritchett, D. B. and Seeburg, P. H. (1990). $GABA_A$ receptor $\alpha 5$-subunit creates novel type II benzodiazepine receptor pharmacology. *J. Neurochem.* **54**, 1802–1804.

Pritchett, D. B., Lüddens, H. and Seeburg, P. H. (1989). Type I and type II $GABA_A$-benzodiazepine receptors produced in transfected cells. *Science* **245**, 1389–1392.

Randall, L. O., Schallek, W., Heise, G. A., Keith, E. F. and Bagdon, R. E. (1960). The psychosedative properties of methaminodiazepoxide. *J. Pharmacol. Exp. Ther.* **129**, 163–197.

Reid, L. D. (1985). Endogenous peptides and regulation of feeding and drinking. *Am. J. Clin. Nutrition* **42**, 1099–1132.

Richards, J. C. and Möhler, H. (1984). Benzodiazepine receptors. *Neuropharmacology* **23**, 233–242.

Roache, J. D. and Zabik, J. E. (1986). The effects of benzodiazepine on taste aversions in a two-bottle choice paradigm. *Pharmacol. Biochem. Behav.* **25**, 431–437.

Sanger, D. J. and McCarthy, P. S. (1980). Differential effects of morphine on food and water intake in food-deprived and freely-feeding rats. *Psychopharmacology* **72**, 103–106.

Saper, C. B. and Loewy, A. D. (1980). Efferent connections of the parabrachial nucleus in the rat. *Brain Res.* **197**, 291–317.

Sarter, M., Nutt, D. J. and Lister, R. G. (eds) (1995). *Benzodiazepine Receptor Inverse Agonists.* Wiley–Liss, New York.

Shivers, B. D., Killisch, I., Sprengel, R., Sontheimer, H., Köhler, M., Schofield, P. R. and Seeburg, P. H. (1989). Two novel GABA$_A$ receptor subunits exist in distinct neuronal subpopulations. *Neuron* **3**, 327–337.

Sigel, E., Stephenson, F. A., Mamlaki, C. and Barnard, E. A. (1983). A GABA/benzodiazepine receptor complex of bovine cerebral cortex. *J. Biol. Chem.* **258**, 6965–6971.

Sigel, E., Baur, R., Trube, G., Möhler, H. and Malherbe, P. (1990). The effect of subunit composition of rat brain GABA receptors on channel function. *Neuron* **5**, 703–711.

Spector, A. C., Norgren, R. and Grill, H. J. (1992). Parabrachial gustatory lesions impair taste aversion learning in rats. *Behav. Neurosci.* **106**, 147–161.

Squires, R. F. and Braestrup, C. (1977). Benzodiazepine receptors in rat brain. *Nature* **266**, 732.

Ticku, M. K. (1991). Drug modulation of GABA$_A$-mediated transmission. *Semin. Neurosci.* **3**, 211–218.

Touzani, K., Tramu, G., Nahon, J. L. and Velley, L. (1993). Hypothalamic melanin-concentrating hormone and alpha-neoendorphin-immunoreactive neurons project to the medial part of the rat parabrachial area. *Neuroscience* **53**, 865–876.

Treit, D. and Berridge, K. C. (1990). A comparison of benzodiazepine, serotonin, and dopamine agents in the taste-reactivity paradigm. *Pharmacol. Biochem. Behav.* **37**, 451–456.

Treit, D., Berridge, K. C. and Schultz, C. E. (1987). The direct enhancement of positive palatability by chlordiazepoxide is antagonized by Ro 15-1788 and CGS 8216. *Pharmacol. Biochem. Behav.* **26**, 709–714.

Turkish, S. and Cooper, S. J. (1984). Enhancement of salt intake by chlordiazepoxide in thirsty rats: antagonism by Ro 15-1788. *Pharmacol. Biochem. Behav.* **20**, 869–873.

Turner, D. M., Sapp, D. W. and Olsen, R. W. (1991). The benzodiazepine/alcohol antagonist Ro 15-4513: binding to a GABA$_A$ receptor subtype that is insensitive to diazepam. *J. Pharmacol. Exp. Ther.* **257**, 1236–1242.

Von Blankenfield, G., Ymer, S., Pritchett, D. B., Sontheimer, H., Ewart, M., Seeburg, P. H. and Kettenmann, H. (1990). Differential benzodiazepine pharmacology of mammalian recombinant GABA$_A$ receptors. *Neurosci. Lett.* **115**, 269–273.

Wise, R. A. and Dawson, V. (1974). Diazepam-induced eating and lever-pressing for food in sated rats. *J. Comp. Physiol. Psychol.* **86**, 930–941.

Yerbury, R. E. and Cooper, S. J. (1987). The benzodiazepine partial agonists, Ro 16-6028 and Ro 17-1812, increase palatable food consumption in nondeprived rats. *Pharmacol. Biochem. Behav.* **28**, 427–431.

Yerbury, R. E. and Cooper, S. J. (1989). Novel benzodiazepine receptor ligands: palatable food intake following zolpidem, CGS 17867A, or Ro 23-0364, in the rat. *Pharmacol. Biochem. Behav.* **33**, 303–307.

Ymer, S., Draguhn, A., Wisden, W., Werner, P., Keinanen, K., Schofield, P. R., Sprengel, R., Pritchett, D. B. and Seeburg, P. H. (1990). Structural and functional characterisation of the γ1 subunit of GABA$_A$/benzodiazepine receptors. *EMBO J.* **9**, 3261–3267.

Young, W. S. III and Kuhar, M. J. (1980). Radiohistochemical localization of benzodiazepine receptors in rat brain. *J. Pharmacol. Exp. Ther.* **212**, 337–346.

17

Neurochemical Interactions in the Control of Ingestive Behaviour

ELIZABETH M. SOMERVILLE and PETER G. CLIFTON

School of Biology, University of Sussex, Brighton BN1 9QG, UK

1 Introduction

In this chapter we hope to provide a broad framework into which some of the specific material of earlier chapters might be integrated. In doing this we shall first review the behavioural organization of feeding, then provide a neuro-anatomical model, and finally give some examples of how specific neuro-chemical data might be accommodated within such a model.

2 Feeding: the behavioural context

A central feature of the organization of motivated behaviour is its tendency to occur in relatively concentrated bouts of performance. In the case of the rat this tendency is seen with feeding, drinking, grooming, sexual behaviour and rest. In addition, for some of these behaviour patterns, there is relatively clear regulation of the total performance of behaviour. Such regulation is evident, at least, for feeding and drinking in which body mass and fluid balance are regulated in part by modification of food and fluid intake. Thus, when examining the patterning of behaviour such as feeding over time, two overlapping questions must be answered. First, what factors lead to the initiation, termination and rate of performance of behaviour during a bout (or meal)? Second, what factors influence performance, both at the level of individual meals and over the longer term, to maintain food intake appropriate to body size, metabolism and environmental conditions?

In many circumstances ingestion of food will be preceded by a complex behavioural sequence that serves to gain access to that food. In a natural situation, a rat may emerge from its burrow, at an appropriate time of day, and then make its way towards locations in which food and water have previously been available. Water will be taken at the appropriate location, and food may

DRG RECEPTOR SUBTYPES AND INGESTIVE BEHAVIOUR
ISBN 0-12-187620-9

also be consumed. Additional food may be brought back to the burrow and hoarded for future use or, in other rodents, may be cached in locations that are subsequently visited when food availability is reduced. At least some of this complexity can be observed in the laboratory, and in addition some surprising experimental dissociations may be demonstrated following drug or central nervous system manipulations. A rat may easily be trained to perform a response, such as lever-pressing or chain-pulling, for food reward. Animals who obtain all of their food in this way will continue to respond on schedules as weak as fixed ratio 1280, if this is the cost of initiating a complete meal (Collier et al., 1972). Under these circumstances meal size greatly increases, with a corresponding decrease in meal frequency, thus minimizing the overall cost of food intake. Increasing the cost of each item, by contrast, has only limited effects on meal patterning which are probably explained by the reduction in feeding rate that results from the interposed instrumental requirement (Clifton et al., 1984).

Curiously, when animals are given access to short sessions in which they lever-press for a distinctive food, whose value is subsequently reduced (for example, by induction of a conditioned taste aversion), then lever-pressing is reduced only after the animal has been given the opportunity actually to ingest the devalued food (Balleine and Dickinson, 1991). The implication of this finding is that the links between performance of a learned response which delivers food, and consumption of the food itself, may be weaker and less direct than might otherwise have been anticipated. Similar results have been obtained in situations where pharmacological manipulations have been used to produce short-term changes in the value of food. If benzodiazepine treatment is given, which plausibly may enhance the palatability of food (see Chapter 16), then operant responding for that food increases only after the animal has experienced it under that drug state (Balleine et al., 1994). A more complex result is obtained if cholecystokinin (CCK), which may act as a satiety signal (see Chapter 1), is used to lower the value of food (Balleine and Dickinson, 1994). Prior experience has no effect on bar-pressing during extinction, although it does reduce rewarded bar-pressing. The authors suggest that this outcome supports the idea that CCK acts as a satiety-specific incentive signal.

Recent studies in our laboratory suggest that these findings, which apply to performance of an instrumental response such as lever-pressing, may not extend to Pavlovian responding. A rat may easily be conditioned to approach and spend time in a distinctive location that was previously associated with the presence of a nutritive sucrose solution; it is usually assumed that the distinctive stimuli associated with the location substitute for the sucrose through Pavlovian conditioning. However, the resulting conditioned place preference is immediately sensitive to a reduction in the value of the sucrose, again achieved using a conditioned taste aversion (S. M. Perks, personal communication). Thus different constraints may operate on instrumental and Pavlovian responses for which food has acted as a reinforcer.

Hoarding behaviour also shows interesting dissociations, both within itself and from more direct measures of ingestive behaviour. Rats may carry food from the location where food is supplied, eat it elsewhere and then return for more. This pattern of behaviour becomes much more likely as the size of food items is increased. A rat may use essentially the same sequence of behaviour, but now hoard the food items rather than eat them. Whishaw and Kornelson (1993) reported that excitotoxic lesions of the nucleus accumbens impair carrying of food to hoard, but have no effect on carrying of food to eat. They suggested that this implies the lesion has little effect on consummatory actions associated with feeding but does impair actions that depend on secondary features of the food. However, although rats with accumbens lesions respond normally to food deprivation cues and show no abnormalities in food intake or weight gain, they do show substantial changes in meal patterning; accumbens lesions result in animals that feed on smaller meals taken more frequently (Clifton and Somerville, 1994). Thus the accumbens may also play a role in the temporal organization of spontaneous feeding behaviour.

During a single meal of either solid or liquid food there are likely to be complex adjustments in the rate of intake which may give insights into changing motivational state. However, during free feeding in undisturbed animals it has been hard to demonstrate such changes; for example, Burton et al. (1981) examined feeding rate in the early and late phases of freely initiated meals but could not demonstrate any reduction in rate towards the end of a meal. This is surprising in the context of studies of intake rate during meals of palatable fluids (e.g. Davis et al., 1978), in which intake gradually slowed during the meal. Modifications in the palatability of the fluid produced clear changes in the initial rate of intake whereas manipulations of the rate at which the fluid cleared the intestine simply affected asymptotic consumption. More recently Lee and Clifton have shown that, with a slight modification of the original situation of Burton et al. (1981), there is a clear slowing of feeding rate during the progression of a conventional solid meal (M. D. Lee and P. G. Clifton, unpublished results). This suggests that measures of feeding rate may be a useful measure of motivational state during a meal.

One important message from this brief selection of studies is that, in trying to understand the neurochemical basis of ingestion, we must remember its behavioural complexity. Simple intake studies are never likely to provide this understanding, although they are an essential prerequisite to be followed by studies of meal patterning, satiety sequences, hoarding and operant studies that allow a separation of incentive and preparatory from consummatory aspects of ingestion, and may also delineate the motivational changes that occur during ingestion. However, such studies also need to be conducted within a theoretical framework that attempts to describe the neural mechanisms that mediate ingestive behaviour, and it is to this that we next turn our attention.

3   A neural model for feeding

If asked about the neural substrate for feeding, any physiological psychologist would place the hypothalamus, particularly the paraventricular nucleus and lateral hypothalamus towards the top of a list of brain areas involved. Nauta's definition of the 'limbic system' in terms of its relationship with the hypothalamus (e.g. Nauta and Feirtag, 1986, p. 121) places this 'system' firmly within the list of brain areas to be considered when considering the organization of behavioural outputs defined as feeding behaviour. This can include the exploratory behaviour before the discovery of food, species-specific consummatory behaviours, the reaction to hedonic properties of the food and the temporal organization of the behaviour such that animals feed in distinct meals. Such a wide variety of motor acts may well be under the control of a number of different neural systems, and thus the question of interest becomes how these are activated in an integrated fashion.

Normal motor output is the result of activity in a number of neural systems, and the sequences of behaviour that characterize particular motivated behaviours are often seen as the final output of such a network. The dorsal striatum is considered to work via the activation of a number of parallel loops (e.g. Alexander and Crutcher, 1990) which link the cortex, basal ganglia and thalamus. Fig. 1 shows a very simplified version of this circuit, which in the rat includes the entopeduncular nucleus. The excitatory, glutamatergic projections to the striatum from the cortex are generally regarded as the input to this circuit. The striatum also has a high rate of spontaneous discharge and thus exerts a tonic γ-aminobutyric acid (GABA)-mediated inhibitory outflow on its targets. Since the input to the thalamus is also inhibitory, the loop effectively works by mediating disinhibition of the thalamus and thus allowing excitatory thalamocortical connections to fire and facilitate or gate cortically initiated movements.

The striatum contains both dorsal and ventral areas, which have similar systems of overlapping loops (Witter and Groenewegen, 1992; Joel and Weiner, 1994). Distinguishing between these two areas of the striatum can be difficult and is possibly best done by considering the connections of these areas. Even so there are some ambiguities and, in the context of feeding behaviour, a particularly intriguing case is that of the ventrolateral striatum, which lies above the lateral wing of the anterior commissure and thus appears to be within the dorsal area of the striatum, and indeed receives input from the supplementary motor area (McGeorge and Faull, 1989). However, this area also receives 'limbic' input (Beckstead, 1979; Kelley et al., 1982).

Recent research implicates the dorsal striatum, in particular, in the integration of individual actions into an orchestrated output during grooming (Berridge and Whishaw, 1992). It is this integration, rather than the performance of the separate movements, that is permanently damaged by lesions of the dorsal striatum. In contrast, the ventral striatum has long been considered to be

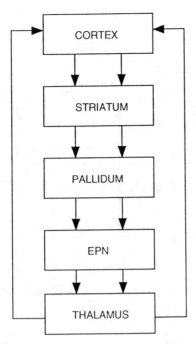

Fig. 1 A simplified corticostriatothalamocortical (CSTC) loop (after Alexander and Crutcher, 1990), expanded to show the entopeduncular nucleus (EPN) in the rat.

part of the limbic system and possibly to function as an interface between this and the motor system (Mogenson *et al.*, 1980; Heimer *et al.*, 1993). It has not been clear, however, how such an interface would function in terms of affecting the motor output of the brain and, in particular, the organization of the overall patterning that characterizes motivated behaviours. In addition, this area of the brain, as may be expected of part of the limbic system, has extensive connections to the hypothalamus (Pennartz *et al.*, 1994). These aspects of its neuroanatomy are of considerable interest in trying to understand how feeding and other motivated behaviours are controlled.

Fig. 2 shows a simplified version of the corticostriatothalamocortical (CSTC) loop in which the ventral striatum is incorporated (Heimer *et al.*, 1985). Although this has obvious parallels, as shown, with the motor loop(s), it does not give the ventral striatum an immediately obvious motor output. At this point it is important to reconsider just what may be involved in the central control of a motivated behaviour such as feeding. If the claim is that such a central control area directly influences motoneurons, thereby making the animal perform an individually choreographed movement, then the ventral striatum, or any other part of its CSTC loop, clearly does not qualify. However, if the central control is thought to be achievable through less direct

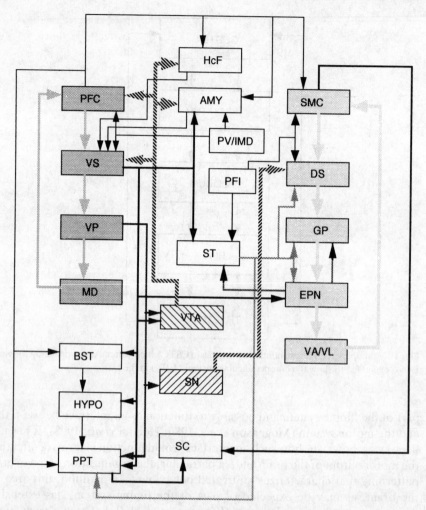

Fig. 2 Selected pathways surrounding the CSTC loop(s) through the ventral (VS) and dorsal striatum (DS). Many of the pathways shown are reciprocal. AMY, (extended) amygdala; BST, bed nucleus of the stria terminalis; EPN, entopeduncular nucleus; GP, globus pallidus; HYPO, hypothalamus; HcF, hippocampal formation; MD, mediodorsal nucleus of the thalamus; PFC, prefrontal cortex; PFI, parafascicular intralaminar nucleus of the thalamus; PPT, pedunculopontine nucleus of the tegmentum; PV/IMD, paraventricular–intermediodorsal thalamic nuclei; SC, spinal cord; SMC, sensorimotor cortex; SN, substantia nigra; ST, subthalamic nucleus; VA/VL, ventroanterior and ventrolateral nuclei of the thalamus; VP, ventral pallidum; VTA, ventral tegmental area.

connections, and indeed to be possibly neuromodulatory in its action, then such a central control area (or areas) may be encompassed within the connections shown in Fig. 2. This concept of central control is close to Holstege's 'third motor system', whereby the limbic system in general, including the hypothalamus, is considered to influence behavioural output via descending pathways that synapse within the somatomotor areas of the brainstem (e.g. Holstege, 1991). The ventral striatum can be seen as the origin of a number of possible routes which could influence motor output in this more general way. First, there is the connection to the hypothalamus, including the lateral hypothalamus; second, there is the output to substantia nigra, which would allow for modulation of the ascending dopaminergic input to the dorsal (motor) striatum; third, there are connections into CSTC motor loops via the entopeduncular nucleus, globus pallidus and the subthalamic nucleus; and finally the cortical target of the limbic loop may itself access motor output via either corticocortical connections or hindbrain structures such as the pedunculopontine nucleus, or via connections to the hypothalamus. These different routes fall into two main groups. First, there are connections that tap into both pyramidal and extrapyramidal motor systems, which could control the expression of ongoing activity, possibly particularly the intensity (or emotionality) of its expression (Pennartz et al., 1994). This group includes all input to the CSTC motor loops and also the input to the pedunculopontine nucleus. The second set of connections are those that depend on a hypothalamic link to brainstem areas such as the lateral tegmental field of the caudal pons and medulla as well as possible links through to the spinal cord, which can access autonomic and motor systems as well as links via the hypothalamus to the locus coeruleus and raphe which have modulatory descending (i.e. spinal) projections, as well as the better-known ascending projections (Holstege, 1991).

The arguments made so far about the neural substrate involved in the control of feeding behaviour have referred simply to broadly defined brain areas. Although for some of these areas it is possible to define subdivisions with their own patterns of connectivity, which are effectively subdivisions of those described, it is not yet possible to do so for all areas. However, it is probably only by considering this finer scale of organization that we can begin to understand the way in which pharmacological manipulation of various neurotransmitters has behavioural sequelae. Fig. 3 shows some of the efferent projections from part of the ventral striatum, the nucleus accumbens, which, like the dorsal striatum, can be subdivided into 'patch' and 'matrix' components. There is a striking overall similarity, in that the output to the mesencephalic dopaminergic cell groups is compartmentally organized, although the details are equally clearly different (Gerfen, 1985; Berendse et al., 1992a). As well as the fine-grained differentiation into compartments, the nucleus accumbens can be divided into core and shell areas (Heimer et al., 1991), which intermingle at the rostral pole (Zahm and Heimer, 1993). The possibility of multiple pathways through this area is clear, even from this very simplified diagram. Of particular interest is the way in which these subdivisions have subtly different, although possibly partially overlapping, sets of connections, with the core area appearing to be very similar in terms of its efferents to the dorsal striatum, whereas the shell area also includes elements in its

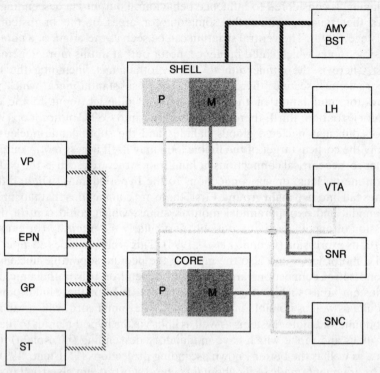

Fig. 3 Partial diagram of the pattern of efferent projections from the nucleus accumbens to show the possibility of multiple pathways from this area. LH, lateral hypothalamus; M and P, matrix and patch component of the nucleus accumbens; SNC, substantia nigra pars compacta, including dopamine cell group A9; SNR, substantia nigra pars reticulata, including dopamine cell group A10; for other abbreviations see legend to Fig. 2.

projection patterns that resemble the amygdala (Heimer *et al.*, 1993; Zahm and Brog, 1992). There is a similar diversity in terms of the inputs to these areas (Brog *et al.*, 1993), and the prefrontal corticostriatal projections show a particularly complex relationship with the neurochemical compartments within the ventral striatum (Berendse *et al.*, 1992b). It is relevant to any consideration of hedonic influences on behaviour that the patch and matrix compartments are distinguishable histochemically by the distribution of enkephalin and other peptides (Jongen-Relo *et al.*, 1993), as well as by acetylcholinesterase, substance P and calcium binding protein (Jongen-Relo *et al.*, 1994).

An important issue still to be resolved is the extent to which these compartments reflect genuinely separated streams of connections through the ventral striatopallidal system. There seems to be much greater respect for compartmental boundaries in the ventral than in the dorsal striatum (Arts and Groenewegen, 1992), but this does not preclude interactions between the compartments or even more widely within the ventral striatum. It seems most probable that interactions which involve the recurrent collaterals of projection neurons would be GABAergic, whereas those involving striatal interneurons would be both GABAergic and cholinergic. There is a distinct possibility that the larger cholinergic interneurons may cross internal boundaries within the ventral striatum (Pennartz et al., 1994).

The ventral striatum is both a target for and a source of pathways that involve a number of the neurotransmitters currently considered to be relevant to feeding behaviour (or at least whose manipulation affects feeding behaviour); this should not be taken to imply that this area is necessarily the site at which the pharmacological manipulations are effective, but it needs to be considered as a possible candidate. With respect to this issue, an interesting fact to emerge from the extended map of the interconnections of the ventral striatum (Fig. 2) is that this area could influence not just the ascending dopaminergic projections to the basal ganglia as a whole, but also, via either the habenula (Li et al., 1993) or the hypothalamus, both the ascending 5-hydroxytryptamine (5-HT) projection from the raphe (Holstege, 1991) and possibly also the noradrenergic projections to the forebrain from the locus coeruleus (Luppi et al., 1995).

The rich connectivity between many brain regions indicated in the figures makes it difficult to determine which of the many possible routes for connecting any two or more areas is functionally the most important. Further experimentation is required to elucidate this. Fig. 2 also shows that some of the targets of the ventral striatum are shared between this area and the areas to which it projects. This clearly allows for a degree of 'parallel processing', which may be a means by which modulation effective against a changing background level of activation can be achieved.

So far, inputs to the extended CSTC loops, which include the ventral striatum, have been taken to be cortical in a broad sense, i.e. also including the main limbic forebrain structures in the forebrain: the amygdala and the hippocampal formation. Fig. 2 also shows the inputs to the striatum from two subdivisions of the midline–intralaminar thalamic complex (Groenewegen and Berendse, 1994). The information from these nuclei may be of a non-discriminative or affective nature, and may serve to prepare the striatal circuits for appropriate action depending on the cortical input. The paraventricular–intermediodorsal subdivision, which projects to the ventral CSTC loop, receives input from limbic and visceral-related cortical and subcortical sources including the parabrachial nucleus and the nucleus of the solitary tract (NST). These hindbrain structures are known to play an important role in the control of feeding. Both of these also have connections to the bed nucleus of the stria terminalis and the hypothalamus, and the NST also projects to the amygdala (Bystrzycka and Nail, 1985; Alden et al., 1994). Thus any signals concerning physiological state from these brainstem nuclei could enter the CSTC loop(s) discussed here via a number of possible routes.

It is now possible to give a brief sketch of a possible sequence of neural events underlying the central coordination of feeding behaviour in the normal, undeprived animal. In the absence of any signal of physiological need it would seem likely that, as an animal moves about the environment, the amygdala may be activated by the recognition and evaluation of the food-related stimulus and/or the hippocampus may signal that the animal is in a place where it has previously found food. These stimulus-related events, together possibly with prefrontal cortical activity, would activate the common target of these three forebrain regions, the ventral striatum. This could set up a diffuse motor activation through both the dorsal striatal CSTC loops as well as activation of the hypothalamus and midbrain motor areas. Contact with a food item under these circumstances would produce sensory input which, relayed to the hypothalamus via the NST and parabrachial nucleus, may further sculpt the motor output into the precise pattern of feeding behaviour.

It is clearly as important to terminate behaviour as it is to initiate it, but it is less obvious how the neural model described here would accomplish this. Feedback from the periphery is certainly involved. Sensory information can enter the CSTC loop in many ways, but for cessation the most relevant information may be that from the NST and parabrachial nucleus, possibly relayed by the paraventricular–intermediodorsal nuclei of the thalamus and/or the amygdala. It is possible that this information acts simply by decreasing activation of feeding behaviour, allowing the animal to switch to a different behaviour. It is also possible that decreased hedonic feedback from the food is responsible for switching from feeding to behaviours, such as exploration, grooming and sleep, that are typical of the satiety sequence (Antin *et al.*, 1974).

4   Neurochemical modulation of feeding behaviour

4.1   Glutamate

In Chapter 14, Stanley reviewed the evidence that either systemic administration of glutamate or intracranial administration to the lateral hypothalamus, but not a wide variety of other anatomically close sites, can enhance food intake. In non-deprived animals he noted that, although feeding occurs with a shorter latency and is intense, the resulting meal is within the size range of normal meals and is followed by the usual postprandial satiety sequence. Within the context of the model outlined above, such data might be explained in terms of enhanced output from the lateral hypothalamus to structures including midbrain motor areas, amygdala and NST (Swanson, 1987). This should produce, respectively, general behavioural activation (hence shortened latency), enhanced responsiveness to stimuli associated with food reward and, in the general context of forebrain control of peripheral input, enhanced responsiveness to the sensory properties of food. There should be no interference with the mechanisms that underlie satiation of response. Studies in which cell firing in the lateral hypothalamus has been correlated with ingestive behaviour suggest further tests of the nature of lateral glutamate-induced feeding. For example, the cells do not resp(after induction of a conditioned aversion to its taste (Alekssany glutamatergic enhancement of food intake should also be sensit aversion.

4.2 GABA

There is relatively little evidence for direct effects of GABA modulation on ingestion, although the potent hyperphagic effects of benzodiazepines such as midazolam and bretazenil are assumed to depend on their action at subtypes of the $GABA_A$ ionotrophic receptor complex (see Chapter 16). Several older studies indicate that $GABA_A$ agonists, such as muscimol, when injected into the ventromedial, dorsomedial or paraventricular nuclei of the hypothalamus can enhance food intake (e.g. Kelly *et al.*, 1979). In addition Minano and co-workers (1992) showed that injection of the $GABA_A$ agonist muscimol into the central nucleus of the amygdala could produce dose-dependent increases in food intake in sated rats; this effect was attenuated by the $GABA_A$ antagonist bicuculline. The authors suggest that their data are most easily explained by connections from the amygdala to the hypothalamus via the stria terminalis. Redgrave *et al.* (1984) showed that bilateral injection of muscimol into the substantia nigra can elicit enhanced feeding between 0 and 120 min after injection; earlier than this, stereotyped sniffing is common and probably interferes with the expression of feeding. These data suggest a stimulation of the dopaminergic input to the striatum.

Ebenezer and Pringle (1992) have provided direct evidence for effects of baclofen, an agonist at the metabotrophic $GABA_B$ receptor, on ingestion. Food intake was increased and water intake decreased in a dose-related fashion after systemic administration. More recently, Wirtschafter *et al.* (1993) showed that injection of baclofen directly into the median raphe nucleus produces hyperactivity, together with increased food and water intake. One obvious interpretation of such effects would be in terms of inhibition of serotonergic input to the hypothalamus and/or nucleus accumbens. However, this is made less likely by the finding that pretreatment with the serotonin synthesis inhibitor *p*-chlorophenylalanine does not modify the effect of baclofen in these experiments. The authors suggest that activation of a non-serotonergic projection to the ventral tegmental area from the dorsal raphe led to the increases in dopamine turnover, locomotor activity and ingestive behaviour.

4.3 Serotonin

Although much of the literature on feeding and serotonin has been concerned with the extent to which this neurotransmitter can be assigned a specific role in developing satiation to food, there are several alternative points of view. First, ι is possible that manipulations that enhance serotonergic tone interfere with feeding responses in one of a number of non-specific ways. A series of studies recording satiety sequences after treatment with drugs that enhance serotonergic activity are relevant to this idea. Blundell and Latham (1980) originally reported that fenfluramine simply 'advances' the satiety sequence, i.e. shortens the duration of feeding, and also leads to earlier onset of exploring, grooming and sleep. By contrast, Montgomery and Willner (1988) reported that fenfluramine produces behavioural disruption in the satiety sequence; however, recent studies by Halford (1995) have essentially confirmed the conclusion of Blundell and Latham's original 1980 study.

Lee and Clifton have taken a slightly different approach to the same question. They reasoned that changes in feeding rate during a meal should provide a good index of satiation. Using an adapted meal-patterning technique in which meals were presented in the home cage at intervals not very different to those at which they might be spontaneously initiated, they were able to show that feeding rate decreases towards the end of the meal (M. D. Lee and P. G. Clifton, unpublished results). This result contrasts with the earlier report of Burton et al. (1981) that no change in feeding rate can be observed as a meal progresses. Intermediate dose levels of fluoxetine were shown to have no effect on feeding rate at the beginning of a meal, but caused a proportionately greater reduction in feeding rate as the meal progressed. Higher doses, by contrast, reduced feeding rate even at the beginning of a meal. Data of this type are compatible with enhancement of satiation by moderate doses of fluoxetine as the meal progresses.

Much of the data presented elsewhere in this volume suggests multiple actions of serotonin, both through separate receptor subtypes and at anatomically separate locations. For example, in meal-patterning studies with fenfluramine or similar compounds, meal size is reduced, intermeal duration, relative to meal size, is increased, and finally feeding rate is reduced. It seems likely that each of these behavioural changes depends on interactions at different 5-HT receptors. Ritanserin (a potent $5\text{-HT}_{2A/C}$ antagonist) can reduce the fenfluramine-induced decrease in feeding rate (Grignaschi and Samanin, 1992), whereas metergoline (a relatively non-selective drug with 5-HT_1 antagonism) reverses the effect on meal size. In addition, Clifton and Cooper (1992) and Grignaschi et al. (1993) have independently reported that the CCK antagonist devazepide can reverse the effect of fenfluramine on meal size, but leaves the ratio of meal size to intermeal interval unaffected. Thus meal-patterning studies reveal at least three aspects to the effects of fenfluramine on feeding. Data showing differential development of tolerance to the effects of fenfluramine on feeding rate and meal size (Grignaschi et al., 1992) are also consistent with this view. Studies with fluoxetine are not yet so complete, but suggest a similar general picture since metergoline actually potentiates the decrease in feeding rate produced by fluoxetine (Lee and Clifton, 1992), yet returns meal size towards its control level.

Central neurochemical studies, by contrast, have not provided clear evidence for multiple actions of serotonin on ingestive behaviour. Leibowitz *et al.* (1990) showed that infusion of 5-HT into the paraventricular hypothalamus and nearby hypothalamic nuclei could reduce food intake, meal size and feeding rate. They later showed that similar effects could be obtained with indirect serotonin agonists such as D-fenfluramine, sertraline and fluoxetine (Weiss *et al.*, 1991). In addition, they reported that metergoline, a non-selective serotonin agonist, could increase consumption of the carbohydrate and fat components of a self-selected diet by increasing meal size (Leibowitz *et al.*, 1993). However, several recent studies have suggested that further exploration of hypothalamic and extrahypothalamic sites would be worthwhile; for example, Fletcher and colleagues (1992) have shown that radiofrequency lesions of the paraventricular hypothalamus fail to reduce the anorectic action of systemically administered TFMPP, fenfluramine and fluoxetine, suggesting that an action outside this site mediates their effects.

Although the effects of serotonergic drugs are often presented as selective to food intake, the data are also compatible with the concept that serotonin may be involved in processes leading to satiation in other motivational systems. Fenfluramine and other indirect serotonergic agonists reduce consumption of ethanol (Sellers *et al.*, 1992) and self-administration of opiates (Higgins *et al.*, 1994) or cocaine (Peltier and Schenk, 1993). This suggests that serotonin may have a general role in satiation of motivated behaviour, rather than one that is limited to feeding. In the above model effects of serotonin at either hypothalamic or extra hypothalamic sites such as the amygdala might mediate such satiety effects.

4.4 Dopamine

Terry has fully reviewed the effects of dopamine agonists and antagonists on ingestive behaviour in Chapter 11; here we restrict our attention to studies relevant to the general arguments outlined above. Lesions and other manipulations of the striatum affect feeding behaviour. For example, Salamone *et al.* (1993) showed that dopamine-depleting lesions of the ventrolateral striatum impair the coordinated execution of oral and forepaw movements during consumption of large food pellets that have to be gnawed while being held in the front paws. The animals can maintain normal bodyweight when provided with a diet that is easy to ingest, such as wet mash. In the same study similar lesions of anteroventromedial striatum and nucleus accumbens had little effect. In a more complex situation, in which rats could feed either on small pellets obtained by lever pressing or on larger pieces of standard chow scattered in the cage, lesions of the ventrolateral striatum reduced intake of both food types whereas lesions of the nucleus accumbens reduced intake of pellets but increased intake of chow (Cousins *et al.*, 1993). A broadly similar pattern of results was obtained from two studies in which either dopamine antagonists (Bakshi and Kelley, 1991a) or dopamine agonists (Bakshi and Kelley, 1991b) were infused into ventrolateral striatum, nucleus accumbens or dorsal striatum. Infusion of haloperidol into the ventrolateral striatum reduced food intake and time spent feeding, but when infused into the nucleus accumbens tended to increase food intake and increased the duration of feeding bouts. The former effect was attributed to direct interference with oral activity involved in ingestion, whereas the latter was attributed to a deficit in switching away from feeding behaviour once it was initiated. A similar effect with respect to the accumbens might account for the results obtained by Cousins *et al.* (1993), although a differential effect on preparatory and consummatory aspects of ingestive behaviour would provide an alternative explanation (e.g. Blackburn *et al.*, 1987). Infusion of amphetamine into the ventrolateral striatum also interfered with feeding due to the production of competing oral stereotypes, whereas accumbens infusion of amphetamine tended to reduce feeding because of induction of locomotor and other competing responses. At least one aspect of these studies is puzzling, when compared with the effects of systemically administered dopamine antagonists. Although the effects of dopamine D2 antagonists on food intake are variable, a reduction in feeding rate is commonly observed. Bakshi and Kelley (1991b) found no striatal site in which centrally administered dopamine antagonists affected the local rate of eating.

4.5   Neuropeptide Y

Neuropeptide Y (NPY) is known for its potent orexigenic response when injected into either the third or fourth ventricle (Steinman *et al.*, 1994). In addition, food deprivation causes an increase in hypothalamic NPY content, which is reversed after ingestion of food (Sahu *et al.*, 1988). In Chapter 15 Corp has reviewed the evidence suggesting that third ventricular administration is likely to be effective through an area broadly localized to the perifornical hypothalamus (Stanley *et al.*, 1993), whereas the fourth ventricular effect probably occurs via action at a hindbrain site which may be the central grey pontine nucleus. Many authors have commented that the eating behaviour evoked by NPY has a frantic and ravenous character, and several recent studies have contributed to the behavioural description of this effect. Lynch *et al.* (1994) recorded patterns of licking for a diluted condensed milk solution after lateral ventricular administration of NPY. The peptide produced a clear increase in milk intake together with distinctive changes in behavioural microstructure. There was little effect on the rate of intake at the beginning of the test session, but the asymptotic intake in the session was increased by about 50%. The primary microstructural change appeared to be a decrease in the size and duration of bouts of licking together with a substantial increase in the number of bouts. Food deprivation, by contrast, increased both the initial intake rate as well as asymptotic consumption, and increased the duration of individual bouts of licking, but had no effect on the number of bouts observed during the 60-min test session. Clearly the effects of food deprivation and NPY are quite different in this paradigm. The results suggest that, at least at the forebrain site of action, a desatiating action rather than an increase in hunger may be critical. However, it is also possible to see how the combination of short bouts followed by short intervals of non-licking might give the impression of 'ravenous' eating. Stricker-Krongrad *et al.* (1994) described the microstructure of intake patterns on a semisolid pastry diet, again after lateral ventricular injection of NPY. They reported dose-related increase in intake over the range 0.5–5.0 μg NPY. A similar enhancement of intake was observed in lean compared with obese Zucker rats, although the minimally effective dose of NPY was lower. Changes in meal patterning were particularly pronounced in lean animals. Meal size increased significantly, consistent with the liquid diet study described above, but there was no change in either meal frequency or the local rate of eating within a meal. Again, the authors argued that their results were consistent with an 'anti-satiety' interpretation.

4.6 Opioid peptides

In Chapter 8 Carr has reviewed evidence, derived from the paradigm of electrical stimulation-induced feeding, that opioid peptides modify the expression of ingestive behaviour. His conclusions fit well with the broader literature concerning systemic and central administration of opioid receptor agonists and antagonists reviewed by Gosnell and Levine in Chapter 7, suggesting that agonists, especially at μ and κ receptors, can enhance food intake, whereas antagonists at these receptors will reduce food intake. They concluded that the critical brain sites mediating the action of opiates on food intake are likely to include the hypothalamus, including the paraventricular nucleus, central nucleus of the amygdala, bed nucleus of the stria terminalis, parabrachial nucleus, ventral tegmental area and nucleus accumbens. The structures listed in Chapters 7 and 8 are all components of the model outlined above, the amygdala is an input structure to the ventral CSTC loop whereas the bed nucleus of the stria terminalis is one of the structures that receives output from that loop. The parabrachial nucleus may feed into the loop by a number of routes.

It is of particular interest that subregions of the striatum can mediate a hyperphagic response after microinjection of opioids. Bakshi and Kelley (1993a) infused morphine sulfate into one of five regions of the striatum (nucleus accumbens, ventromedial, ventrolateral, anterior dorsal, posterior dorsal) of sated rats and recorded ingestive behaviour over the succeeding 4 h. Injection of 5 μg morphine into the accumbens or ventromedial striatum led to a 4–5-fold increase in intake, with non-significant effects at this dose from other sites. It is unclear from the data whether, in individual animals, eating was concentrated into meals followed by the usual postprandial sequence, or whether the natural structure of the behaviour was lost. Drug administration into the accumbens, but not the ventromedial striatum, was associated with an increase in activity; the results from these two sites strongly imply that the increase in eating was not consequent on some general increase in arousal. In a second study Bakshi and Kelley (1993b) reported that injection of selective agonists into a subset of the regions examined in the first study can also enhance food intake. The μ-selective agonist DAMGO (D-Ala^2,N-Me-Phe^4,Gly-ol^5-enkephalin) (at doses of 2.5 μg and above) produced a substantial effect but the δ agonist DPEN (D-Pen^{2,5}-enkephalin) was much less effective, and the κ agonist U50 488H was without effect. Bakshi and Kelley (1993b) suggested that one interpretation of their results is that the opioid is potentiating the rewarding effect of food and hence increasing consumption. While this is certainly a plausible suggestion, the differences in enkephalinergic expression in patch and matrix within the striatum mentioned above indicate an alternative. It may be that the parallel pathways running through striatum have differential neurochemical coding that maps on to their behavioural role, and that enkephalinergic expression is characteristic of particular circuits responsible for the organization of feeding.

5 Conclusion

In this chapter we have tried to interpret some data on the neurochemistry of feeding in the context of a broader neuroanatomical model than has traditionally been used. This arises, in part, from viewing feeding as a convenient exemplar of motivated behaviour. Such a viewpoint immediately raises the question of how the neural substrate for feeding behaviour is linked into the more general circuits that underlie motivated behaviour (Mogenson et al., 1980). Our description of these circuits has mainly been based on neuroanatomical studies, which need to be integrated with the rapidly increasing information concerning the anatomical localization of neurotransmitter receptor subtypes. In the particular case of feeding, the precise central administration of selective agonists and antagonists, which has been extensively reviewed elsewhere in this volume, provides one of the best ways of investigating the function of these circuits. In general terms this has been a classical problem in behavioural neuroscience, and in thinking about this issue we took encouragement from re-reading parts of Grossman's text of 1967. The final paragraph of his chapter on 'Hunger and the Regulation of the Organism's Energy Balance', which is an area of research to which he had already made a notable contribution, suggested that 'Future research in this field will have to concentrate on the physiological mechanisms that excite or inhibit the hypothalamic centers and *on the integrative processes that translate the resultant hypothalamic activity into overt behaviour*' (p. 384, our italics). This remains an ambitious research programme for the next decade and more.

References

Alden, M., Besson, J.-M. and Bernard, J.-F. (1994). Organisation of the efferent projections from the pontine parabrachial area to the bed nucleus of the stria terminalis and neighbouring regions: a Pha-L study in the rat. *J. Comp. Neurol.* **341**, 289–314.

Alekssanyan, Z. A., Buršová, O. and Bureš, J. (1976). Modification of unit responses to gustatory stimuli by conditioned taste aversion. *Physiol. Behav.* **17**, 173–179.

Alexander, G. E. and Crutcher, M. D. (1990). Functional architecture of basal ganglia circuits: neural substrates of parallel processing. *Trends Neurosci.* **13**, 266–271.

Antin, J., Gibbs, J., Holt, J., Young, R. C. and Smith, G. P. (1974). Cholecystokinin elicits the complete behavioral sequence of satiety in rats. *J. Comp. Physiol. Psychol.* **89**, 784–790.

Arts, M. P. A. and Groenewegen, H. J. (1992). Relationships of the dendritic aborizations of ventral striatomesencephalic projection neurons with boundaries of striatal compartments. An *in vitro* intracellular labelling study in the rat. *Eur. J. Neurosci.* **4**, 574–588.

Bakshi, V. P. and Kelley, A. E. (1991a). Dopaminergic regulation of feeding behaviour: I. Differential effects of haloperidol microinfusion into three striatal subregions. *Psychobiology* **19**, 223–232.

Bakshi, V. P. and Kelley A. E. (1991b). Dopaminergic regulation of feeding behaviour: I. Differential effects of amphetamine microinfusion into three striatal subregions. *Psychobiology* **19**, 233–242.

Bakshi, V. P. and Kelley, A. E. (1993a). Striatal regulation of morphine-induced hyperphagia: an anatomical mapping study. *Psychopharmacology* **111**, 207–214.

Bakshi, V. P. and Kelley A. E. (1993b). Feeding induced by opioid stimulation of the ventral striatum: role of opiate receptor subtypes. *J. Pharmacol. Exp. Ther.* **265**, 1253–1260.

Balleine, B. and Dickinson, A. (1991). Instrumental performance following reinforcer devaluation depends upon incentive learning. *Q. J. Exp. Psychol.* **43B**, 279–296.

Balleine, B. and Dickinson, A. (1994). Role of cholecystokinin in the motivational control of instrumental action in rats. *Behav. Neurosci.* **108**, 590–605.

Balleine, B., Ball, B. and Dickinson, A. (1994). Benzodiazepine-induced outcome revaluation and the motivational control of instrumental action in rats. *Behav. Neurosci.* **108**, 573–589.

Beckstead, R. M. (1979). An autoradiographic examination of cortico-cortical and subcortical projections of the mediodorsal–projection (prefrontal) cortex in the rat. *J. Comp. Neurol.* **84**, 43–62.

Berendse, H. W., Galis-de Graaf, Y. and Groenewegen, H. J. (1992a). Topographical organization and relationship with ventral striatal compartments of prefrontal corticostriatal projections in the rat. *J. Comp. Neurol.* **316**, 314–347.

Berendse, H. W., Groenewegen, H. W. and Lohman, A. H. M. (1992b). Compartmental distribution of ventral striatal neurons projecting to the mesencephalon in the rat. *J. Neurosci.* **12**, 2079–2103.

Berridge, K. C. and Whishaw, I. Q. (1992). Cortex, striatum and cerebellum: control of serial order in a grooming sequence. *Exp. Brain Res.* **90**, 275–290.

Blackburn, J. R., Phillips, A. G. and Fibiger, H. C. (1987). Dopamine and preparatory behaviour: I. Effects of pimozide. *Behav. Neurosci.* **101**, 352–360.

Blundell, J. E. and Latham, C. J. (1980). Characterisation of adjustments to the structure of feeding behaviour following pharmacological treatment: effects of amphetamine and fenfluramine and the antagonism produced by pimozide and methergoline. *Pharmacol. Biochem. Behav.* **12**, 717–722.

Brog, J. S., Salyapongse, A., Deutch, A. Y. and Zahm, D. S. (1993). The patterns of afferent innervation of the core and shell in the 'accumbens' part of the rat ventral striatum: immunohistochemical detection of retrogradely transported fluoro-gold. *J. Comp. Neurol.* **338**, 255–278.

Burton, M. J., Cooper, S. J. and Popplewell, D. A. (1981). The effect of fenfluramine on the microstructure of feeding and drinking in the rat. *Br. J. Pharmacol.* **72**, 621–633.

Bystrzycka, E. K. and Nail, B. S. (1985). Brainstem nuclei associated with respiratory, cardiovascular and other autonomic functions. In *The Rat Brain Vol. II, Hind Brain and Spinal Cord*. (G. Paxinos, ed.), pp. 95–110. Academic Press, London.

Clifton, P. G. and Cooper, S. J. (1992). 5-HT/CCK interactions influence meal size in free feeding rats. In *Multiple Cholecystokinin Receptors in the CNS* (C. T. Dourish, S. J. Cooper, S. D. Iversen and L. L. Iversen, eds), pp. 286–289. Oxford University Press, Oxford.

Clifton, P. G. and Somerville, E. M. (1994). Disturbance of meal patterning following nucleus accumbens lesions in the rat. *Brain Res.* **667**, 123–128.

Clifton, P. G., Popplewell, D. A. and Burton, M. J. (1984). Feeding rate and meal patterns in the laboratory rat. *Physiol. Behav.* **32**, 369–374.

Collier, G. H., Hirsch, E. and Hamlin, P. (1972). The ecological determinants of reinforcement in the rat. *Physiol. Behav.* **9**, 705–716.

Cousins, M. S., Sokolowski, D. and Salmone, D. (1993). Different effects of nucleus accumbens and ventrolateral striatal dopamine depletions on instrumental response selection in the rat. *Pharmacol. Biochem. Behav.* **46**, 943–951.

Davis, J. D., Collins, B. J. and Levine, M. W. (1978). The interaction between gustatory stimulation and gut feedback in the control of the ingestion of liquid diets. In *Hunger Models* (D. A. Booth, ed.), pp. 109–143. Academic Press, London.

Ebenezer, I. and Pringle, A. K. (1992). The effect of systemic administration of baclofen on food-intake in rats. *Neuropharmacology* **31**, 39–42.

Fletcher, P. J., Ming, Z. H., Zack, M. H. and Coscina, D. V. (1992). A comparison of the effects of the 5-HT$_1$ agonists TFMPP and RU 24969 on feeding following peripheral or medial hypothalamic injection. *Brain Res.* **580**, 265–272.

Gerfen, C. R. (1985). The neostriatal mosaic. I. Compartmental organization of projections from the striatum to the substantia nigra in the rat. *J. Comp. Neurol.* **236**, 454–476.

Grignaschi, G. and Samanin, R. (1992). Role of serotonin receptors in the effect of D-fenfluramine on feeding patterns in the rat. *Eur. J. Pharmacol.* **212**, 287–289.

Grignaschi, G., Neill, J. C., Petrini A., Garattini S. and Samanin R. (1992). Feeding pattern studies suggest that D-fenfluramine and sertraline specifically enhance the state of satiety in rats. *Eur. J. Pharmacol.* **211**, 137–142.

Grignaschi, G., Mantelli, B., Fracasso, C., Anelli, M., Caccia, S. and Samanin, R. (1993). Reciprocal interaction of 5-hydroxytryptamine and cholecystokinin in the control of feeding patterns in rats. *Br. J. Pharmacol.* **109**, 491–494.

Groenewegen, H. J. and Berendse, H. W. (1994). The specificity of 'nonspecific' midline and intralaminar thalamic nuclei. *Trends Neurosci.* **17**, 52–57.

Grossman, S. P. (1967). *A Textbook of Physiological Psychology*. John Wiley, New York.

Halford, J. C. (1995). *Analysis of the behaviour associated with feeding in drug-induced anorexia in the rat*. PhD thesis, University of Leeds.

Heimer, L., Alheid, G. F. and Zaborsky, L. (1985). Basal ganglia. In *The Rat Brain Vol. I. Forebrain and Midbrain* (G. Paxinos, ed.), pp. 37–86. Academic Press, London.

Heimer, L., Zahm, D. S., Churchill, L., Kalivas, P. W. and Wohltmann, C. (1991).

Specificity in the projection patterns of accumbral core and shell in the rat. *Neuroscience* **41**, 89–125.

Heimer, L., Alheid, G. F. and Zahm, D. S. (1993). Basal forebrain organization: an anatomical framework for motor aspects of drive and motivation. In *Limbic Motor Circuits and Neuropsychiatry* (P. W. Kalivas and C. D. Barnes, eds), pp. 1–43. CRC Press, Boca Raton.

Higgins, G. A., Wang, Y. P., Corrigall, W. A. and Sellers, E. M. (1994). Influence of 5-HT_3 receptor antagonists and the indirect 5-HT agonist, dexfenfluramine, on heroin self-administration in rats. *Psychopharmacology* **114**, 611–619.

Holstege, G. (1991). Descending motor pathways and the spinal motor system: limbic and non-limbic components. *Prog. Brain Res.* **87**, 307–421.

Joel, D. and Weiner, I. (1994). The organization of the basal ganglia–thalamocortical circuits: open interconnected rather than closed segregated. *Neuroscience* **63**, 363–379.

Jongen-Relo, A. L., Groenewegen, H. J. and Voorn, P. (1993). Evidence for a multi-compartmental histochemical organization of the nucleus accumbens in the rat. *J. Comp. Neurol.* **337**, 267–276.

Jongen-Relo, A. L., Voorn, P. and Groenewegen, H. J. (1994). Immunohistochemical characterization of the shell and core territories of the nucleus accumbens in the rat. *Eur. J. Neurosci.* **6**, 1255–1264.

Kelley, A. E., Domesick, V. B. and Nauta, W. J. H. (1982). The amygdalostriatal projection in the rat—an anatomical study by anterograde tracing methods. *Neuroscience* **7**, 615–630.

Kelly, J., Rothstein, J. and Grossman, S. P. (1979). GABA and hypothalamic feeding systems: I. Topographical analysis of the effects of microinjections of muscimol. *Physiol. Behav.* **23**, 1123–1134.

Lee, M. D. and Clifton, P. G. (1992). Partial reversal of fluoxetine anorexia by the 5-HT antagonist metergoline. *Psychopharmacology* **107**, 359–364.

Leibowitz, S. F., Weiss, G. F. and Suh, J. S. (1990). Medial hypothalamic nuclei mediate serotonin's inhibitory effect on feeding behaviour. *Pharmacol. Biochem. Behav.* **37**, 735–742.

Leibowitz, S. F., Alexander, J. T., Cheung, W. K. and Weiss, G. F. (1993). Effects of serotonin and the serotonin blocker metergoline on meal patterns and macronutrient selection. *Pharmacol. Biochem. Behav.* **45**, 185–194.

Li, Y. G., Takada, M. and Mizuno, N. (1993). Demonstration of habenular neurons which receive afferent fibers from the nucleus accumbens and send their axons to the midbrain periaqueductal gray. *Neurosci. Lett.* **158**, 55–58.

Luppi, P.-H., Aston-Jones, G., Akaoka, H., Chouvet, G., and Jouvet, M. (1995). Afferent projections to the rat locus coeruleus demonstrated by retrograde and anterograde tracing with cholera-toxin B subunit and *Phaseolus vulgaris* leucoagglutinin. *Neuroscience* **65**, 119–160.

Lynch, W. C., Hart, P. and Babcock, A. M. (1994). Neuropeptide-Y attenuates satiety—evidence from a detailed analysis of patterns of ingestion. *Brian Res.* **636**, 28–34.

McGeorge, J. A. and Faull, R. L. M. (1989). The organisation of the projection from the cerebral cortex to the striatum in the rat. *Neuroscience* **29**, 503–537.

Minano, F. J., Sancho, M. S. M., Sancibrian, M., Salinas, P. and Myers, R. D. (1992). GABA(A) receptors in the amygdala—role in feeding in fasted and satiated rats. *Brain Res.* **586**, 104–110.

Mogenson, G. J., Jones, D. J. and Yim, C. Y. (1980). From motivation to action: functional interface between the limbic system and motor system. *Prog. Neurobiol.* **14**, 69–97.

Montgomery, A. M. J. and Willner, P. (1988). Fenfluramine disrupts the behavioural satiety sequence in rats. *Psychopharmacology*) **94**, 397–401.

Nauta, W. J. H. and Feirtag, M. (1986). *Fundamental neuroanatomy*. W. H. Freeman, New York.

Peltier, R. and Schenk, S. (1993). Effects of serotonergic manipulations on cocaine self-administration in rats. *Psychopharmacology* **110**, 390–394.

Pennartz, C. M. A., Groenewegen, H. J. and Lopes da Silva, F. H. (1994). The nucleus accumbens as a complex of functionally distinct neuronal ensembles: an integration of behavioural, electrophysiological and anatomical data. *Prog. Neurobiol.* **42**, 719–761.

Redgrave, P., Dean, P. and Taha, E. B. (1984). Feeding induced by injection of muscimol into the substantia nigra of rats—unaffected by haloperidol but abolished by large lesions of the superior colliculus. *Neuroscience* **13**, 77–85.

Sahu, A., Kalra, P. S. and Kalra, S. P. (1988). Food deprivation and ingestion induce reciprocal changes in neuropeptide Y concentrations in the paraventricular nucleus. *Peptides* **9**, 83–86.

Salamone, J. D., Mahan, K. and Rogers, S. (1993). Ventrolateral striatal dopamine depletions impair feeding and food handling in rats. *Pharmacol. Biochem. Behav.* **44**, 605–610.

Sellers, E. M., Higgins, G. A. and Sobell, M. B. (1992). 5-HT and alcohol abuse. *Trends Neurosci.* **13**, 69–75.

Stanley, B. G., Magdalin, W., Seirafi, A., Nguyen, M. M. and Leibowitz, S. F. (1993). The perifornical area: the major focus of (a) patchily distributed hypothalamic neuropeptide Y-sensitive feeding system(s). *Brain Res.* **604**, 304–317.

Steinman, J. L., Gunion, M. W. and Morley J. E. (1994). Forebrain and hindbrain involvement of neuropeptide-Y in ingestive behaviors in rats. *Pharmacol. Biochem. Behav.* **47**, 207–214.

Stricker-Krongrad, A., Max, J. P., Musse, N., Nicolas, J. P., Burlet, C. and Beck, B. (1994). Increased threshold concentrations of neuropeptide-Y for a stimulatory effect on food-intake in obese Zucker rats—changes in the microstructure of the feeding-behavior. *Brain Res.* **660**, 162–166.

Swanson, L. W. (1987). The hypothalamus. In *Handbook of Chemical Neuroanatomy. Vol. 5: Integrated Systems of the CNS, Part 1*. (A. Björklund, T. Hôkfelt and L. W. Swanson, eds), pp. 1–124. Elsevier, Amsterdam.

Weiss, G. F., Rogacki, N., Fueg, A., Buchen, D., Suh, J. S., Wong, D. T. and Leibowitz, S. F. (1991). Effect of hypothalamic and peripheral fluoxetine injection on natural patterns of macronutrient intake in the rat. *Psychopharmacology* **105**, 467–476.

Whishaw, I. Q. and Kornelson, R. A. (1993). Two types of motivation revealed by ibotenic acid nucleus accumbens lesions: dissociation of food carrying and hoarding and the role of primary and incentive motivation. *Behav. Brain Res.* **55**, 283–295.

Wirtschafter, D., Stratford, T. R. and Pitzer, M. R. (1993). Studies on the behavioral activation produced by stimulation of GABA(B) receptors in the median raphe nucleus. *Behav. Brain Res.* **59**, 83–93.

Witter, M. P. and Groenewegen, H. J. (1992). Organizational principles of hippocampal connections. In *The Temporal Lobes and the Limbic System* (M. R. Trimble and T. G. Bolwig, eds), pp. 37–60. Wrightson Biomedical Publishing, Petersfield.

Zahm, D. S. and Brog, J. S. (1992). On the significance of subterritories in the 'accumbens' part of the rat ventral striatum. *Neuroscience* **50**, 751–767.

Zahm, D. S. and Heimer, L. (1993). Specificity in the efferent projections of the nucleus accumbens in the rat: comparison of the rostral pole projection patterns with those of the core and shell. *J. Comp. Neurol.* **327**, 220–232.

Index

Entries in **bold** are main discussions; entries in *italic* indicate reference to illustrations and tables